COMMON SCREENING TESTS

David M. Eddy, MD, PhD
Editor

Published by the American College of Physicians
Philadelphia, Pennsylvania

Printed in the United States of America

Library of Congress Cataloging-in-Publication Data

Common screening tests / David M. Eddy, editor.
    417 pp.   cm.
    Collection of papers originally published in Annals of in-
ternal medicine.
    Includes bibliographical references.
    ISBN 0-943126-19-3 : $37.00 ($31.00 to ACP members)
    1. Medical screening.   I. Eddy, David M., 1941-
II. Annals of internal medicine.
    [DNLM: 1. Mass Screening—methods—collected works. WA 245 C734]
RA427.5.C65   1991
616.07'5—dc20
DNLM/DLC
for Library of Congress   91-4566
                                           CIP

CONTENTS

Contributors vii

Preface
      David M. Eddy. xi

1. How to Think About Screening
      David M. Eddy. 1

2. Screening for Hypertension
      Benjamin Littenberg, Alan M. Garber,
      and Harold C. Sox, Jr. 22

3. The Resting Electrocardiogram as a Screening Test:
   A Clinical Analysis
      Harold C. Sox, Jr., Alan M. Garber, and
      Benjamin Littenberg 47

4. The Role of Exercise Testing in Screening for
   Coronary Artery Disease
      Harold C. Sox, Jr., Benjamin Littenberg, and
      Alan M. Garber 81

5. Screening Asymptomatic Adults for Cardiac
   Risk Factors: The Serum Cholesterol Level
      Alan M. Garber, Harold C. Sox, Jr., and
      Benjamin Littenberg 113

6. Screening for Diabetes Mellitus
      Daniel E. Singer, Jeffrey H. Samet, Christopher
      M. Coley, and David M. Nathan 154

7. Screening for Thyroid Disease
      Mark Helfand and Lawrence M. Crapo 179

8. Screening for Osteoporosis
      L. Joseph Melton III, David M. Eddy, and
      C. Conrad Johnston, Jr. 202

9. Screening for Breast Cancer
      David M. Eddy. 229

10. Screening for Cervical Cancer
      David M. Eddy. 255

11. Screening for Colorectal Cancer
      David M. Eddy. 286

12. **Screening for Lung Cancer**
    David M. Eddy. 312

13. **Preventive Care Guidelines in 1990**
    Robert S. A. Hayward, Earl P. Steinberg, Daniel E.
    Ford, Michael F. Roizen, and Keith Roach. 326

Appendixes

Introduction to the Guidelines
Douglas S. Peters. 394

Guidelines

Screening for Hypertension 396

Screening for Asymptomatic Coronary Artery
Disease: The Resting Electrocardiogram 398

Screening for Asymptomatic Coronary Artery
Disease: Exercise Stress Testing 400

Screening Low Risk, Asymptomatic Adults for
Cardiac Risk Factors: Serum Cholesterol
and Triglycerides 402

Screening for Diabetes Mellitus in Apparently
Healthy, Asymptomatic Adults 404

Screening for Thyroid Disease 406

Screening for Osteoporosis in Perimenopausal
Women 409

Screening for Breast Cancer 411

Screening for Cervical Cancer 413

Screening for Colorectal Cancer 415

Screening for Lung Cancer 417

CONTRIBUTORS

Christopher M. Coley, MD
Instructor in Medicine
Harvard University School of Medicine
Cambridge, Massachusetts

Lawrence M. Crapo, MD, PhD
Associate Professor of Medicine
Stanford University School of Medicine
Stanford, California
and
Chief of Endocrinology
Santa Clara Valley Medical Center
San Jose, California

David M. Eddy, MD, PhD
Professor of Health Policy and Management
Center for Health Policy Research and Education
Duke University
Durham, North Carolina

Daniel E. Ford, MD, MPH
Assistant Professor of Medicine, of Epidemiology, and
   of Health Policy and Management
Welch Center for Prevention, Epidemiology, and
   Clinical Research
Johns Hopkins University
Baltimore, Maryland

Alan M. Garber, MD, PhD
Assistant Professor of Medicine
Stanford University School of Medicine
Stanford, California

Robert S. A. Hayward, MD, FRCPC
Program for Medical Technology and Practice
   Assessment
and
Welch Center for Prevention, Epidemiology, and
   Clinical Research
Division of Internal Medicine
Johns Hopkins University
Baltimore, Maryland

Mark Helfand, MD, MS
Assistant Professor of Medicine
Division of General Internal Medicine
Portland Veterans Affairs Medical Center
Portland, Oregon

C. Conrad Johnston, Jr., MD
Professor of Medicine and Chief
Division of Endocrinology and Metabolism
Indiana University School of Medicine
Indianapolis, Indiana

Benjamin Littenberg, MD
Assistant Professor
Department of Medicine
Dartmouth-Hitchcock Medical Center
Hanover, New Hampshire

L. Joseph Melton III, MD
Professor of Epidemiology
Department of Health Sciences Research
Mayo Clinic
Rochester, Minnesota

David M. Nathan, MD
Director
Diabetes Research Center and Diabetes Clinic
Massachusetts General Hospital
Boston, Massachusetts

Keith Roach, MD
Department of Medicine
University of Chicago
Chicago, Illinois

Michael F. Roizen, MD, FACP
Professor and Chairman
Department of Anesthesia and Critical Care
Professor of Internal Medicine
University of Chicago
Chicago, Illinois

Jeffrey H. Samet, MD
Assistant Professor of Medicine
General Internal Medicine Section
Boston City Hospital
Boston University School of Medicine
Boston, Massachusetts

Daniel E. Singer, MD
Associate Professor of Medicine
and
Associate Professor of Clinical Epidemiology
Department of Health Care Policy
Harvard University School of Medicine
Cambridge, Massachusetts

Harold C. Sox, Jr., MD, FACP
Professor of Medicine and Chairman
Department of Medicine
Dartmouth-Hitchcock Medical Center
Hanover, New Hampshire

Earl P. Steinberg, MD, MPP, FACP
Associate Professor of Medicine and of Health Policy
    and Management
and
Director
Program for Medical Technology and Practice
    Assessment
Johns Hopkins University
Baltimore, Maryland

The chapters in this book analyze screening for hypertension; coronary artery disease; cardiac risk factors (serum cholesterol); diabetes; thyroid disease; osteoporosis; and cancers of the breast, cervix, colon, and lung. Also included are a background chapter on how to think about screening tests, a survey of screening recommendations made by various organizations, and screening recommendations from the American College of Physicians.

The work described here evolved out of a project initiated by the Blue Cross and Blue Shield Association. Each of the analyses was originally commissioned by the Association for use by individual Blue Cross and Blue Shield Plans to cover the costs of screening in their indemnity plans and HMOs. However, from its beginning, the project was closely coordinated with the American College of Physicians. Each paper was submitted to *Annals of Internal Medicine*, and each was used as a background paper by the College's Clinical Efficacy Assessment Subcommittee of the Health and Public Policy Committee to develop the recommendations for screening for common diseases presented in the appendix.

The review of these papers was extraordinary. Each was reviewed at least five times—by the authors' personal reviewers, by the Blue Cross and Blue Shield Association, by *Annals of Internal Medicine*, by the Clinical Efficacy Assessment Subcommittee, by the Health and Public Policy Committee, and by the Board of Regents of the College. Given this, it is remarkable that any of the papers could have survived, much less that a consistent set of policies could have been developed. The reason for this success is that all parties in this process shared a firm commitment to certain principles.

The first principle was that screening recommendations should be based on evidence—not on tradition, not on hope, and not on personal or professional interests. This commitment to evidence provided a rudder that steered debates and kept all parties on a common course. A second principle was that, to the greatest extent possible, recommendations should be based on an explicit understanding of the benefits, harms, and costs of screening to patients. While this greatly increased the work required to analyze a screening policy, it also helped focus debates and resolve conflicts. The third principle is that, in the end, recommendations for screening should be based on the needs and desires of patients. The fourth principle concerned the purpose of this effort. The ultimate goal was not to force particular practices, not to squash individual clinical judgment, and not to save money. Rather, the goal was to help practitioners make decisions with their patients about screening.

Any decision about screening involves value judgments—weighing evidence; comparing benefits, harms, and costs; and tailoring general lessons to very individualized people. For some screening tests, the benefits are clear and blanket recommendations are obvious. For other tests, however, the evidence is not clearcut and the desirability of the outcomes is not obvious. For these tests, a blanket recommendation might not be possible. Rather, the appropriate recommendation is for individual decision-making—the appropriate recommendation is "Talk to your doctor." This type of individualized decision-making requires sensitivity, insight, and compassion. It also requires information. You, the reader, bring the first three qualities. The goal of this book is to provide you with the information you need to exercise these qualities in the interests of your patients.

David M. Eddy, MD, PhD
Duke University
Durham, North Carolina

How to Think About Screening

DAVID M. EDDY, MD, PhD

Making recommendations about screening is one of the most difficult problems in clinical medicine. Screening, by definition, involves testing persons, usually in large numbers, who have no symptoms of the condition being searched for. Most persons who are screened will receive no benefit because they do not have the target condition. But many persons will suffer risks, and all will face some inconvenience, anxiety, personal cost, and sometimes discomfort. In short, the stakes are high. This fact places a special burden on any individual or group that wants to recommend a screening test. They must determine that screening can in fact deliver benefits and that the potential benefits outweigh the harms and justify the costs.

The main issues in the evaluation of screening tests and the design of screening policies are discussed in this chapter. The issues are described from the point of view of the individual or organization that is designing the screening policy. The purpose of this chapter is to help practitioners who actually do screening to evaluate the rationale for the recommendations offered to them.

Definitions

Screening

Screening is the application of a test to detect a potential disease or condition in a person who has no known signs or symptoms of that disease or condition. There are two main purposes for screening. One is to detect a disease early in its natural history when treatment might be more effective, less expensive, or both. The other purpose is to detect risk factors that put a person at a higher than average risk for developing a disease, with the goal of modifying the risk factor or factors to prevent the disease. Screening for high cholesterol levels to prevent a myocardial infarction is one example. (Hereinafter, the term "condition" will be used in a general sense to describe any disease, risk factor, or other condition that is the target of screening.)

Asymptomatic

For the purpose of defining screening, a person is asymptomatic if, at the time screening is done, he or she has no known signs or symptoms of the target condition. The person might have signs or symptoms of which he or she is unaware, in which case screening might result in discovery of those hidden signs or symptoms. For example, a woman might be unaware of a tiny breast mass that could be found during a breast physical examination. The persons being screened might also have other signs or symptoms suggestive of other conditions. The crucial point is that, at the time of screening, neither the patient nor the practitioner is aware of any signs or symptoms of the target condition.

Patient

In a physician's practice many if not most of the persons being screened will have other medical problems. The term "patient" therefore will be used in a general sense to describe the persons being screened.

Practitioner

Many types of health care professionals, for example, physicians, nurses, and specially trained assistants, can do screening. For simplicity, the term "practitioner" will be used to include anyone who does the screening test.

Screening Tests

A condition can be detected by a variety of methods, including patient history, blood tests, physical examinations, invasive procedures, and imaging tests. The term "test" will be used in a general sense to include any screening method.

Policymaker

An individual, a group of individuals, or an organization can develop a recommendation for screening. Frequently, as was the case for this book, the process will require all three: Individual authors will draft papers for review by one or more committees and final approval by an organization. In this chapter, the term "policymakers" will be used to describe the collection of persons that produced a screening recommendation. "Policymaking" will refer to the process.

Steps

Once a condition has been selected for analysis, designing a screening recommendation for that condition has two main steps. The first is to estimate the health and economic outcomes of the proposed screening strategy—the benefits, harms, and costs. The second step is to compare those outcomes to determine whether the benefits outweigh the harms and whether the health outcomes (benefits and harms combined) are worth the costs.

It is important to keep the two steps separate. The first step is a question of science and is anchored to evidence. Different parties should be able to agree on the evidence and on the estimated outcomes of screening. In contrast, the second step is not a question of science but a question of personal values. It is anchored not to evidence but to the preferences and desires of the persons receiving the screening tests. Different persons have different preferences, and it might well be that no single screening recommendation is best for everyone. When designing a screening policy, policymakers must take into account not only the evidence of benefits and harms, but also the range of patients' preferences about the outcomes.

Both of these main steps can be divided into several smaller steps. To estimate the outcomes, policymakers must formulate the screening problem; identify the health outcomes that are important to the persons who will be screened (hereinafter called "patients"); search for evidence for the effect of screening on each health outcome; interpret the pieces of evidence; and synthesize or combine the evidence to estimate the effect of the test on health and economic outcomes. When making value judgments, policymakers must determine who should compare the benefits, harms, and costs; actually make the comparisons; and design the policy.

Important issues arise in the performance of these steps. These issues, which will be discussed in turn, include the formulation of a screening strategy; the types of outcomes affected by screening tests; the types of evidence commonly used to evaluate screening tests; biases that typically affect evidence for screening tests; techniques used to synthesize the evidence; the comparison of benefits, harms, and costs; and techniques for incorporating uncertainty about outcomes and variability of preferences in the design of a policy.

Formulating a Screening Strategy

Before the appropriateness of a screening program can be analyzed, the program must be defined. Variables to be considered include which persons will be targeted for screening (for example, groupings based on gender, age, risk factors, geographic regions, or socio-economic status); which tests will be used; the order and frequency of testing; and the setting in which screening will be offered (for example, who will do the screening, where, and under what circumstances). Defining variables of the program in advance is important because the benefits, harms, and costs of screening depend acutely on these factors. For example, the outcome of screening high-risk women 50 to 65 years of age with an annual breast physical examination and mammography in practitioners' offices is very different from the value of screening average-risk women 40 to 50 years of age with biennial "low-cost" mammography. Indeed, the category of "screening with mammography" is so general that it cannot be evaluated without further specification.

When identifying screening strategies, it is important not to be limited by tradition or convention. For example, many screening tests have been offered annually based on no better logic than the fact that the earth circles the sun every year. The frequency of screening depends on the natural history of the condition—how long it takes to develop from first detectability to signs or symptoms—not on astronomy, and it might be that frequencies other than once a year are more appropriate. Similarly, just because two or more tests are available to screen for a condition does not mean they all have to be used. Decisions about combinations of tests depend on the properties and dependencies of the tests, not on their availability.

Frequently, it will be appropriate to identify several different screening strategies so that they can be compared. Decisions about a particular screening strategy should be based on the strategy's benefits, harms, and costs compared with those of adjacent strategies (what economists call "marginal" benefits, harms, and costs). The benefits, harms, and costs of a screening strategy should not be evaluated in comparison with no screening (what economists call "average" benefits, harms, and costs). For example, screening for hypertension every 5 years should be compared with 4-year screening and 6-year screening, not with no screening. To ensure that the proper strategies are being compared, several adjacent strategies must be identified and analyzed.

Types of Outcomes

Health Outcomes

The purpose of screening, indeed the purpose of all medical interventions, is to improve health outcomes.

Health outcomes are outcomes that patients experience and care about. These outcomes can affect length and quality of life and may cause pain, anxiety, death, or functional disability and affect appearance or peace of mind.

Screening typically affects several types of health outcomes, such as the immediate side effects of screening: the inconvenience, anxiety, and possible discomfort associated with the test. These outcomes are experienced by everyone who gets the screening test, although different patients might react to them differently. Another type of health outcome affected by screening is any potential risks of the tests (for example, perforation of the colon by a sigmoidoscope or the potential radiation effects of mammography).

Other outcomes affected by the performance of the test are outcomes associated with the test results. When a screening test is done on a patient, four results are possible: The test might correctly indicate the presence of the target condition (a true-positive result); it might incorrectly indicate that the condition is absent when in fact it is present (a false-negative result); it might correctly indicate the absence of the condition (a true-negative result); or it might falsely indicate that the condition is present when in fact it is absent (a false-positive result). Each of these results affects health outcomes. A true-positive result controls the potential benefits of screening—the possible reduction in morbidity and mortality. However, the other three test results can also affect health outcomes. A false-negative result can lead to a false sense of security. A false-positive result can cause great anxiety, can label a patient, and can require that additional testing be done, with its attendant side effects, risks, and costs. A true-negative result can provide reassurance, which for many people is the main reason to be screened. It is important to recognize that the first result—the benefit from detecting an existing condition—is experienced by only a few of the people who are screened, those who happen to have the condition. In contrast, the harms of screening are experienced by many more people.

Intermediate Outcomes or Measures

In addition to health outcomes, screening tests have intermediate outcomes or measures that policymakers might use to help evaluate screening. Intermediate outcomes and measures cannot be directly experienced by patients and are important to patients only to the extent that they provide information about the probabilities or magnitudes of health outcomes. Examples of intermediate outcomes and measures frequently used to help evaluate screening tests include the probability that the screening test will detect a condition if it is present (the sensitivity or true-positive rate of the test); the proportion of screened people who are found to have the condition (the "yield" of screening in a population); the predictive values of the test (the probability that patients who test positive actually have the condition, and the probability that people who test negative do not actually have the condition); and the shift in the state of the condition at the time of detection (for example, an increase in the proportion of patients who have cancer detected in the early stages).

When information about intermediate outcomes is used as the basis for decisions about screening, some assumptions must be made about how the intermediate outcomes and measures affect the health outcomes. For example, finding a condition in 5% of a population does not by itself determine whether screening is good or bad. To decide that, assumptions must be made about whether the discovery of the condition changes management, whether the change in management changes health outcomes, and whether the magnitude of the expected change in health outcomes is worth the side effects, risks, and costs.

Types of Evidence

It is rare that all the outcomes of screening can be learned from a single source. More commonly, a policymaker must examine many sources and types of evidence to document the benefits of screening and to estimate the magnitude of benefits, harms, and costs.

The harmful outcomes of a screening test—side effects, risks, and false-positive results—are usually learned by simply observing what happens when a large population is tested. Patients can be asked about anxiety and discomfort; the frequency of short-term risks such as perforations can be noted; and the frequency of false-positive test results can be counted. For some screening tests, the potential risks are more difficult to estimate, particularly when they occur with low frequency or over long periods of time, or both. An example of this type of outcome is the potential radiation hazard of mammography. For this type of risk, indirect evidence and mathematical models are usually required.

Given that virtually all screening tests have potential for harm, it is essential to determine that the test can also yield benefit. Documenting the benefits of screening can be extremely difficult, far more difficult than for a treatment. The effect of screening on health outcomes is inherently indirect, requiring a sequence of actions and outcomes. The primary effect of screening is to provide information about the probability a patient has the targeted condition. A positive test result increases the probability that the patient has the condition; a negative result decreases the probability. In order for the screening test to have any effect on health outcomes, a positive test result must lead to a diagnostic workup to confirm the presence of the condition; which in turn must cause a change in the choice or timing of treatment; which in turn must cause a change in health outcomes. Thus, many links must be in place to connect screening to an improvement in health outcomes (Figure 1).

If any of these links is broken, the value of screening to a patient can be nullified. For example, the screening center might neglect to follow up a positive result; a patient might decline to return for a diagnostic workup; the practitioner might not choose the correct treatment; or the treatment might not change health outcomes. To document that screening will in fact improve health outcomes, there must be evidence for all of these links. That evidence can be either direct or indirect.

Direct Evidence

The most desirable type of evidence directly connects the application of the screening test with the occurrence of health outcomes. (That is, direct evidence spans from one end of Figure 1 to the other.) The prototype for direct evidence is the randomized controlled trial. Because exposure to the screening tests is determined by the investigator and because both the screened and control groups are essentially similar in all other respects, any differences in health outcomes between the two groups can be attributed to screening. Unfortunately, this type of evidence is rare, usually because huge numbers of people must be screened to generate a sufficient number of outcomes for statistical analysis, and because many of the outcomes are chronic and require long follow-up times. Examples of conditions

Figure 1.

Apply the screening test	→	Detect the possible presence of the condition	→	Confirm the presence of the condition	→	Change the timing of treatment	→	Change the health outcomes

for which randomized controlled trials have been done are screening for cancers of the breast, colon, and lung (Chapters 9, 11, and 12). Each of these trials followed tens of thousands of patients over decades.

Occasionally, nonrandomized controlled trials are used to provide evidence for screening. These trials usually involve comparisons of convenience. For example, screening might be offered to persons who live in one town, with persons who live in an adjacent town serving as controls. The value of this design depends on the similarities between the two groups and the extent to which any differences in outcomes can be attributed to screening as opposed to other uncontrollable factors (for example, differences in the population or differences in the available treatments). Statistical techniques can sometimes be used to adjust for such differences. The Edinburgh trial of breast cancer screening is an example (Chapter 9).

Another type of direct evidence used to evaluate screening tests is the case-control study. In this design, the investigators identify patients, or "cases," who have had the outcome of interest (for example, who have died of breast cancer). The investigators also identify a group of persons (the "controls") who have not had the outcome (for example, who have not died of breast cancer), but who are similar in other respects such as age and socioeconomic status. The investigators then retrospectively review the histories of both the cases and controls to determine what proportion of persons in each group had received the screening test. From these proportions, an odds ratio can be calculated to compare the odds of the outcome (for example, the odds of dying of breast cancer) in screened as opposed to unscreened people. This design has several advantages: It does not require randomization; it can take advantage of natural experiments; and it can be conducted more quickly and less expensively than randomized controlled trials. A major disadvantage is the high potential for patient-selection biases and errors in retrospectively determining screening histories. Case-control studies have been used to evaluate screening for cervical cancer (Chapter 10), breast cancer (Chapter 9), and osteoporosis (Chapter 8).

The uncontrolled study is a fourth type of direct evidence. A typical design is to offer screening to a population, follow the patients who are screened, and observe the outcomes. Uncontrolled studies of screening are common because they are the easiest and least expensive type of design. This design is useful for determining outcomes that can occur only with screening,

matically increase the time between the moment of detection and the occurrence of some outcome, such as death. This increase occurs whether or not the outcome has actually been postponed. Thus, the observation of a longer survival time from diagnosis might be due only to advancing the time of diagnosis, not to postponing the time of death. Because of this, a comparison of survival rates in screened or unscreened populations can be misleading. A randomized controlled trial of lung cancer screening illustrates the potential for this bias and shows how a randomized design can correct for it (Chapter 12).

Another problem affecting the interpretation of uncontrolled studies that follow patients with conditions detected by screening is the so-called "length bias." Conditions detected by a test in a periodic screening program tend to have longer preclinical intervals than average. The preclinical interval is the interval between the time a screening test *could* detect a condition and the time a patient would seek care for signs or symptoms in the absence of screening. The duration of this interval is related to the growth rate and other biological characteristics of the condition, the effectiveness of the screening test, and the patient's awareness of signs or symptoms. Several of these factors can influence how long a patient survives from the time of diagnosis. For example, conditions with longer preclinical intervals might have slower growth rates, be less aggressive, and have inherently better prognoses. Thus, observations of longer survival times in uncontrolled studies might be due to the selection of patients with longer preclinical intervals rather than to any real improvement in survival. This bias can be overcome by tracking *all* patients offered screening, not just those whose conditions were detected through screening.

A third problem that can confuse the interpretation of data from uncontrolled studies is overdiagnosis. The purpose of screening is to find conditions in their earliest stages. Unfortunately, there is often no sharp boundary between normal findings and the earliest stages of a condition, and it is possible to overdiagnose an atypical but essentially normal finding as a very early case of the condition. As well as increasing the number of "conditions" detected, overdiagnosis can inflate the number of conditions thought to be detected in the earliest stages. Because these cases would never have become clinically significant, this can inflate survival statistics.

Adjusting for Biases

When any of these biases is believed to exist, policymakers must determine the potential effect of each bias on the results of the study. If the policymakers intend to estimate the actual magnitudes of benefits and harms, they must go on to make quantitative estimates of how the biases affect the studies' results. At present, the most common approach for dealing with biases is the "all or nothing" approach; the policymaker determines either that the biases are so great that the study should be discarded or that the biases are sufficiently small that they can be ignored and the study can be taken at face value. Obviously, both choices are oversimplifications. A second approach is to attempt to adjust subjectively for the biases. This approach is not only difficult technically, but introduces the possibility of professional or personal biases. A third approach is to use formal statistical techniques to adjust for biases, but these techniques are still relatively new and not widely available. Currently, the most common approach is to estimate a range of uncertainty for important variables. The range of uncertainty should incorporate both the design of the trial (for example, sample size) and the presence of biases. Then sensitivity analyses are done to explore the impact of uncertainty about specific variables on the outcomes of interest.

Synthesizing Evidence

After the experimental evidence has been identified and pieces of evidence have been interpreted, the evidence must be synthesized. For any variable—whether it is a health outcome that can be estimated directly from the evidence or a variable to be used in a model of indirect evidence—there are frequently multiple pieces of evidence that show slightly different, sometimes conflicting results. The policymaker must reconcile these differences to develop a "best" estimate of the health outcome or variable based on the combined results. The most common approach is to calculate a weighted average of the results of separate pieces of evidence or to combine the evidence subjectively. In the latter, the policymaker surveys all of the evidence and attempts to "sense" the best estimate and an appropriate range of uncertainty. As with techniques for adjusting for biases, formal statistical techniques for synthesizing evidence from multiple sources are becoming available (called "meta-analysis").

After the evidence has been interpreted and synthesized, the resulting estimates can then be used directly to estimate the benefits, harms, and costs of the screening program (if the evidence is direct) or to execute a model that in turn estimates the health and economic outcomes (if the evidence is indirect). The ranges of uncertainty are used to do sensitivity analyses.

Comparing Benefits, Harms, and Costs

Three main issues arise when comparing benefits, harms, and costs: obtaining estimates of benefits, harms, and costs; making the comparisons; and avoiding pitfalls.

The Importance of Estimating Outcomes

Ideally, a decision to recommend a screening test will be based on an explicit comparison of the test's benefits, harms, and costs. Making such a comparison obviously requires estimates of the magnitudes of the benefits, harms, and costs. Without such estimates of health outcomes, there is no solid basis for the comparison. In particular, when an analysis of a screening test describes only intermediate outcomes, such as the sensitivity, yield, or predictive values of the screening test, a truly informed comparison of benefits and harms is not possible. In such cases, judgments about the desirability of screening based on intermediate outcomes require making many assumptions, usually unstated, about what the detection of a disease (an intermediate outcome) implies about the morbidity and mortality of the disease (the health outcomes). To the extent that the actual magnitudes of health and economic outcomes are not explicitly estimated, there is greater uncertainty about the appropriateness of a screening recommendation.

Who Should Make the Comparisons?

Comparison of the benefits, harms, and costs of screening should ideally be done by the people who will actually receive the benefits and harms and pay the costs—that is, the patients themselves. Information about their preferences could be learned through such methods as polls, interviews, focus groups, or even experiments. At present, these methods are virtually never used. For screening recommendations (or recommendations about any health intervention, for that matter), representatives of patients are not systematically surveyed for their preferences. Rather, policymakers commonly use their own personal judgments to weigh the benefits and harms of screening. The implicit as-

sumption is either that the policymaker's personal preferences match the preferences of patients, or that the
policymakers are separating their personal values from
the values of patients, are trying to represent patients
(act as their agents), and accurately know how patients
feel about the benefits, harms, and costs. Both of these
assumptions are questionable, and some day the standard practice will be to consult representatives of patients for their preferences before developing recommendations for a screening test. Learning the spectrum
of preferences by surveying representatives of patients
differs from the individualized decision-making described below. In the spirit of market research, these
surveys would provide essential information about how
patients, in general, value the benefits, harms, and costs
of a screening test.

Psychological Biases

Comparing the benefits and harms of any intervention
can be affected by many psychological traps. This comparison involves not only processing complex information, but explicitly addressing issues that have powerful
emotional connotations. In addition, few people readily
want the responsibility of making a decision that will
affect the lives of hundreds of thousands of people. As
a consequence policymakers have a powerful psychological drive to find some simplifying principle that will
make the decision obvious and minimize the need for
personal exposure. Unfortunately, most of the simplifying principles are misleading. Some examples of common traps are the following: picking a single outcome
and using it as the sole basis for a decision, and ignoring the other outcomes such as harms ("Screening reduces mortality, therefore it should be recommended");
using statistical significance as a proxy for the desirability of an outcome ("The benefits of screening were
statistically significant, therefore it should be recommended," or conversely, "There is no randomized controlled trial proving the test is effective, therefore it
cannot be recommended"); ignoring costs; using spuri-
ous tricks to tip the balance ("I cannot decide if this
screening test is desirable for average-risk people; but if
it is a tossup for average-risk people, it must be desirable for high-risk people"); ignoring the actual magnitude of an outcome ("If there is *any* benefit, screening
must be worthwhile," or "If *only one* life is saved, the
effort will have been worthwhile"); retreating to gener-
alities ("Cancer is bad, therefore any intervention that
combats cancer must be worthwhile"); or following the

tional Health and Nutrition Examination Survey (1976 to 1980) found that 21.7% of adults have blood pressures at or above 160/95 mm Hg. Prevalence increases from less than 2% for white women who are 18 to 24 years old to over 70% for elderly black women. Another 12% of adults have diastolic blood pressures ranging from 90 to 94 mm Hg (1, 2). Most hypertensive subjects detected by community surveys already know they have an elevated blood pressure. However, during 1976 to 1980, at least 16% of the adult population had hypertension that was not adequately controlled, and 6.3% had hypertension that had never been diagnosed (1).

Natural History and Impact

The risk for stroke, myocardial infarction, and renal dysfunction increases with even mildly elevated pressures (3, 4). High blood pressure contributes to a large percentage of deaths in the United States (5). The higher the pressure, the higher the incidence of heart disease, stroke, and death, especially when other risk factors are present (6). Even among normotensive persons, an increase in blood pressure is associated with an increase in the rate of cardiovascular complications.

Conclusion

Hypertension is common among Americans and is associated with substantial morbidity and mortality. A significant proportion of Americans are hypertensive, and a significant proportion of the hypertensive population is not under adequate treatment. These persons are at risk for devastating complications that often occur without warning.

Is Hypertension Detectable?

The Accuracy of Sphygmomanometry

The test characteristics of routine sphygmomanometry are not precisely known because there is no obvious reference criterion with which to compare it. Cuff pressures tend to overestimate "true" arterial pressures as measured by arterial cannulation, especially in elderly and obese persons (7, 8). However, most of what is known about the natural history of hypertension (for example, the Framingham study) is based on cuff pressures taken under conditions that approximate those of a medical clinic or doctor's office. Therefore, indirect sphygmomanometry is the appropriate method for estimating prognosis and monitoring therapy. In a certain sense, there is no standard for comparison at all; arterial hypertension measured by sphygmomanometry in the doctor's office is essentially the definition of the condition. Community standards of care are based on this definition.

Application and Interpretation

Significant errors in diagnosis are possible if sphygmomanometry is not properly done and interpreted. Recent guidelines from the World Health Organization (9) specify that the patient should be seated comfortably for several minutes before pressures are measured, a cuff of appropriate size should be used, and care should be taken to inflate the cuff to a pressure greater than systolic before slowly releasing the pressure. Disappearance of the Korotkoff sounds (phase V) indicates diastolic pressure. The mean of at least two measurements should be recorded. A diastolic blood pressure at screening of over 90 mm Hg indicates that repeat visits are necessary. Mild hypertension should not be diagnosed unless the diastolic blood pressure recorded in the office or clinic is above 90 mm Hg on at least three occasions over several weeks. Treatment should be individualized; a pressure of 90 mm Hg does not necessarily mandate drug therapy (10).

Alternatives

Sphygmomanometry is the only reasonable method currently available to screen for hypertension. Automated ambulatory blood pressure recording may someday provide superior diagnostic accuracy. At present, however, information is not sufficient to assert that this relatively expensive technique offers any added benefit for the patient (11). Direct measurement of intra-arterial blood pressure by the introduction of a catheter into the bloodstream has the advantage of identifying a subset of patients with falsely elevated cuff pressures (pseudohypertension) (7, 12). However, this invasive procedure is expensive, painful, dangerous, time-consuming, and not generally available outside special facilities. Furthermore, long-term epidemiologic follow-up of hypertension is based on sphygmomanometry, not on direct pressure recording. A shift in the diagnostic standard away from sphyg-

Risks and Costs

The direct risks of sphygmomanometry are nil. A diagnosis of hypertension, however, has several indirect risks for the patient. First, a normotensive patient may be misdiagnosed because of a spuriously elevated pressure. These patients are subject to the adverse effects of antihypertensive therapy with little potential for benefit. The diagnosis of mild hypertension should be based on repeated measures at each of several encounters, with careful attention given to cuff size and other confounding variables (9, 10).

Treatment of a correctly diagnosed hypertensive patient also includes risks, the most important of which are the adverse effects of drug therapy. Antihypertensive medications cause many adverse effects, ranging from headache and constipation to hemolytic anemia and sudden death. There is evidence that some antihypertensive preparations can have a harmful effect on cardiac risk factors such as cholesterol level (22). In addition, treatment can be expensive. The lifelong direct costs of medications alone can reach thousands of dollars. Especially for patients with mild hypertension, these risks and costs might exceed the potential benefits of treatment.

Labeling a patient as hypertensive may induce an unwanted change in the patient's behavior (23). There is some evidence that the patient's sense of well-being may deteriorate and that his or her absenteeism from work may rise after diagnosis (24). There are controversial, but disturbing, data that the incomes of persons labeled "hypertensive" are lower than those of their normotensive peers (25).

The search for treatable secondary causes of hypertension can be costly and dangerous. Invasive tests such as intravenous pyelography, renal arteriography, and selective adrenal-vein sampling are sometimes advocated for selected patients. These tests have substantial risks, including contrast reactions, local vascular damage, and the ever-present possibility of misinformation (26).

Previous Work

Weinstein and Stason (27) estimated the cost-effectiveness of both screening for hypertension and treating known hypertension. The unit of measure for this type of analysis is the dollar cost of changing to a new procedure (the marginal cost) divided by the resultant change in life expectancy. The authors modified the value of years of life to account for pain, disability, or other morbidity. The analysis yielded estimates of quality-adjusted life expectancy. For instance, they assumed that having a stroke is equivalent to losing 1.5 years of healthy life span on average. They also assumed that a treated subject would be better off than an untreated person with hypertension but would not attain the full benefit of being naturally normotensive. This "fraction of benefit" analysis was done before most of the trials of treatment for hypertension had been completed; the efficacy estimates used by Weinstein and Stason (27) were based on their own subjective judgments.

Weinstein and Stason (27) found that the cost per quality-adjusted life-year (QALY, a measure of life expectancy corrected to account for morbidity) saved by screening depended on the blood pressure before treatment and on age and sex. Under their central assumptions (especially that compliance with treatment is imperfect) and varying the treatment threshold according to age, sex, and diastolic pressure, they estimated the marginal cost-effectiveness of community-wide screening to be $20 077/QALY. Case-finding (the testing of patients who present to the provider for other reasons) had lower marginal costs than mass screening because fewer patients are lost to follow-up and the cost of case-finding itself is simply added to an existing episode of care. The authors found case-finding to cost $15 818/QALY. Both these estimates are in the range of the estimated cost-effectiveness for other widely accepted health interventions.

New Information

Since Weinstein and Stason's report in 1976 (27), dramatic changes have occurred in both the prevalence of undetected hypertension and therapy for mild hypertension. Because of a major nationwide detection effort, many Americans have become aware of their blood pressure and the prevalence of untreated hypertension has fallen (1, 2). The treatment of hypertension has been refined dramatically. Dozens of new antihypertensive preparations are available. Physicians have become more adept at diagnosing and treating hypertension. Interest in non-drug modalities has risen. At least eight major trials since 1979 have contributed information on the risks and benefits of treating mild hypertension. Although these trials have not reproduced the striking reduction in mortality shown by the earlier trials in patients with severe and moderate hypertension, they have shown substantial reductions in the costly and disabling morbidity of stroke. Because these factors may modify the net benefit of screening for hypertension, we were prompted to re-estimate the cost-effectiveness.

Cost-Effectiveness Analysis

We estimated the costs and effects on life expectancy of screening with sphygmomanometry for diastolic blood pressures in the range of 90 to 105 mm Hg. Under this strategy, adults are screened and treated if they have persistent mild hypertension. For this model, the initial assumptions (Table 2) are based on the best available data. We subjected our estimates to sensitivity analysis by varying them over the ranges shown in Table 2.

Population under Consideration
We used published data on life expectancy, morbidity, and response to therapy in adults. Life-table data for men and women of all races in the United States in 1986 are the basis for our estimates of the expected survival of treated hypertensive subjects (28). We estimated cost-effectiveness for men and women separately; they were assumed to be 20, 40, or 60 years of age at the time of screening.

Effect of Therapy
We relied on a previous meta-analysis (16) for estimates of the effect of therapy. This analysis used the Mantel-Haenszel method to estimate the reduction in relative risk for nonfatal myocardial infarction, nonfatal stroke, and all-cause mortality from eight community-based trials of hypertension therapy. These estimates are expressed as the odds ratio for having an event in the treatment group compared with the control group. The results of this analysis did not differ substantially from a previous analysis that used a slightly different population of trials (15). We allowed the baseline estimates to vary by two standard deviations (the approximate 95% confidence intervals) for upper and lower estimates of efficacy in the sensitivity analysis. The risk-ratio estimates for some complications of hypertension are not significantly different from 1.0. There are trends, however, and they represent the best available estimates of the true efficacy. We used confidence intervals around these estimates in our sensitivity analysis. This method allows us to recognize uncertainty in our data but does not force us to

Table 2. *Assumptions for the Cost-Effectiveness Analysis of Screening Asymptomatic Adults for Hypertension*

Variable	Base Case	Range for Sensitivity Analysis
Age at screening or treatment, y	40	20 to 60
Prevalence of hypertension		
Women	0.051	0.013 to 0.095
Men	0.105	0.052 to 0.134
Yearly heart attack rate for untreated persons	0.0041	0.0020 to 0.0082
Yearly stroke rate for untreated persons	0.0024	0.0012 to 0.0048
Relative risk for death with treatment	0.88	0.79 to 0.97
Relative risk for heart attack with treatment	0.91	0.82 to 1.01
Relative risk for stroke with treatment	0.6	0.51 to 0.71
Compliance with follow-up	1.0	0.5 to 0.9
Cost of screening, $	5	0 to 50
Cost of death, $	1000	100 to 10 000
Cost of heart attack, $	10 000	1000 to 100 000
Cost of stroke, $	5000	500 to 50 000
Cost of treatment per year, $	300	50 to 500
Discount rate, %	5	3 to 8
Quality adjustment for heart attack, y	0.5	0 to 1.0
Quality adjustment for stroke, y	1.5	0 to 3.0
Mortality in treated hypertension*	1.0	0.85 to 1.15

* As a fraction of U.S. age- and sex-adjusted mortality.

assume that a small, statistically insignificant effect does not exist.

To estimate death rates in untreated hypertensive persons we multiplied the 5-year age-specific mortality rates in the general U.S. population by the relative risk for mortality of untreated hypertensive subjects. The treated group was assumed to have the same mortality as the general U.S. age- and sex-matched population. In the sensitivity analysis, we allowed the mortality in treated hypertensive patients to vary from 15% below to 15% above the reported mortality in the age- and sex-matched U.S. population.

Incidence and Cost of Complications
We referred to the eight community-based trials of hypertension therapy (16) for estimates of the inci-

dence of myocardial infarction and cerebrovascular accident in untreated hypertensive subjects. We took the sum of fatal events of each type and divided it by the total number of subjects at risk, correcting for the length of observation. In the sensitivity analysis, we allowed these values to range from one half to twice the base-case estimates.

We obtained our base-case estimates of the direct medical cost of death, myocardial infarction, and cerebrovascular accident from a previous study (29). According to this study, death costs $1000; myocardial infarction, $10 000; and cerebrovascular accident, $5000. We varied these estimates over a wide range in the sensitivity analysis.

Cost of Treatment

We estimated the costs of therapy from the average wholesale cost of various common medication regimens (30). Annual drug costs vary from $2.92 for reserpine (0.1 mg daily) to $220.10 for enalapril (10 mg daily). A commonly prescribed regimen combining atenolol, triamterene, and hydrochlorothiazide has an average wholesale cost of $180.67 yearly. There is often a substantial mark-up by the retail pharmacist. The cost of repeat visits to monitor blood pressure and observe for adverse reactions must also be included. In addition, many physicians order laboratory tests to monitor therapy, especially when diuretics are used. Taking all these factors into account, we estimated a cost of approximately $300 per year for care of mild hypertension. We varied this estimate over the range from $50 to $500 per year in the sensitivity analysis.

Discount Rate

As a base-case estimate, we used a discount rate of 5%. Discounting compensates for the fact that dollars paid in the future are worth less than dollars spent in the present (27). We discounted both costs and benefits and varied the rate from 3% to 8% in the sensitivity analysis.

Cost of Screening

We estimated that the direct cost of screening is $5 and varied this estimate from zero to $50. The figure of $5 estimates the marginal cost of screening done during a doctor visit or in a community screening program. The upper figure may be more appropriate for a physician visit solely for health maintenance.

Prevalence of Undetected Hypertension
We used age- and sex-specific data from the second National Health and Nutrition Examination Survey (1976 to 80) (1). This survey defined definite hypertension as "diastolic pressure greater than 95 mm Hg or systolic pressure greater than 160 mm Hg" and defined undiagnosed hypertension as "definite hypertension in a subject who had not been told of the diagnosis." If a more liberal definition of undetected hypertension (including diagnosed but untreated subjects and the lower threshold of 90/140 mm Hg) were used, then a somewhat more favorable estimate of cost-effectiveness would result because more screened subjects would be diagnosed and treated.

Compliance
Imperfect adherence to the medical regimen is included in the estimates of efficacy from the literature. All eight trials included subjects who showed less than perfect compliance with therapeutic advice. We assumed that patients offered treatment would be as adherent as those enrolled in the eight clinical trials. We also assumed that compliance with the recommendation to initiate follow-up and treatment after screening would be perfect in the base case. In the sensitivity analysis, we assumed that 10% to 50% of subjects would not have follow-up.

Quality Adjustment
We assumed that some of the value of treatment lies in averting the morbidity associated with the hypertensive complications of myocardial infarction and stroke. To quantify this value, we followed the method of Weinstein and Stason (27), who calculated that the morbidity, pain, inconvenience, and suffering associated with the average stroke is equivalent, in terms of patient utility or sense of well-being, to avoiding the stroke but suffering a loss of 1.5 years of healthy life expectancy. Likewise, they valued a heart attack at 0.5 life-year equivalents. These estimates include discounting from the time of the occurrence of the complication until the subject's death. Discounting from the time of screening to occurrence of the complication was also done. This quality adjustment is arbitrary. In the sensitivity analysis, we varied the values from zero (no quality adjustment) to twice the values used by Weinstein and Stason (27).

Results

Table 3 reports the base-case cost-effectiveness of a screening program. The cost per QALY saved by screening is $29 291 for men at age 20 years, $16 280 at 40 years, and $8374 at 60 years. For women, the corresponding figures are $44 412, $23 216, and $12 404. The absolute benefits of screening are quite small. Under our base-case assumptions, the average screenee can expect to save between 1 and 20 days of quality-adjusted life at a cost per screenee (including treatment of hypertensive screenees) of between $76 and $491. Our estimates of cost-effectiveness are higher than those of Weinstein and Stason (27), in part because we had access to the results of clinical trials that showed smaller benefits than the projections available in 1976. Of note, our analysis considered the financial costs of drug therapy but not the side effects or noncardiovascular morbidity.

Sensitivity Analyses

Table 3 summarizes the results of the sensitivity analyses. The cost-effectiveness of screening for hypertension varies greatly with gender and age at screening. Older subjects and men, because they are more likely to have high blood pressure, receive a greater benefit. Wide variation in some of the assumptions have only a small effect on the estimated cost-effectiveness of screening. For example, a fourfold change in the estimated rate of heart attacks in untreated hypertensive subjects has a minuscule effect on the cost per QALY saved (Figure 1). The effect of therapy on heart attacks and strokes, the costs of complications, the compliance with follow-up, the cost of screening, and the estimated mortality in normotensive subjects receiving treatment (as a fraction of U.S. mortality rates) also have little effect. There is a moderate effect on cost-effectiveness from varying the estimated rate of strokes in the untreated population or the degree of quality adjustment for complications of hypertension. Cost-effectiveness is highly sensitive to the discount rate, the effect of treatment on the death rate (Figure 2), and especially the annual cost of therapy (Figure 3). Because the annual cost of treating identified patients is a continuing expense and the cost of screening a person is relatively low, the cost-effectiveness of a screening policy can best be controlled by attention to the type of therapy prescribed rather than the method of screening.

Table 3. The Cost-Effectiveness of Screening Asymptomatic Adults for Hypertension: Results*

Variable	Men			Women		
	Age 20	Age 40	Age 60	Age 20	Age 40	Age 60
Marginal cost, $	281	491	456	76	255	363
Marginal life expectancy, y	0.0096	0.0302	0.0544	0.0017	0.0110	0.0293
Marginal life expectancy, d	4	11	20	1	4	11
Cost-effectiveness, $/QALY†	29 291	16 280	8374	44 412	23 216	12 404
Sensitivity analysis‡						
Yearly heart attack rate in untreated persons						
0.002	29 768†	16 458	8431	45 345	23 536	12 516
0.0082	28 387	15 937	8265	42 664	22 605	12 187
Yearly stroke rate in untreated persons						
0.0012	33 669	17 651	8768	54 302	25 944	13 216
0.0048	23 048	14 013	7659	32 212	19 046	10 997
Relative risk for death with treatment						
0.79	17 452	9138	4507	28 151	13 371	6764
0.97	68 075	47 588	29 223	85 673	59 895	39 591
Relative risk for heart attack with treatment						
0.82	28 105	15 787	8176	42 198	22 390	12 069
1.01	30 412	16 736	8556	46 548	23 990	12 712
Relative risk for stroke with treatment						
0.51	26 176	15 187	8031	38 097	21 171	11 730
0.71	32 624	17 351	8693	51 787	25 316	13 047
Compliance with follow-up						
90%	29 813	16 445	8466	47 328	23 671	12 574
50%	29 349	16 298	8384	44 736	23 267	12 422

Cost of screening						
$0	28 770	16 114	8282	41 495	22 761	12 233
$50	33 986	17 770	9201	70 657	27 310	13 941
Cost of death						
$100	29 476	16 494	8606	44 568	23 415	12 626
$10 000	27 440	14 142	6059	42 848	21 229	10 178
Cost of heart attack						
$1000	29 628	16 451	8444	44 914	23 474	12 525
$100 000	25 927	14 563	7677	39 391	20 634	11 192
Cost of stroke						
$500	30 001	16 672	8569	45 441	23 775	12 698
$50 000	22 192	12 360	6422	34 116	17 626	9459
Cost of treatment						
$50 per year	4176	2131	1013	8269	3308	1619
$500 per year	49 348	27 599	14 263	73 326	39 143	21 031
Discount rate						
3%	19 644	12 174	7175	29 279	17 301	10 591
8%	46 467	24 254	10 538	70 276	34 541	15 698
Quality adjustment						
None	39 334	18 934	8994	70 617	29 044	13 857
Double baseline	23 334	14 278	7834	32 391	19 336	11 226
Treated mortality rate						
1.15 × U.S. mortality	27 298	14 943	7575	38 784	20 901	11 043
0.85 × U.S. mortality	31 846	17 857	9350	48 004	25 674	14 002

* Using base-case assumptions.
† Dollars per quality-adjusted life-year saved.
‡ Effects of varying assumptions on cost-effectiveness.

Comparisons with Other Health Programs

The cost-effectiveness of screening for hypertension compares favorably with other interventions used in health care. (To facilitate comparisons, we express all the cost-effectiveness figures in this section in 1988 U.S. dollars adjusted for inflation.) A review of cost-effectiveness (also called cost-utility) analysis (31) found that surgery for left main coronary artery disease cost $4500/QALY, neonatal intensive care for infants weighing under 1000 g cost $35 300/QALY, and hospital hemodialysis cost $57 300/QALY. More recently, an analysis (32) of the use of non-ionic radiologic contrast media found the cost per QALY to be $56 700. An analysis (33) of another screening program (exercise electrocardiography) for cardiovascular disease in asymptomatic subjects found that cost-effectiveness ranged from $24 600/life-year (without quality adjustment) for 60-year-old men to more than $200 000 for 40-year-old women.

Balancing Risks, Costs, and Benefits: Conclusions

The cost-effectiveness analysis provides an estimate of the balance among the risks, costs, and benefits of screening for hypertension. Where the data are uncertain, we make assumptions that disfavor screening. Despite this practice, the analysis supports screening adults for hypertension. Men should be screened at a younger age than women. The cost-effectiveness of screening for hypertension depends greatly on the cost of treatment.

Frequency of Screening

Because hypertension is common, measuring blood pressure in previously unscreened adults will frequently show new cases of hypertension. Repeat screening, however, has a much lower yield. Because the number of undiagnosed cases in the population is lower after the initial screen, the cost of finding an undiagnosed case goes up. The most critical question, therefore, is not should we screen but how often should we screen. A rational answer depends in part on the yield of hypertensive subjects in a previously screened population and the consequences of a delay in treatment. What is the chance that a normotensive (or borderline) subject will develop hypertension during the screening interval? What is the damage done by not treating during that interval? These basic aspects of the natural history of hypertension and the effect of hypertensive

The Resting Electrocardiogram as a Screening Test: A Clinical Analysis

HAROLD C. SOX, Jr., MD; ALAN M. GARBER, MD, PhD; and BENJAMIN LITTENBERG, MD

The most commonly done screening test for coronary artery disease is undoubtedly the resting electrocardiogram (ECG). Many physicians include a resting ECG when they do a complete health appraisal. There are several reasons to question this practice. The annual probability that a previously asymptomatic man at average risk will have angina pectoris, myocardial infarction, or sudden cardiac death is less than 4 per 1000 at 40 years of age and 18 per 1000 at 60 years of age (1). The annual incidence of coronary artery disease in men with no cardiovascular risk factors, calculated using the Framingham risk score, is only 1.4 per 1000 and 7.4 per 1000 at 40 and 60 years of age, respectively. Furthermore, the incidence of coronary artery disease has fallen since these data were obtained by the Framingham Study. Second, the resting ECG is an imperfect reflection of existing coronary artery disease and a poor predictor of future heart disease. Third, the effect of early detection on the outcome of coronary artery disease is not known. Very little is known of the prognosis of coronary artery disease in asymptomatic persons.

Many experts have recommended against using a resting ECG to screen for coronary artery disease. The Canadian Task Force on the Periodic Health Examination (2) concluded that there was strong evidence against obtaining resting ECGs as part of the periodic health examination of asymptomatic patients. The Institute of Medicine (3) did not list a resting ECG among its recommended preventive services for well persons. Frame (4) did not recommend a resting ECG because of its low sensitivity for coronary artery disease and the lack of treatment, other than risk-factor reduction, for ECG abnormalities in asymptomatic persons. Breslow and Somers (5) did not include the resting ECG among recommended preventive services for healthy people. These authors did not present the

▶ This chapter was originally published in *Annals of Internal Medicine*. 1989;**111**:489-502.

47

evidence on which their recommendations were based. The purpose of this paper is to analyze the evidence that a resting ECG should be done in ambulatory, asymptomatic men who do not have hypertension or other risk factors for coronary artery disease.

Definitions and Scope

We define *screening* as testing for a disease in a person who has no evidence for the condition. Using this definition of screening, we assume that a clinician has taken a brief cardiac history and done a physical examination that includes cardiac auscultation and sphygmomanometry. If this examination is abnormal, if a serum cholesterol screening test is abnormal, or if the patient has diabetes mellitus or smokes cigarettes, many physicians would obtain an ECG. We will not discuss the diagnostic value of the ECG in persons with risk factors for coronary artery disease or clinical evidence of heart disease. We are concerned with the patient who has no clinical evidence of heart disease and does not have risk factors for developing heart disease. Our topic is the use of the screening ECG in ambulatory adults in a primary-care setting. The ECGs done before surgery and at hospital admission have been discussed by Goldberger and O'Konski (6). We will not discuss diseases that are rarely seen in primary-care practice.

A good screening test detects disease before the occurrence of symptoms and at a reasonable cost, and is done because a patient can benefit more from early treatment than if treatment were delayed until symptoms occurred. Therefore, the following questions are pertinent: First, what is the prognosis of the ECG finding in such persons? Second, how prevalent is the ECG finding in persons without other evidence of heart disease? Finally, can early detection of the ECG finding lead to treatments that are more effective because they are used early?

We first discuss the use of the ECG to identify persons who are especially likely to have a serious outcome that could be prevented by early treatment. In this discussion, we consider many ECG findings, posing two questions: First, does a person with the particular finding have an increased probability of a serious cardiac event? Second, will early detection of this person's risk status reduce the chance of having the cardiac event? To answer the second question, we examine the evidence on whether treatment is effective and, if so, whether there is an advantage to starting treatment before symptoms of heart disease have occurred. Our second topic is the baseline ECG. We ask if an ECG obtained during good health might improve health outcomes by helping a physician to interpret a subsequent ECG. After reviewing this evidence, we discuss the value of using an ECG to screen for heart disease and make recommendations.

Detecting Silent Heart Disease

Table 1 gives an overview of ECG abnormalities in asymptomatic persons. A six-lead ECG and a heart-disease questionnaire were obtained from 18 403 British male civil servants, 40 to 64 years of age (7). After 5 years, the vital status of 99% of the cohort was obtained from the National Health Service Central Registry. Based on their responses to the baseline questionnaire, most of the cohort had no evidence of coronary artery disease. Table 1 shows the prevalence of ECG findings and the associated mortality rates for subjects with symptoms of coronary artery disease and for asymptomatic persons. The prevalence of the ECG findings in asymptomatic men is much lower than in men with symptoms. Furthermore, when these ECG findings are present, the risk of dying from coronary artery disease is still quite low. Potentially significant ECG findings occur in 10 to 15 persons per 1000 asymptomatic persons. When these findings are present, the death rate from coronary artery disease is only 30 per 1000 per 5 years. Thus, ECG findings occur much less commonly in healthy people than in patients with heart disease, and they have a better prognosis. The British report underscores the importance of avoiding conclusions that are based on studies of a heterogeneous population. Whenever possible, we base our conclusions on studies of patients with no clinical evidence for heart disease and no cardiovascular risk factors.

Ventricular Premature Beats

Risk Factor

The risk for death is increased when a person with known coronary artery disease has frequent ventricular premature beats. The role of ventricular premature beats as a prognostic factor in persons without known coronary artery disease is less clear. There have been several population studies (7-12) of ventricular premature beats in apparently healthy persons; these

Table 1. *Prevalence of Electrocardiographic Abnormalities and Death Rate from Coronary Artery Disease in Asymptomatic and Symptomatic Men*

Finding	Asymptomatic		Symptomatic	
	Prevalence	5-yr CAD Death Rate	Prevalence	5-yr CAD Death Rate
Q wave				
Large	0.4	420	8.6	70
Medium	3.6	50	15.6	90
Small	11.8	30†	20.2	90
Left axis deviation	28.9	20†	44.1	80†
ST depression				
Major	0.9	0	5.8	390†
Intermediate	3.7	20	26.3	110†
Minor	3.6	30	18.1	110†
Upward sloping	0.9	0	2.1	0
T-wave inversion				
Major	0.1	0	0.8	0
Intermediate	5.1	30	42.4	210†
Minor or flattening	27.9	30†	60.1	80†
AV conduction defect				
2:1 block	0.1	0	0.05	450
First-degree block	22.9	10	30.5	40
WPW syndrome	0.3	0	0	0
Left bundle branch block	13.7	30†	27.6	80
Rhythm disturbance				
> 10 VPBs per minute	12.5	30	20.2	40
Atrial fibrillation	2.1	70†	15.2	30
Rate > 100/minute	24.3	10	20.2	120†
Rate < 50/minute	13.5	0	11.9	70
Entire population	15 974	10	2429	50

* Adapted from a table in Fisher and Tyroler (10). All prevalence and mortality rates are expressed as number per 1000 subjects. CAD = coronary artery disease; AV = atrioventricular; VPBs = ventricular premature beats; WPW = Wolff-Parkinson-White syndrome.

† Denotes a coronary artery disease death rate in men with the ECG finding that is higher ($P < .05$) than the death rate in men without the ECG finding.

studies are summarized in Table 2. Some studies used total mortality from coronary artery disease as an endpoint, whereas others used sudden death. By definition, sudden death is unexpected and occurs within an hour of the onset of the terminal illness (some studies

Table 2. *(Continued)*

Rose (7)	Fisher (10)†‡	Knutsen (12)	Total
5	11	12	...
194	78	54	584
6	4	6	21
5.0	4.4	8.3	...
15 620	1099	7435	35 939
154	33	187	447
1.9	2.6	2.0	...
3.4	1.9	4.7	3.6¶
1.5 to 7.5	0.7 to 5.2	2.1 to 10.8	2.3 to 5.6
0.013	0.068	0.008	0.016

§ Mortality rate is expressed as number of deaths per 1000 subjects.
‖ Relative risk was calculated by adding 0.5 to each cell before taking the cross product. Pooled relative risk is 3.6 (95% CI, 2.3 to 5.6) and was determined by taking the mean weighted by the reciprocal of the variance.
¶ Pooled relative risk was determined by taking the mean weighted by the reciprocal of the variance.

nary artery disease in men who had frequent ventricular premature beats was 4.7 (95% CI, 2.1 to 10.8).

A different form of evidence about the prognosis of ventricular premature beats is provided by a longitudinal study of 73 asymptomatic persons who had been referred to cardiologists because of complex ventricular ectopy (14-16). Multiform ventricular ectopic beats were present in 63% of the patients, ventricular couplets in 60%, bigeminy in 96%, and three-to-four-beat runs of ventricular tachycardia in 26%. Because of risk factors for coronary artery disease, 25 patients had coronary arteriography, and 6 (24%) had at least 50% stenosis of at least one vessel. After 6.5 years of observation, 5 of the 73 patients had had angina, nonfatal myocardial infarction, or cardiac arrest, and 1 patient had died suddenly. The survival curve for this cohort was similar to that of a normal population of the same age.

Table 2 summarizes the five longitudinal studies in which patients with and without ventricular premature beats were observed concurrently. With one exception, the range of annual mortality rates for coronary artery disease in patients with ventricular premature beats was 4.4 to 8.3 per 1000. The studies are homogeneous, as judged by the similar annual mortality rates, study designs, and patient populations. All but one study used the same definition of frequent ventricular premature beats (at least 10% of all beats).

The studies were statistically homogeneous by the chi-square test (17). We therefore pooled the studies. The prevalence of ventricular premature beats in the pooled sample is 1.6%. The relative risk of death from coronary artery disease in the pooled sample is 3.6 (95% CI, 2.3 to 5.6). In these healthy populations, frequent ventricular premature beats are a risk factor for death from coronary artery disease. The attributable risk from ventricular premature beats (the mortality rate in people with ventricular premature beats minus the mortality rate in people with no ventricular premature beats) ranged from 1.8 to 6.3 deaths per 1000 per year.

The prevalence of frequent ventricular premature beats in the population studies was as low as 0.008 and as high as 0.041. The prevalence in the pooled sample was 0.016.

Treatment
There have been many studies showing that antiarrhythmic drugs reduce the frequency of ventricular premature beats. As discussed by Reid (18), there is no placebo-controlled evidence that antiarrhythmic drugs prolong life, with the single exception of long-term therapy with beta-adrenergic blocking agents after myocardial infarction. We did a MEDLINE search of the English-language literature from 1966 to 1987 and found no studies on the effect of antiarrhythmic therapy on survival in people without clinical evidence of heart disease. Effective antiarrhythmic drugs have significant side effects, including death. The mortality rate in people who have ventricular premature beats but do not have evidence of coronary artery disease is quite low (Table 2). For these reasons, treatment of ventricular premature beats is not generally recommended in people without evidence of heart disease (19).

Bifascicular Block

The three pathways for electrical activation of the ventricles are the right bundle branch and the anterior and posterior branches of the left bundle branch. When one of these pathways is interrupted, the sequence in which the ventricles are activated is abnormal. This condition is not serious in itself but is a marker for heart disease, especially coronary artery disease, and may be a precursor of complete heart block, which is a cause of sudden death.

In bifascicular block, two of the three main branch-

es of the ventricular conduction pathway are interrupted. Bifascicular block includes left bundle branch
block and right bundle branch block in association
with left anterior hemiblock (the anterior fascicle ot
the left bundle) or left posterior hemiblock (the posterior fascicle of the left bundle). (Unlike some authors,
we follow the convention of including left bundle
branch block in bifascicular block). Each of the forms
of bifascicular block is recognizable on a resting ECG.
Interruption of the remaining fascicle results in complete heart block and possibly sudden death. If this
sequence were common, early detection of bifascicular
block followed by the insertion of a prophylactic cardiac pacemaker might save many lives. Is detecting
bifascicular block a valid reason for doing an ECG in
a healthy person?

Risk Factor
There are two approaches to measuring the prognosis
of bifascicular block. Population studies have compared the mortality rate in apparently healthy middle-
aged men with left bundle-branch block (LBBB) with
the mortality rate in men without LBBB. None of 39
people with LBBB died in 4 years in Tunstall Pedoe's
study (11). There were too few enrollees in the Honolulu Heart Study with LBBB to study its prognosis.
The age-adjusted mortality rate in people with LBBB
was 6 per 1000 per year in the study of British civil
servants; this rate was significantly higher ($P < .05$)
than the rate in those without LBBB (7). Thus, the
prognosis of LBBB in healthy people is not yet clear,
although the mortality rate has been low.

When LBBB occurs in a person with clinically apparent cardiac disease, the prognosis is relatively poor.
Of a cohort of 5209 persons in the Framingham Study
(20), 55 persons developed LBBB. The mean age at
onset was 62 years. Most of the 55 patients (73%)
had other clinical evidence of cardiac disease before
developing LBBB. Within 10 years of the appearance
of LBBB, 50% of the patients died of cardiovascular
disease compared with only 11.6% of age-matched
subjects who did not have LBBB. The causes of death
from coronary artery disease were not reported, so
that the proportion who died from sequellae of LBBB,
such as complete heart block, is unknown.

In these populations, LBBB, which is one of the
forms of bifascicular block, was an infrequent finding.
In these populations, only 2 of 7682 enrollees (0.02%)
in the Honolulu Heart Study had complete LBBB

(12). In two British studies (7, 11), the prevalence of LBBB was 1.2% and 0.5%, respectively.

Treatment
Studies in large populations have not evaluated the prognostic importance of other forms of bifascicular block. The prognosis of right bundle-branch block in association with left anterior hemiblock or left posterior hemiblock, as well as LBBB, has been studied in cohorts of persons who were referred to a medical center because of these findings. Most of the cohort studies indicated how many patients developed complete heart block, an outcome that is potentially preventable by a cardiac pacemaker. Thus, the cohort studies provide important insight into the potential value of early detection and treatment of bifascicular block.

McAnulty and colleagues (21) followed 554 patients who had all types of bifascicular block for a period that averaged 42 months. The mean age of the patients was 63 years, and 74% had associated heart disease. Almost 30% of the cohort died during an observation period that averaged 42 months. Forty-two percent of the deaths were sudden, 73% of which were due to causes other than bradyarrhythmias. Only two deaths were known to be associated with a bradyarrhythmia. Each year, 1% of the cohort developed complete heart block. All but 2 of the 19 patients with complete heart block were successfully treated with a cardiac pacemaker. Complete heart block was preceded by symptoms of cardiac disease in 18 of the 19 patients.

DePasquale and Bruno (22) contrasted the prognosis of acute and chronic bifascicular block. He followed 115 patients with bifascicular block who presented either as admissions to the coronary care unit or to an office setting. One quarter of the patients admitted to the coronary care unit developed complete heart block, and the patients in the coronary care unit as a group had a very high in-hospital mortality rate. The 83 office patients with bifascicular block were followed for a mean of 3.1 years. Only 2 patients developed complete heart block; syncope preceded heart block in both patients. Chronic bifascicular block had a good prognosis in this study.

The prognosis of bifascicular block in asymptomatic persons was studied in 86 patients who were followed for an average of 3.31 years (23). The mean age of this cohort was 62 years. The cumulative incidence of sudden death was 11% in those who were monitored for 5 years. Only 1 patient developed complete heart block independent of other cardiac disease, and that person had premonitory syncope.

Bifascicular block occurs in apparently healthy persons but progresses to complete heart block relatively infrequently and almost always after warning symptoms (usually syncope). Preventive treatment of bifascicular block is not indicated. Sudden death is relatively common in patients with bifascicular block but is usually related to underlying heart disease rather than to bradyarrhythmias and complete heart block.

Left Axis Deviation

Defined as a shift in the electrical axis of the heart, left axis deviation is usually due to an interruption in the anterior division of the left bundle branch. By definition, left axis deviation is a mean QRS vector of less than −30 degrees in the frontal plane.

Risk Factor

Left axis deviation is associated with heart disease. Elliot and colleagues (24) compared 195 members of the armed forces who had left axis deviation as their only ECG finding with a control group of 100 men who had a normal ECG and clinical examination. Subjects with left axis deviation had hypertension, angina pectoris, latent diabetes, and hypercholesterolemia much more frequently than the subjects in the control group, both at the start of the study and during the 22-month follow-up period. The association of left axis deviation with other evidence of cardiac disease was confirmed by Corne and colleagues (25) in a study of 413 insurance applicants who were compared with an age-matched control group.

There have been several studies (Table 3) of left axis deviation in persons without other evidence of heart disease (isolated left axis deviation). In the Tecumseh study (8, 9), the age-adjusted death rate in 105 persons with isolated left axis deviation was the same as in the Tecumseh cohort as a whole. The relative risk of death from coronary artery disease was 1.1 (95% CI, 0.3 to 4.1). In the study (7) of British civil servants, the coronary artery disease mortality rate for isolated left axis deviation was 4 per 1000 per year. The relative risk for death from coronary artery disease was 2.1 (95% CI, 1.1 to 4.1).

The Honolulu Heart Study (27) measured the prognosis of isolated left axis deviation in a cohort of 5754 Japanese-American men between 45 and 69 years of age. None of the patients had hypertension, overt cardiac disease, or other ECG abnormalities. People with abnormal axis deviation were subdivided into those with left axis deviation (axis between –30 and –44 degrees) and those with left anterior hemiblock (axis between –45 and –90 degrees). All subjects were monitored for primary coronary events during a period that averaged 4.75 years. The rate of fatal coronary artery disease was 0.7% in the 138 men with isolated left axis deviation, 1.4% in the 70 men with isolated left anterior hemiblock, and 0.25% in 5446 men with neither finding. The relative risk of death from coronary artery disease with isolated left axis deviation was 4.1 (95% CI, 0.8 to 22.1). The number of events was too small to justify strong conclusions.

We pooled these three studies on the natural history of isolated left axis deviation (Table 3). The pooled relative risk was 2.0 (95% CI, 1.2 to 3.5). Left axis deviation, even in people without evidence of coronary artery disease, is a predictor of death from coronary artery disease. However, the attributable risk from left axis deviation is very low, ranging from 0.1 to 2.7 deaths per 1000 per year. The prevalence of left axis deviation in the population studies ranged from 0.022 to 0.029. The prevalence in the pooled sample was 0.027.

Other than those of coronary artery disease, for which it is a marker, left axis deviation has no management implications. The implications of treating coronary artery disease in asymptomatic persons are discussed in the section on myocardial ischemia.

First-Degree Atrioventricular Block

On the electrocardiogram, the PR interval is longer than 0.20 seconds in first-degree atrioventricular block. First-degree atrioventricular block does not cause symptoms and is of interest because it might reflect atrioventricular node disease that could progress to complete heart block. Several studies have examined the prognosis of first-degree atrioventricular block.

Perlman and colleagues (28) monitored the outcome of first-degree atrioventricular block in 63 members of the Tecumseh study cohort. The frequency of other cardiovascular disease and of risk factors for coronary artery disease was similar in case-subjects and in controls who did not have atrioventricular block. At the end of the 47-month follow-up period, 46 of the case-subjects had shorter PR intervals than

Table 4. *Data from Longitudinal Studies on the Prognosis of Q Waves**

	Rose (7)	Pedoe (11)	Higgins (46)	Total
Follow-up, *y*	5	4	8	. . .
With Q waves, *n*				
Lived	244	82	21	347
Died	10	2	4	16
Annual mortality rate†	7.8	5.9	20.0	. . .
Without Q waves, *n*				
Lived	15 573	8086	2224	25 883
Died	157	49	87	293
Annual mortality rate†	1.9	1.5	4.7	. . .
Relative risk	4.2	5.0	5.3	4.6‡
95% CI	2.3 to 8.0	1.4 to 18.0	1.9 to 15.0	2.8 to 7.6
Prevalence of finding	0.016	0.01	0.01	0.014

* Definition of Q waves was based on Minnesota codes 1.1-1.3.
† Mortality rate is expressed as number of deaths per 1000 subjects.
‡ Pooled relative risk.

the relative risk do not include 1.0, indicating a statistically significant association. In the pooled sample, the relative risk of dying from coronary artery disease is 2.6 if T-wave inversion is present (95% CI, 2.0 to 3.3). The attributable risk from T-wave inversion ranged from 1.0 to 4.7 deaths per 1000 per year.

Abnormalities of the ST segment at rest increase the probability of dying from coronary artery disease. Whether or not the definition of an abnormal ST segment includes ST-segment elevation, the relative risk for dying from coronary artery disease is 3.4. The attributable risk from ST-segment depression ranged from 0 to 8.4 deaths from coronary artery disease per 1000 per year.

Prevalence
The ECG indicators of myocardial ischemia occur infrequently in apparently healthy men. The prevalence of Q waves was similar in the three population studies, and the prevalence in the pooled sample was 0.014. The prevalence of T-wave inversion ranged from 0.033 to 0.074; the prevalence in the pooled sample was 0.043. The prevalence of ST-segment changes was similar in all four studies, ranging from 0.009 to 0.02.

Diagnostic Significance
The resting ECG has been an imperfect indicator of

Table 5. *Data from Longitudinal Studies on the Prognosis of T-Wave Inversion*

	Rose (7)	Pedoe (11)	Higgins (46)	Knutsen (12)	Total
Follow-up, y	5	4	8	12	. . .
With T-wave inversion, n					
Lived	514	481	166	270	1431
Died	16	10	8	31	65
Annual mortality rate†	6.0	5.0	5.7	8.5	. . .
Without T-wave inversion, n					
Lived	15 290	7648	2079	7327	32 344
Died	154	41	83	355	633
Annual mortality rate†	1.9	1.3	4.7	3.8	. . .
Relative risk	3.2	4.0	1.3	2.4	2.6‡
95% CI	1.9 to 5.3	2.0 to 8.0	0.6 to 2.6	1.6 to 3.5	2.0 to 3.3
Prevalence of finding	0.033	0.060	0.074	0.038	0.043

* Definition of T-wave inversion was based on Minnesota codes 5:1-3.
† Mortality rate is expressed as number of deaths per 1000 subjects.
‡ Pooled relative risk.

coronary artery disease in patients referred for angiographic studies. Many patients with coronary artery disease do not have the resting ECG abnormalities of ischemia. In the Coronary Artery Surgery Study (42), 29% of the angina patients who took part in the randomized study had a normal resting ECG. A Q-wave myocardial infarction pattern occurred in 29%, T-wave inversion was present in 38%, and ST-segment depression occurred in only 10%. Therefore, when these findings are absent, the probability of having coronary artery disease changes very little.

Persons whose coronary arteries are angiographically normal can have Q waves, ST-segment abnormalities, and T-wave changes. In the study by Cohn and colleagues (49), 32% of 38 patients with normal coronary arteriograms had Q waves, ST-segment changes, or T-wave inversion (as compared with 53% of 62 patients with coronary artery disease). Of 37 patients with anginal chest pain but normal coronary arteriograms (50), 9 (24%) had nonspecific ST-T wave changes, and 7 (19%) had ischemic changes. These patients had an excellent prognosis. In the study by Kemp and colleagues (51) of 129 patients with chest pain and normal coronary arteriograms, 69 (53%) had ST-T wave abnormalities, but only 6 (4.6%) had a myocardial infarction pattern. The prevalence of these findings in patients who had normal coronary arteriograms may be deceptively high because the ECG finding might have influenced the decision to refer the patient. Nonetheless, these studies confirm the claim that, as predictors of coronary artery disease, ST-segment and T-wave abnormalities are nonspecific.

Therapeutic Implications

If a patient has an ECG finding that indicates an adverse prognosis, a physician must decide on an intervention strategy. One possibility would be to try to make a diagnosis of coronary artery disease by doing exercise tests followed by angiography if the tests are abnormal. This topic is discussed in another article in this series on screening tests (52). The cost-effectiveness of screening depends critically on the prevalence of severe coronary artery disease and on the assumption that coronary bypass surgery for left main stenosis prolongs life as much in asymptomatic persons as it does in people with angina pectoris. The prevalence of

Table 6. *Data from Longitudinal Studies on the Prognosis of ST-Segment Depression*

	Minnesota Codes 4:1-4			Minnesota Codes 4:1-3		
	Rose (7)	Pedoe (11)	Total	Higgins (46)	Knutsen (12)	Total
Follow-up, *y*	5	4	. . .	8	12	. . .
With ST-segment depression, *n*						
Lived	143	187	330	22	131	153
Died	3	4	7	0	23	23
Annual mortality rate*	4.1	5.3	. . .	0	12.4	. . .
Without ST-segment depression, *n*						
Lived	15 690	7648	23 318	2223	7165	9388
Died	158	41	199	91	363	454
Annual mortality rate*	2.0	1.3	. . .	5.1	4.0	. . .
Relative risk	2.4	4.4	3.4†	0.5	3.5	3.4†
95% CI	0.8 to 7.0	1.7 to 11.8	1.6 to 6.9	.03 to 9.0	2.2 to 5.5	2.2 to 5.2
Prevalence of finding	0.009	0.024	0.014	0.009	0.020	0.018

* Mortality rate is expressed as number of deaths per 1000 subjects.
† Pooled relative risk.

Table 7. *Data from Longitudinal Studies on the Prognosis of Major Electrocardiographic (ECG) Abnormalities**

| | Definition A | | |
| | Knutsen (12) | Cedres (53)† | |
		Gas Co.	Western Electric
Follow-up, *y*	12	11	20
With major ECG abnormalities, *n*			
Lived	401	28	32
Died	33	11	13
Annual mortality rate‖	5.4	16.5	20.3
Without major ECG abnormalities, *n*			
Lived	7088	992	1511
Died	160	179	130
Annual mortality rate‖	1.9	8.9	4.0
Relative risk	3.7	2.2	4.8
95% CI	2.5 to 5.4	1.1 to 4.5	2.5 to 9.3
Prevalence of finding	0.056	0.032	0.027

* Major ECG abnormalities were defined as follows: Definition A = Minnesota codes: 4.1-4.2; 5.1-5.3; 6.1-6.2; 7.1-7.2, 7.4; 8.1-8.3; Definition B = Minnesota codes: 1.1-1.3; 2.1-2.2; 3.1-3.3; 4.1-4.4; 5.1-5.3; 6.1-6.5; 7.1-7.2, 7.4; 8.1-8.8; Definition C = Minnesota codes: 1.1-1.3; 2.1-2.2; 3.1-3.3; 4.1-4.3; 5.1-5.3; 6.1-6.8; 7.1-7.8; 8.1-8.6; 9.1-9.2; right axis deviation greater than 120 degrees.

† The report by Cedres and colleagues analyzes the results of the Gas Company study, the Western Electric study, and the Chicago Electric study.

high-risk coronary artery disease is very low in asymptomatic persons in the general population (52). The prevalence of high-risk coronary artery disease when asymptomatic persons have Q waves, abnormal ST segments, or T-wave abnormalities is not known. The effect of bypass surgery on asymptomatic coronary artery disease is unknown.

Other possible treatments of asymptomatic persons include anti-anginal drugs and risk-factor reduction. This topic was discussed in the section on ECG-LVH, which concluded that aside from cardiovascular risk-factor reduction, there is no good evidence that pharmacologic or surgical treatment of coronary artery disease prolongs life in asymptomatic persons; and that cardiovascular risk-factor reduction is indicated only when these risk factors are present and not simply because of ECG-LVH. The same conclusions apply to Q waves, abnormal ST segments, and T-wave inversion.

Although associated with increased mortality from

Table 7. *(Continued)*

Definition A		Definition B	Definition C
Cedres (cont.)†		Pedoe (11)	MRFIT (38)‡
Chicago Electric§	Total		
5	. . .	4	7
592	461	1747	1149
43	57	13	26
13.5	. . .	1.8	3.2
7346	9591	6430	3625
72	469	38	54
2.0	. . .	1.5	2.1
7.4	3.6¶	1.3	1.5
5.1 to 10.9	2.6 to 4.8	0.7 to 2.4	1.0 to 2.5
0.079	0.049	0.21	0.24

‡ MRFIT = Multiple Risk Factor Intervention Trial.
§ This study was not pooled with the other Definition A studies because its results deviated so much from those of the others.
‖ Annual mortality rate is expressed as number of deaths per 1000 subjects.
¶ Pooled relative risk.

coronary artery disease, Q waves, abnormal ST segments, and T-wave inversion do not indicate a poor prognosis in apparently healthy men. In most of the population studies, the annual mortality rate was less than 10 deaths per 1000 men with these ECG findings (Tables 4, 5, and 6). These findings are uncommon, occurring in 1% to 4% of middle-aged men with no clinical evidence of coronary artery disease, and most people who are destined to die of coronary artery disease do not have these findings. There is no convincing evidence that detecting these abnormalities with a screening ECG would alter their prognosis.

The study populations for these studies of prognosis included persons with risk factors for coronary artery disease. Prognosis in persons who did not have risk factors was not reported. If there is a strong association between risk factors, ECG findings of myocardial ischemia, and death from coronary artery disease, much of the risk attributed to the ECG findings could be due to the risk factors for coronary artery disease.

Thus, the risk that these studies appear to attribute to these ECG findings represents an upper bound on the true risk.

A Global Definition of an Abnormal ECG

In a search for findings that would serve as a rationale for doing a screening ECG, this analysis has focused on the implications of individual ECG findings. In practice, physicians do a screening ECG because they hope to detect or exclude any one of several prognostically significant ECG findings. Several studies address this issue (Table 7). In these studies, an ECG was considered abnormal if any of several findings ("major ECG findings") were present. The definition of a major ECG finding varies, but four studies (7, 11, 12, 53) used the same definition (Definition A in Table 7). We applied the chi-square test for homogeneity to this pool of four studies. We found that the Chicago Electric study (53) had a significantly higher mortality rate than the other studies, and we did not include it in the pooling procedure.

If a study subject had at least one of the Definition A findings, the relative risk of dying from coronary artery disease was 3.6 (95% CI, 2.6 to 4.8). The risk attributable to a major ECG finding varied among the studies, ranging from 3.5 to 16.3 deaths from coronary artery disease per 1000 men per year. Nearly 5.0% of the pooled population of men with no clinical evidence of coronary artery disease had at least one of the major ECG findings. If the definition of abnormal is enlarged to include additional ECG findings (Definitions B and C), up to 25% of men had an abnormal ECG. However, the risk that was attributable to having at least one of these ECG findings was only 0.3 and 1.1 deaths per 1000 men per year for Definition B and Definition C, respectively (Table 7).

The populations for these studies of prognosis included persons with hypertension, hypercholesterolemia, a smoking habit, and diabetes. They did not report the risk attributable to major ECG findings in persons without these risk factors for coronary artery disease. However, there were two studies that tested the hypothesis that major ECG findings help to predict death from coronary artery disease in persons with similar risk factors (12, 53). Major ECG findings were an independent predictor of coronary artery disease mortality in both studies. However, the articles did not report the magnitude of risk that was attributable to the ECG findings. A global definition of an abnormal ECG provides a useful perspective on the yield of a screening ECG. The hypothesis that early detection can alter the prognosis of patients with these findings has not been tested.

The Value of a Baseline Electrocardiogram

The second rationale for doing an ECG in a healthy person is to help a physician decide if findings on a subsequent ECG are due to an acute process, such as myocardial infarction, or represent chronic abnormalities. If the ECG abnormalities represent change, an acute process is more likely, and hospitalization may be indicated. The logic of this rationale depends on several steps.

1. The baseline ECG must be available to the emergency physician on short notice. A baseline ECG that is in the patient's office record may not be available in an emergency situation.

2. The baseline ECG must have been done recently enough so that the patient's ECG pattern does not change during the period between the baseline ECG and presentation at the emergency department. If change occurred in the interim, the ECG in the emergency department might he interpreted incorrectly as representing an acute process, and the patient would be admitted needlessly.

3. The baseline ECG can aid in interpreting ECG findings that could represent acute myocardial ischemia. The ECG changes in patients with myocardial infarction can be quite subtle and require a baseline ECG to interpret them correctly. Approximately 67% of patients with proven myocardial infarction have the classic findings, which are usually unmistakable, of new Q waves, ST-segment elevation, and deep T-wave inversion; 10% of patients with myocardial infarction have a normal ECG. The remainder have findings that are probably nonspecific but could represent ischemia. A baseline ECG might be helpful in interpreting these subtle findings.

Several investigators have tried to assess the value of the baseline ECG in emergency-room decision making. Rubenstein and Greenfield (54) evaluated the role of the ECG in the emergency rooms of a university medical center and a community hospital. They reviewed each of 236 patients' emergency·room records, including the emergency-room ECG, and decided whether a baseline ECG could have improved the accuracy of the decision to admit the patient. A baseline ECG was available for 7% of the patients. The authors made a home visit to do an ECG on all patients who were discharged from the emergency room. The results are shown in Figure 1. The history and physical examination were sufficient to make an admission decision for 37.3% of the patients. The clinical examination was equivocal for 45.4% of the patients, but the ECG findings were indisputably normal or indicative of infarction.

A baseline ECG might have been valuable in the 41 patients whose clinical examination and emergency-room ECG were both equivocal. In 26 patients, a baseline ECG was not available, but the patient was discharged anyway. In 4 patients, comparison with a baseline ECG led to admission. None of these patients had an infarction, so that the baseline ECG did not improve the accuracy of the admission decisions. The baseline ECG was possibly useful in 11 patients (4.7%). Nine patients did not have a baseline ECG and were admitted; a baseline ECG might have prevented what the authors called an unnecessary admission. Two patients were discharged after a baseline ECG showed the emergency-room ECG to be unchanged. Thus, a baseline ECG could have been useful, if available, in only 5% of the patients.

Hoffman and Igarashi (55) asked emergency-department house officers and faculty if a baseline ECG would have been helpful in a series of patients with suspected myocardial infarction. They studied 84 consecutive adults who had a comparison ECG and were seen in the emergency room of a university hospital because of chest pain. Study data forms were filled out on all patients by at least one physician. After taking the patient's history but before seeing any electrocardiograms, the physicians were asked if a current ECG would be helpful to them in the admission decision. After seeing the current ECG, they were asked if a baseline ECG would influence their decision about admission. They were also asked to commit themselves temporarily to a course of action at three stages in their evaluation of the patient: before seeing any ECGs, after seeing a current emergency-room ECG, and after seeing the current ECG and a baseline ECG.

The house officers often stated that a comparison ECG would be useful. After seeing the current ECG, the house officer felt that a baseline ECG could influence the admission decision in 20% of the 39 admitted patients and in 30% of the 37 discharged patients. The number of faculty questionnaires was too small to draw any conclusions about differences between facul-

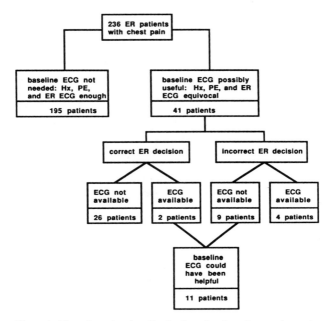

Figure 1. Flow sheet showing distribution of patients in a study on the effect of a baseline ECG on decision making in patients with suspected myocardial infarction (54). ER = emergency room; ECG = electrocardiogram; HX = history; PE = physical examination.

ty and house staff. In contrast to what the physicians said, they never changed their minds about a decision to admit or discharge a patient after seeing a comparison ECG.

These studies have significant shortcomings. The study by Rubenstein and Greenfield (54) used only two reviewers to make the judgments about the usefulness of the ECG. Their findings would have been far more convincing if they had been obtained using a panel of randomly chosen, experienced physicians. In both studies, a larger sample of cases would have been necessary to measure the frequency of uncommon but catastrophic errors of judgment that might have been prevented by a baseline ECG. Neither report included a description of the baseline ECG results and the patients. There have been no studies of a related problem: the use of a baseline tracing when interpreting ECG findings obtained before surgery.

Conclusions

Two studies of the effect of a baseline ECG on decision making in cases of patients with suspected myocardial infarction reached similar conclusions. One study

(54) showed that the baseline ECG does not improve diagnostic accuracy, and the other study (55) showed that the baseline ECG seldom affects decisions about hospital admission. These conclusions may surprise many physicians who find that the cognitive task of making these decisions is easier when a baseline ECG is available. A study with a surprising result should be repeated, and the role of the resting ECG as a baseline for interpreting other ECG findings, such as arrhythmias, should be evaluated. Nonetheless, current evidence indicates that physicians can make good interpretative judgments without a baseline ECG and seldom change their minds when they see a baseline ECG.

Summary

There is a sharp contrast between physicians' use of a resting ECG for screening and the recommendations of expert panels. Many physicians routinely do a resting ECG in asymptomatic adults with no risk factors for coronary artery disease. The Canadian Task Force on the Periodic Health Examination is just one of the groups that have recommended against doing a resting ECG as part of a comprehensive health evaluation. We have re-examined the evidence, hoping to reconcile past recommendations with the beliefs of thoughtful clinicians. We found that some ECG findings increase the probability that an apparently healthy person will die from coronary artery disease. However, these findings are uncommon, and the risk for death attributable to them is small. We do not know what happens when physicians take action based on these findings, nor do we know the consequences of watchful waiting. Despite many years of routinely doing a resting ECG, we know almost nothing about the health effects of this practice.

What should one do when there is no positive evidence for the value of a health intervention, yet one's clinical intuition indicates that it ought to have some value? We believe that additional study is needed. A randomized study of the resting ECG as a screening device might provide a measure of its health effects but events that can be attributed to the ECG findings will be infrequent and far in the future. Consequently, many interventions other than the resting ECG might be responsible for the outcome in a patient. Studies in people over 65 years of age would be particularly valuable because the prevalence of coronary artery disease in asymptomatic persons increases with age (56).

differently, a baseline ECG was associated with a small but signficant reduction in inappropriate admissions to the hospital. The impact of a baseline ECG was most striking in patients in whom the ECG done in the emergency department showed ischemia or old infarction. When the current tracing showed ischemia or old infarction and there was a baseline tracing, the relative risk that a patient without infarction would be sent home was 2.11 (95% CI, 1.57 to 2.83). Thus, the baseline ECG was most helpful when the findings on the current ECG would ordinarily lead to admission, presumably because the findings on the current ECG showed no change from the baseline ECG. Stated differently, when the current ECG showed ischemia or infarction, the probability that a patient without infarction would avoid admission to the hospital was 26% when the baseline ECG was available and 12% when it was not.

This study is a signficant advance over the studies cited in the analysis of the resting ECG for two reasons. First, the number of patients was very large, minimizing the chance of failing to detect an important difference. Second, the authors studied real decision making, unlike the two studies cited in the ACP analysis of the resting ECG.

How should this information affect our recommendations about doing a resting ECG? In our opinion, the recommendations depend on the probability that a patient will have a myocardial infarction.

Patients with an above average probability of having a myocardial infarction: Given the low cost of a resting ECG and the high cost of an inappropriate admission for suspected acute myocardial infarction, a resting ECG would appear to be a good use of resources in patients who have an above average probability of having a myocardial infarction. We recommend strongly that physicians obtain a resting ECG on such patients and send a copy of it to the hospitals where they practice. Age over 60 years, risk factors for coronary artery disease, and symptoms of coronary artery disease are all indications for a baseline resting ECG.

Patients with a below average probability of having a myocardial infarction: What about patients whose chance of a myocardial infarction is lower than average because they have neither coronary artery disease symptoms nor risk factors for coronary artery disease? In our opinion, there is not enough evidence to warrant a strong recommendation for doing a resting ECG in low risk patients. A myocardial infarction is an uncommon event in low risk patients, and many resting ECGs might be required to avoid a single inappropriate admission from the emergency department.

Thus, the primary recommendation of this paper stands: Do not do a resting ECG in a person whose history, physical examination, and laboratory findings disclose no evidence of increased risk of coronary artery disease.

Reference

1. **Lee TH, Cook EF, Weisberg MC, Rouan GW, Brand DA, Goldman L.** Impact of the availability of a prior electrocardiogram on the triage of the patient with acute chest pain. *J Gen Intern Med.* 1990;**5**:381-8.

Table 1. *(Continued)*

With CAD		Annual Incidence of CAD		Risk Ratio
Abnormal E-ECG	Normal E-ECG	Abnormal E-ECG	Normal E-ECG	
n				
15	14	2.2	0.19	11.6
15	11	8.2	0.8	10.3
14	23	3.1	0.94	3.3
21	13	2.5	0.5	5.0
13	29	0.88	0.24	3.7
85	356	1.65	1.15	1.43

main equivalent disease as significant stenosis in both the proximal left anterior descending and the proximal left circumflex coronary arteries (17). Each anatomic subset was associated with a life expectancy that could be calculated from reported studies of medically treated patients. We used the declining exponential approximation of life expectancy to convert survival data into life expectancy (18). A sample calculation is shown in the Appendix. The patient's life expectancy was calculated as follows: Life expectancy = probability (no coronary artery disease) × life expectancy (no coronary artery disease) + probability (one-vessel coronary artery disease) × life expectancy (one-vessel coronary artery disease) + ... + probability (left main coronary artery disease) × life expectancy (left main coronary artery disease). To obtain the average cost, substitute the cost for life expectancy in this equation. In this model, we considered only the costs of care that are a direct consequence of screening. Therefore, the costs of not screening are zero.

Do a Screening Exercise Test

We used the structural abnormalities of the coronary arteries as the basis of our model so that we could incorporate knowledge of the benefits of coronary bypass surgery (16, 19), which depend on the number of coronary vessels with significant stenosis. The result of exercise testing could have been either abnormal or normal. The consequences of testing depended on the results of the test.

Abnormal Exercise Test: In one version of the model, we assumed that an abnormal exercise electrocardiogram (ECG) was followed by coronary arteriography (Figure 1). In another version (not shown), an abnormal exercise ECG was followed by thallium scintigraphy, and arteriography was done only if both exercise tests were abnormal. If a patient survived arteriography and had left main stenosis, left main equivalent coronary artery disease, or three-vessel coronary artery disease and poor ventricular function ("severe" disease), we assumed that coronary artery bypass sur-

Table 2. *Frequency of Abnormal Exercise Electrocardiograms in Populations Screened for Coronary Artery Disease*

Study*	Type of Test	With an Abnormal Test
		n/n (%)
Giagnoni (52)	Submaximal	135/10 723 (1.3)
Cumming (50)	Maximal	61/510 (12.0)
Froelicher (49)	Maximal	109/1327 (8.2)
Allen (51)	Maximal	104/888 (11.7)
Bruce (40)	Maximal	264/2365 (11.2)
Hollenberg (53)	Maximal	45/377 (11.9)
Rautaharju (14)	Submaximal	734/6008 (12.2)
Gordon (13)	Submaximal	185/3640 (5.1)

* All studies used 1-mm horizontal or downsloping ST-segment depression as the criterion for an abnormal exercise test, with the exception of the study by Rautaharju (area under the ST segment within the first $7/16$ of an abnormally depressed ST segment). In addition, most of the studies used populations from whom patients with evidence of cardiac disease had been excluded, except for that by Cumming (no exclusions), that by Hollenberg (a mixture of high-risk and low-risk men), and that by Rautaharju (the top 15% of patients with cardiac risk by the Framingham risk profile).

gery would be offered. The model included the possibility that the patient would decline arteriography or surgery. If the patient had three-vessel disease and good left ventricular function, two- or one-vessel disease, we assumed that surgery would not be done, because surgery did not prolong survival in these subgroups of patients in CASS. We also assumed that medical therapy for coronary artery disease would not be given to asymptomatic persons.

Normal Exercise Test: If either the exercise ECG or thallium scintigram was normal, we assumed that there was no further intervention.

Assumptions of the Model

When the medical literature contained no information about the structural abnormalities of the coronary arteries in asymptomatic persons, the prognosis of anatomic subsets of the disease, or the effects of treatment, we made assumptions that would maximize the impact of exercise testing.

Prevalence of Disease in Asymptomatic Persons

We used the prevalence of significant coronary stenosis in persons who had an autopsy after accidental death, as summarized by Diamond and Forrester (20). In asymptomatic men, 4.0% of those less than 50 years old (mean age, 41) had coronary artery disease, and 11.0% of those more than 50 years old (mean age, 59) had the disease. In asympto-

Table 2. *(Continued)*

Mean Age	Men	Probability of an Abnormal Test†		Endpoint‡
		Subjects with CAD	Subjects without CAD	
y	%			
45	83	. . .	. . .	A,M,SD
40-65	100	. . .	. . .	None
44	100	0.52	0.07	A,M,SD
?	65	0.31	0.11	A,M,SD
45	100	0.30	0.11	A,M,SD
37	100	. . .	. . .	None
35-57	100	0.19	0.12	M,SD
48	100	0.37	0.05	CV death

† In calculating the probability of an abnormal exercise test in subjects who developed coronary artery disease and the probability of an abnormal exercise test in patients who did not develop coronary artery disease, the diagnostic endpoint was the occurrence of a primary cardiac endpoint. Blank spaces indicate no relevant data. CAD = coronary artery disease.

‡ A = angina pectoris; M = myocardial infarction; SD = sudden cardiac death; and CV death = death from cardiovascular disease.

matic women, 0.7% of those less than 50 years old (mean age, 41) had the disease, and 5.0% of those more than 50 years old (mean age, 59) had the disease.

We wanted to determine the prevalence of coronary artery disease in asymptomatic persons with no risk factors. Because this information was not known directly, we estimated it with the following procedure. The overall prevalence of the disease was derived from a population comprised of persons with no risk factors and persons with at least one risk factor. The overall prevalence of the disease was the sum of its prevalence in each subpopulation, weighted by the proportion of persons in the subpopulation. (The overall prevalence of coronary artery disease = [percent of the population that has risk factors] × [prevalence of coronary artery disease in patients with risk factors] + [percent with no risk factors] × [prevalence of coronary artery disease in patients with no risk factors]. The overall gender-specific and age-specific prevalence of coronary artery disease and the proportion of patients with no risk factors for disease were known. The prevalence of the disease in the general population of persons with no risk factors was unknown. The prevalence of the disease in persons with risk factors was a multiple of its prevalence in persons with no risk factors. We obtained the relative prevalence of the disease in persons with and without risk factors from a study (21) of 255 asymptomatic aircrewmen who had an abnormal exercise ECG. The prevalence of coronary artery disease was 0.29 and 0.10 in those with and without risk factors, respectively. Substitute 2.9 × [prevalence of coronary artery disease in patients with no risk factors for disease] for the prevalence

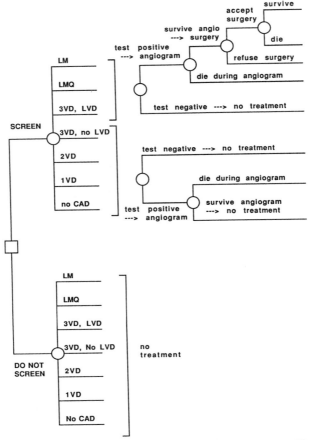

Figure 1. Decision tree for exercise testing in asymptomatic persons. The first chance node represents the true state of the patient's coronary arteries, which is unknown unless angiography is done. The next two levels of nodes represent the results of exercise testing and angiography, which are done only if the result of exercise testing is abnormal. Surgery is offered only if the angiogram shows severe coronary artery disease (CAD). To model of thallium scanning add a chance node after the "test positive" branch of the node for an exercise electrocardiogram; surgery is done only if the result of thallium testing is abnormal. The probabilities at the first chance node are taken from Table 3 and those at the second chance node from Table 4. LM=stenosis of the left main coronary artery; LMQ=left main equivalent coronary artery disease; 3VD, 2VD, and 1VD=triple-vessel, double-vessel, and single-vessel coronary artery disease (without left main stenosis), respectively; LVD=left ventricular dysfunction (35% to 50% ejection fraction measured in patients at rest); and angio=angiography.

of disease in patients with risk factors for disease and solve for the prevalence of disease in patients with no risk factors for disease. We used data from the National Health and Nutrition Examination Surveys (22) on the prevalence of persons with no risk factors (0.40) and at least one risk factor (0.60). According to our method, the prevalence of coronary artery disease in patients with no risk factors is 0.05, and the prevalence in 60-year-old men with at least one risk factor is therefore 0.15.

The results of coronary arteriography in patients catheterized for reasons other than chest pain corroborated the results of the autopsy studies. The prevalence of significant stenosis in one such arteriography study (23) was 6.3% in men and 3.4% in women. Most of the subjects in other arteriographic studies (24, 25) of asymptomatic persons had abnormal exercise test results. These studies provide an upper bound on the probability of coronary artery disease in persons who are candidates for exercise testing.

Severity of Disease in Asymptomatic Persons

There have been no studies in which coronary arteriography was done in persons with no evidence of coronary artery disease. As a proxy, we used arteriographic findings in patients from the CASS Registry who had "atypical chest pain" (17). We reasoned that the severity of disease in patients with atypical chest pain should closely approximate the severity of disease in asymptomatic persons. The only evidence pertaining to this assumption is indirect. The incidence of clinical coronary artery disease in subjects from the Seattle Heart Watch who had atypical chest pain was more than twice the incidence in symptom-free subjects (15). When coronary artery disease occurred, however, asymptomatic persons were more likely to die than persons with atypical chest pain. Overall, the probability of dying from the disease was about the same in the two groups.

Chaitman and colleagues (17) studied the prevalence of anatomic subsets of coronary artery disease in patients from CASS who had atypical chest pain (Table 3). Very few patients had left main stenosis, left main equivalent disease, or three-vessel disease. These authors reported the prevalence of left main and left main equivalent disease. Patients with these forms of coronary artery disease were also included in their tally of patients with three-vessel and two-vessel disease. For Table 3, the prevalence of patients with two-vessel and three-vessel disease who do not have left main stenosis or left main equivalent disease was estimated by removing patients with left main stenosis or left main equivalent disease from the tally of patients with three-vessel and two-vessel disease. Ninety percent of patients with left main stenosis were assumed to have been classified as having three-vessel disease and the others as having two-vessel disease. Therefore, the prevalences of left main and left main equivalent disease were added; 90% of this sum was subtracted from the prevalence of three-vessel disease and 10% of this sum was subtracted from the prevalence of two-vessel disease. For example, 13% of men under 50 years of age had left main stenosis or left main equivalent disease. In their study (17), 31% of men had three-vessel disease (including those with left main stenosis and left main equivalent disease). To estimate the prevalence of three-vessel disease without left main stenosis and left main equivalent disease, 90% of 13%, or 12%, was subtracted from 31% to obtain the prevalence of three-vessel disease alone (12%).

The CASS data are corroborated by a study (24) of 298 asymptomatic aircrewmen (mean age, 42 years) who had arteriography because of electrocardiographic findings sug-

Table 3. *The Effect of Age and Sex on the Prevalence of Anatomic Subsets of Coronary Artery Disease in Patients with Nonanginal Chest Pain**

Disease	Men		Women	
	< 50	> 50	< 50	> 50
LM†	0	0.2	0.007	0.005
LMQ	0.002	0.007	0	0.001
3VD	0.01	0.01	0	0
2VD	0.01	0.05	0.009	0.02
1VD	0.06	0.11	0.03	0.05
No CAD	0.92	0.80	0.96	0.93

    * The data were adapted from those in the study by Chaitman and colleagues (17). Each number is the prevalence of coronary artery disease in the corresponding subgroup. LM = left main; LMQ = left main equivalent; 3VD = three-vessel disease; 2VD = two-vessel disease; 1VD = one-vessel disease; and CAD = coronary artery disease.
    † Stenosis greater than 50%.

gesting coronary artery disease. None of the aircrewmen had left main stenosis, and 87% of those with coronary artery disease had one- or two-vessel disease. These aircrewmen were asymptomatic, and it is unlikely that the patients with three-vessel disease had poor ventricular function. Nevertheless, we assumed that the prevalence of poor ventricular function in three-vessel disease was the same (20%) as in patients from CASS. We did not find any arteriographic studies of asymptomatic women or older men.

We assumed that the severity of coronary artery disease in asymptomatic men and women was the same as in patients with atypical chest pain and arteriographically proven disease. *This assumption may overestimate the prevalence of severe coronary artery disease and may make the effect of screening appear larger than its true effect.*

Test Performance of Exercise Electrocardiography
The decision model (Figure 1) required the frequency of abnormal exercise test results in the anatomic subsets of coronary artery disease. Three studies (10, 11, 26) had large study populations and reported the frequency of several exercise test endpoints in each anatomic subset. We used the study (11) that had the largest number of patients for most of the analyses. We had no information on the frequency of an abnormal exercise test in left main equivalent coronary artery disease and assumed that it was the same as in three-vessel disease. We assumed that a physician would treat an equivocal test in the same way as a negative test when deciding whether to do additional studies. The effect of this assumption is to reduce cost due to false-positive results at the expense of missing a few patients with the disease.

The true-positive rates shown in Table 4 are probably higher than if all patients who had an exercise ECG had been enrolled in the studies. Patients with normal exercise tests are likely to be underrepresented in the study population, because patients with a normal exercise test are less likely to be referred for arteriography. This referral bias decreases the frequency of false-negative results in the study population as compared with all persons who have an exercise test. A study that underestimates false-negative findings must overestimate true-positive findings. *Using these data sources makes exercise testing in asymptomatic persons appear more effective than it really is.*

The false-positive rate of the exercise ECG in a population of healthy persons may be estimated from the frequency of positive tests in a population of healthy persons. We used the data in Table 2 and the methods described in the Appendix. When the criterion for an abnormal exercise ECG was ST-segment depression of 1 mm or greater, the false-positive rate of the exercise ECG in asymptomatic men was 0.09. Then another exercise ECG finding was the criterion for an abnormal test, we used the frequency of the finding in patients with a normal coronary arteriogram as the false-positive rate of the exercise ECG. We assumed that the false-positive rate of the exercise ECG is 0.09 in women, even though there is evidence that the false-positive rate in women is higher than in men (26, 27). *This assumption makes exercise testing in asymptomatic women appear more effective than it really is.*

We assumed that the interpretation of the exercise test in community practice would be as rigorous as in these studies, in which the investigators followed written criteria. If physicians in community practice interpreted the exercise ECG as abnormal more frequently than did the investigators, the true-positive rate and false-positive rate of the test would be larger in community practice than as represented in Table 4. Both measures of test performance would be smaller than shown in Table 4 if community physicians consistently failed to identify exercise ECG abnormalities.

Longevity of Asymptomatic Persons

The purpose of our model was to calculate the effect of screening on the length of patients' lives, which depends on the extent of coronary artery disease. There have been no angiographic studies of persons who did not have any clinical evidence of coronary artery disease, and therefore, the mortality rate of each anatomic subset of the disease is unknown. The best characterization of asymptomatic persons with angiographically defined coronary artery disease is found in the studies by Erikssen and colleagues (28, 29) of 50 men with abnormal exercise electrocardiograms. These men were all instructed to follow a moderate lipid-lowering diet, to exercise, and to stop smoking. During the first 8.5 years of observation, 3 men died from coronary artery disease, and the annual mortality rate was zero, 0.6%, and 0.9% in one-vessel, two-vessel, and three-vessel disease, respectively. By 13.5 years of follow-up, 6 more men had died from coronary artery disease. The overall mortality rate for the entire 13.5-year period was 1.5% per year. Of the 9 men who died from coronary artery disease, 8 had angina before death. Thus, the mortality rate before the first symptoms of the disease is low, and warning symptoms precede death in most patients. From a review of these and other data, Cohn (30) concluded that the mortality rate in asymptomatic persons with coronary artery disease was approximately one half that of treated symptomatic patients.

We used the CASS randomized trial (16, 19) of coronary bypass surgery as the source of mortality rates for asympto-

Table 4. *Test Performance of Exercise Electrocardiography**

Criterion for Abnormal Result	Probability of Result	
	All	1VD
McNeer (11)†		
Patients, *n*	875	408
≥ 1-mm ST depression	0.44	0.32
Indeterminant	0.17	0.18
< 1-mm ST depression	0.39	0.50
≥ 1-mm ST depression and less than 6 min of exercise time	0.24	0.09
Bartel (10)		
Patients, *n*	451	108
≥ 1-mm ST depression	0.48	0.27
Indeterminant	0.26	0.29
< 1-mm ST depression	0.26	0.44
≥ 2-mm ST depression	0.20	0.11
Weiner (25)		
Patients, *n*	350	220‡
≥ 1-mm ST depression	0.71	0.58
Indeterminant	0.11	0.14
< 1-mm ST depression	0.28	0.28

* 1VD = one-vessel disease; 2VD = two-vessel disease; 3VD = three-vessel disease; LM = left main; and CAD = coronary artery disease.

† In this study, patients with single- and two-vessel disease were combined. We assume that the frequency of findings is the same in these two groups. This assumption does not lead to error in our model, because patients with single- and double-vessel disease have the same life expectancy both with and without surgery (16, 19), and they are managed the same way, according to the model (Figure 1).

matic patients with coronary artery disease. In our model, three groups of asymptomatic persons had the disease but did not have surgery: those whose angiogram showed either one- or two-vessel disease, or three-vessel disease and good ventricular function; those who had a normal exercise test; and those who did not have an exercise test. Findings in the medically treated patients in CASS should be congruent with those in the first group, although these patients probably have a higher mortality rate than asymptomatic patients with a normal exercise test. The third group, those who are not screened, are analogous to the 50 asymptomatic patients in the studies by Erikssen and Thaulow (28, 29) described previously. Erikssen and Thaulow (28) measured the mortality rate of coronary artery disease in patients who were asymptomatic when they were diagnosed as having the disease by angiographic means and in patients who were symptomatic when they were first diagnosed as having the disease. The asymptomatic patients had a much lower mortality rate than the symptomatic patients. In the second study (29), done by Erikssen alone, patients who were initially asymptomatic were not compared with patients who were symptomatic. For the entire 13-year period, however, the mortality rate in the initially asymptomatic persons was lower than that reported for the medically treated patients in CASS. *By using medically treated patients in CASS as a*

Table 4. *(Continued)*

	Probability of Result (cont.)		
2VD	3VD	LM	No CAD
. . .	360	107	597
0.32	0.53	0.63	0.07
0.18	0.17	0.14	0.17
0.50	0.30	0.22	0.76
	0.23	0.36	0.008
113	180	31	199
0.50	0.52	0.84	0.06
0.25	0.30	?	0.33
0.25	0.18	0.16	0.61
0.11	0.26	0.52	0.005
. . .	93	37	141
0.58	0.93	0.92	0.16
0.14	0.04	0.05	0.12
0.28	0.03	0.03	0.72

‡ In this study, patients with single- and double-vessel disease were combined. In addition, of their 55 patients with indeterminant tests, only the number of such patients that had left main and three-vessel disease were specified. We assumed that the remaining 49 patients were distributed equally between single-vessel disease, double-vessel disease, and no CAD.

surrogate for unscreened asymptomatic persons with coronary artery disease, we overestimated both the mortality rate in unscreened persons and, therefore, the effect of screening.

Effectiveness of Coronary Artery Surgery in Asymptomatic Persons

No randomized studies have been done on the effect of coronary artery bypass surgery or angioplasty on survival in asymptomatic persons with coronary artery disease. In one nonrandomized study (31) of coronary artery bypass surgery, 18% of the patients were asymptomatic. Unfortunately, the effect of surgery on these patients' survival was not analyzed separately. Therefore, screening for coronary artery disease does not meet an essential requirement for adopting a screening policy: *that there should be good evidence that early detection alters prognosis.* To analyze the case for screening in the most favorable light, we assumed that surgery has the same effect on survival in asymptomatic persons with three-vessel disease and poor ventricular function as it did in the CASS randomized trial. In the case of left main stenosis and left main equivalent coronary artery disease, we assumed that the effect of surgery was the same as in the report (32) from the European Coronary Surgery Study Group and that (33) from the CASS Registry, respectively. For single-vessel and two-vessel disease and for three-vessel disease with good ventricular function, we used survival data from CASS. The conclusions of this study about the effect of surgery were similar to those of the Veterans Administration Cooperative trial. We chose CASS as our source of survival data because the patients appeared to have relatively mild coronary artery disease, angiographically and clinically, as would be expected in asymptomatic persons. The European Cooperative Surgery Study had many more patients with proximal stenosis of the left anterior descending coronary artery and many more patients with severe angina than the two American studies (34, 35). We did not use the European study because its patients seemed so dissimilar to asymptomatic patients.

Unwillingness to Have Surgery
In our model, surgery is offered to patients with high-risk coronary artery disease. Asymptomatic persons would probably decline surgery more frequently than patients with angina. However, we assumed that asymptomatic persons with severe disease would decline surgery at the same rate (11%) as patients with angina in CASS (16). *This assumption makes the effect of screening appear larger than the true effect.*

Mortality of Cardiovascular Procedures
Mortality rates are based on the published literature. Because so few asymptomatic persons have coronary artery disease, we assumed a mortality rate for coronary arteriography in asymptomatic persons (0.1%) that is somewhat lower than that in patients from CASS (0.2%) (36). The mortality of coronary artery bypass surgery is assumed to be 5.0% for patients with left main stenosis (37) and 1.9% for all other patients (38). We did not include the mortality of exercise testing in the model, because it is so small (1 in 10 000 procedures [12]).

An Alternative Screening Strategy
We evaluated an alternative strategy in which a person had thallium myocardial scintigraphy if and only if the exercise electrocardiogram was abnormal. In this strategy, patients would be referred for arteriography only if both exercise tests were abnormal. Two reviews (20, 39) have pooled the results of many studies of the test performance characteristics of myocardial scintigraphy in patients with chest pain. In both reviews, the pooled true-positive rate was 0.72, and the false-positive rate was 0.06. These figures appear to apply to men and to women.

Costs
To calculate average costs, we used the decision tree in Figure 1 but substituted cost for life expectancy. According to the decision model, the costs include exercise testing for everyone, coronary arteriography for patients with an abnormal exercise test, and surgery in some patients. The costs do not include any subsequent procedures, such as coronary arteriography or surgery for patients with coronary artery disease who become symptomatic at a later time.

We used the *lower* end of the range for reimbursement by

Blue Cross-Blue Shield of Northern California for exercise electrocardiography ($165), exercise and rest thallium myocardial scintigraphy ($667), and coronary artery bypass surgery ($31 178). For coronary artery bypass surgery, we used the sum of total hospital charges for scheduled procedures ($21 953) and physicians' hospital fees ($9225) (38). We used the Medicare diagnosis-related group reimbursement for coronary arteriography ($3595). These data represent reimbursement of charges, not the marginal cost of producing the service, which is undoubtedly lower than these charges would suggest.

Results

Cost-Effectiveness

Exercise Electrocardiography

Table 5 shows the results of the cost-effectiveness analysis of screening with an exercise test. In Table 5, the definition of an abnormal exercise ECG is at least 1-mm ST segment depression at least 0.08 seconds beyond the J point. The average cost of screening, which includes the expense of arteriography and surgery when indicated, ranges from $514 per patient in 40-year-old women to $832 in 60-year-old men. Exercise testing adds 2 days to the life expectancy of an asymptomatic 40-year-old man and 12 days to the life expectancy of an asymptomatic 60-year-old man. The additional cost to gain 1 additional year of life (cost-effectiveness) is $80 349 for 40-year-old men and $24 600 for 60-year-old men.

We evaluated the effect of considering risk factors for coronary artery disease in making the decision to screen 60-year-old men. In men with no risk factors, the probability of coronary artery disease is low (0.05), and screening adds only 5 days to life expectancy, at a cost of $44 332 per additional year of life. In men with one or more risk factors, the probability of coronary artery disease is 0.15, and screening prolongs life by 17 days at a cost of $20 504 per additional year of life. The yield of screening men with risk factors might be even greater if such patients had severer disease than patients at average-risk.

Exercise testing in women is less cost-effective than in men. In 40-year-old women, exercise electrocardiography adds 1 day to life expectancy at a cost of $216 496 per additional year of life. In 60-year-old women, exercise testing adds 5 days to life expectancy at a cost of $47 606 per additional year of life gained.

A Sequence of Screening Tests

If persons are referred for coronary arteriography only

when both a thallium myocardial scintigram and an exercise ECG are abnormal, costs are reduced considerably, and there is a small reduction in benefit. This sequential testing strategy costs $536 and adds 9 days to the life expectancy of a 60-year-old man, as compared with a cost of $832 and 12 added days with exercise electrocardiography alone (Table 5).

Sensitivity Analysis

The most questionable assumption in our model is

Table 5. *Marginal Cost-Effectiveness of Using Exercise Testing to Screen for Coronary Artery Disease*

Test	Cost	Life Expectancy	Difference in Cost	Difference in Life Expectancy*	Marginal Cost-Effectiveness
	$	y	$	d	$/y
Exercise ECG					
Men					
40 years old					
Test	538	28.6952	538	2	80 349
No test	0	28.6885			
60 years old					
Test	832	16.7176	832	12	24 600
No test	0	16.6837			
Women					
40 years old					
Test	514	34.8169	514	1	216 496
No test	0	34.8145			
60 years old					
Test	610	21.8469	610	5	47 606
No test	0	21.8340			
Exercise ECG and exercise thallium scan†					
Men					
40 years old					
Test	285	28.6950	285	2	43 768
No test	0	28.6885			
60 years old					
Test	536	16.7090	536	9	21 201
No test	0	16.6885			
Women					
40 years old					
Test	265	34.8183	265	1	70 456
No test	0	34.8145			
60 years old					
Test	351	21.8445	351	4	33 532
No test	0	21.8340			

* Calculated by multiplying the difference in life expectancy in years by 365 days per year.
† An exercise thallium scan was done if the exercise ECG was abnormal.

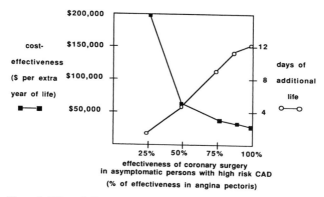

Figure 2. Effect of different assumptions about the effectiveness of coronary bypass surgery in asymptomatic persons. The analysis applies to 60-year-old men. The effectiveness of coronary bypass surgery in asymptomatic men with high-risk subsets of coronary artery disease (left main stenosis, left main equivalent coronary artery disease, or three-vessel disease with poor ventricular function) is expressed as a fraction of its effectiveness in men with angina pectoris and high-risk subsets of coronary artery disease. Open circles denote the gain in life expectancy *(days)* from doing screening, and closed squares, the cost of screening per added year of life gained.

that bypass surgery in asymptomatic persons with high-risk coronary artery disease improves survival as much as if the patients had angina pectoris. We tested the effect of this assumption by postulating that life expectancy in high-risk disease is better in untreated asymptomatic persons than it is in patients with medically treated stable angina, as suggested by the studies by Erikssen and Thaulow of the natural history of asymptomatic, angiographically proven coronary artery disease. Under this assumption, the potential improvement in life expectancy from surgery is reduced. The results are shown in Figure 2. If the effect of surgery on life expectancy in asymptomatic high-risk disease is only 50% of the effect in patients from CASS, screening 60-year-old men adds 5 days to life expectancy. The marginal cost-effectiveness of screening is $59 168 per additional year. If the improvement in life expectancy from surgery were 75% of the gain in patients from CASS, the marginal cost-effectiveness of screening would be $34 737 per additional year. Thus, if early surgical intervention in high-risk disease has a smaller effect in asymptomatic persons than in patients with angina, screening would be less cost-effective.

Reducing the cost of diagnostic procedures and assuming a wide range of values for the probability of events have little effect on the costs or benefits of a screening exercise ECG (Table 6). We analyzed the case of 60-year-old men, the group in which screening might provide the greatest benefit. The only factor that affects cost-effectiveness is the overall prevalence of coronary artery disease, which has a significant effect on the benefits of screening. We also studied the effect of assuming that high-risk coronary artery disease is commoner than is shown in Table 3. If patients with high-risk disease comprised twice the proportion of patients with coronary artery disease as in our baseline assumption, the cost per additional year of life

Table 6. *The Effect of Uncertainty about the Values of the Clinical Variables of the Decision Tree by One-Way Sensitivity Analysis**

Variable†	Values		Range		Cost per Extra Year of Life
	Base-line	Range	Marginal Effec-tiveness‡	Marginal Costs§	
			d	*$/person*	*$ × 10³*
None	NA	NA	12	832	24.6
Probability					
Of LV dysfunction in 3VD	0.20	0-0.4	11-13	816-849	25.9-23.5
Of perioperative death	0.019	0-0.10	13-12	832‖	24.2-26.3
Of perioperative death in left main stenosis	0.05	0-0.10	14-11	832‖	22.4-27.2
Of death during angiography	0.001	0-0.002	13-12	832‖	23.3-26.1
Of CAD in population	0.11	0.05-0.25	2-29	566-1271	87.1-16.1
Of a refusal to do bypass surgery	0.11	0-0.5	14-7	862-729	22.5-40.0
Of a refusal to do angiography	0	0-0.8	12-2	832-298	24.6-44.1
Cost of angiography	3595¶	0-4000¶	12‖	401-881	11.8-26.0
Cost of surgery	31 178¶	10 000-40 000¶	12‖	672-899	17.6-26.6
Cost of exercise ECG	165¶	50-250¶	12‖	717-917	21.2-27.1

* In this analysis, all variables were set at their base values for the case except for the variable being tested (one-day sensitivity analysis). The analysis was done for screening 60-year-old men with exercise electrocardiography only. The definition of an abnormal exercise ECG was at least 1-mm ST segment depression in any stage of the exercise protocol. LV = left ventricular; 3VD = three-vessel disease; CAD = coronary artery disease; NA = not applicable; and ECG = electrocardiogram.

† The value of the parameter was varied over the range shown in the third column.

‡ The range of expected gain in life expectancy (averaged over all screened patients) is given; the value on the left corresponds to the lower end of the range shown in the third column, and the value on the right corresponds to the upper end of the range. The lower end of the range in the third column will sometimes correspond with a larger gain in life expectancy.

§ The range of the average cost per screened patient.

‖ The outcome measure did not change as the parameter in the first column was varied. The analysis was done for 60-year-old men.

¶ Cost in dollars.

would decrease from $24 600 to $22 932. If high-risk disease were one-half as common as in our baseline assumption, the cost per year of life would increase to $44 332.

The operating characteristics of the exercise ECG influence its cost-effectiveness (Table 7). The frequency of positive exercise tests in left main coronary artery disease is a potentially important factor. If we assume that 93% of patients with left main stenosis have a positive exercise ECG, as shown by Weiner and colleagues (25), instead of 63%, as shown in a much larger study by McNeer and colleagues (11), the effect on longevity in 60-year-old men would increase from 12 to 19 days.

Adopting stringent criteria for defining an abnormal screening exercise ECG would increase cost-effectiveness. If the minimum criterion for an abnormal test is 1-mm ST-segment depression, exercise testing in 60-year-old men costs $24 600 per additional year of life gained. When the criterion for an abnormal test is poor exercise tolerance (failing to complete stage II of the Bruce protocol by Bruce and Hornsten) and at least one 1-mm ST-segment depression, the cost is $16 357 per additional year of life. However, a stringent criterion for referring a person for coronary arteriography screening would identify fewer patients with serious disease.

Discussion

Should Physicians Do Exercise Testing to Screen for Disease?

With our present understanding of coronary artery disease in apparently healthy persons, physicians should not feel obliged to do an exercise test in asymptomatic persons who do not have diabetes, hypertension, or hypercholesterolemia and do not smoke cigarettes. Screening is efficacious only if the early detection of disease prolongs the patient's life or improves its quality. There is no direct evidence that screening for coronary artery disease with an exercise test fulfills this condition. Therefore, we studied the effects of screening under the assumption that surgical treatment of high-risk coronary artery disease is as beneficial in asymptomatic persons as in patients with angina pectoris. Despite this assumption and others that were favorable to exercise testing, our model shows that screening adds little to life expectancy. Furthermore, the costs of screening are high, largely because of the costs induced by evaluating disease in patients with positive tests.

Table 7. *The Effect of Different Assumptions about the Operating Characteristics of the Exercise Electrocardiogram by Sensitivity Analysis**

Assumption	p [test result in condition]†		Marginal Effectiveness	Marginal Cost	Cost per Extra Year of Life
	LM	Non-CAD			
			d	*$/person*	*$*
Baseline‡§	0.63	0.09	12	832	24 600
Sensitivity in LM					
As shown by Weiner et al. (25)	0.93	0.09	19	1114	19 552
As shown by Bartel et al. (10)§	0.84	0.09	17	940	17 662
Cut off for abnormal E-ECG					
2-mm ST depression‖	0.52	0.005	9	413	19 060
1-mm ST depression					
In stage I‡	0.13	0	3	220	30 791
In stage II or III‡	0.49	0.008	9	419	16 357
In stage I, II, or III‡	0.60	0.035	12	593	18 444
Sole criterion for abnormal E-ECG					
Failure to complete stage I‡	0.24	0.08	4	541	45 898
Failure to complete stage I or II‡	0.69	0.31	12	1571	46 090
False-positive rate of exercise ECG assumed to be 0.20§	0.63	0.20	12	1184	35 007
Treatment of an equivocal test result as an abnormal result‡§	0.77	0.24	15	1708	41 317

* The analysis was done for the case of 60-year-old men. The screening test was exercise electrocardiography only. LM = left main; CAD = coronary artery disease; E-ECG = exercise electrocardiogram.

† The frequency of the assumed E-ECG result in other forms of CAD is taken from the specified references.

‡ Data taken from McNeer and colleagues (11).

§ The definition of an abnormal exercise ECG was at least 1-mm ST segment depression in any stage of the exercise protocol.

‖ Data taken from Bartel and colleagues (10).

Screening for coronary artery disease is not a good application of exercise testing for several reasons. First, most asymptomatic people do not have the disease. Second, most patients with a positive test have false-positive results. When arteriography is done in asymptomatic persons with a positive exercise ECG, only about 20% have the disease (7, 8). Third, the types of coronary artery disease that might be treated by bypass surgery occur infrequently in asymptomatic persons. The most frequent type of coronary artery disease in such persons is single-vessel or double-vessel disease. Surgery did not prolong life in patients from CASS with these forms of coronary artery disease.

Our findings are similar to a cost-effectiveness analysis that antedated the CASS randomized trial (6).

The authors assumed that surgery would be done for patients with two-vessel disease or worse conditions, that the frequency of abnormal tests is independent of disease severity, and that the false-positive rate for exercise testing was higher. Adjusted for inflation, our results are somewhat more favorable to screening than their results.

Other Ways to Express Results

The units of measure in this analysis (average cost per patient, marginal cost-effectiveness, and additional days of life) may obscure the impact of the widespread adoption of screening. There are approximately 1 million 60-year-old men in the United States. If physicians adopted a policy of doing an exercise test when a healthy man reached his 60th birthday, the annual cost would be approximately $830 million dollars.

The clinical relevance of our findings may be expressed as follows. We found that screening with an exercise ECG would prolong life by an average of at most 12 days in 60-year-old men. If all of the benefit of screening were concentrated in 1 person, 30 men would have to be screened, at a total cost of $24 960 to prolong that person's life by 1 year. For the same benefit, 180 men, who were forty years old, would have to be screened.

Comparison with Other Cardiovascular Disease Interventions

Screening with exercise testing can be placed into perspective by comparing it with other medical interventions (Table 8). Routine angiography, if done in all 60-year-old men with typical angina, would prolong life by an average of 577 days at a cost of $8700 per added year of life (6). The cost-effectiveness of hypertension treatment depends on the degree of patients' adherence to medication. With full adherence, the reduction of diastolic blood pressure from 110 to 90 mm Hg would add 110 days to the life expectancy of 60-year-old men and 1 year to that of 60-year-old women. Incomplete adherence would reduce the gain in life expectancy.

Under the assumptions of our model, screening 60-year-old men at average risk with an exercise test has a much smaller effect on life expectancy and is somewhat less cost-effective than treating hypertensive men or doing angiography in men with angina pectoris (Table 8). Several points should be considered in

Table 8. *Cost-Effectiveness of Cardiovascular Interventions*

Intervention	Marginal Cost per Patient	Marginal Effectiveness*	Cost-Effectiveness†
	$	d	$
Exercise ECG‡	832	12	24 000
Angiography§	13 837	577	8700
Reducing diastolic blood pressure‖			
Men, 60 y	4890	110	16 300
Women, 60 y	5000	365	5000

* Additional days of life.
† Cost per additional year of life.
‡ Average-risk 60-year-old men.
§ In all 55-year-old men with typical angina pectoris (6).
‖ Blood pressure was reduced from 110 to 90 mm Hg. For this intervention, it was assumed that full compliance was obtained. The cost per year of additional life may increase 50% to 100% if compliance is similar to that seen in practice. The reduction of risk was based on the age-varying partial benefit assumption (54).

making these comparisons. First, the assumptions of our model favored screening; therefore, our findings should represent an upper bound on the benefit of screening. Second, there is good evidence for the effectiveness of coronary bypass surgery in patients with angina pectoris and antihypertensive therapy. There is no evidence with which to decide if early intervention can prolong life in patients with angiographically proven asymptomatic coronary artery disease. We altered our model so that early treatment of high-risk disease is less effective in asymptomatic persons than in persons with angina. Under these conditions, screening is even less cost-effective than interventions to treat diastolic hypertension and angina pectoris (Figure 2). Adopting a policy of screening without evidence of the effectiveness of treatment is inadvisable.

There is an emerging consensus that exercise testing in persons with no symptoms or risk factors for coronary artery disease is not worthwhile (2). Our findings further support this view. There are, however, several special situations in which some students of this field advocate screening with an exercise test. As discussed below, we feel that there is insufficient evidence to adopt screening as a routine practice in these situations.

Exercise Testing in Asymptomatic Persons with Other Risk Factors for Coronary Artery Disease

Screening with exercise testing is inefficient in part because coronary artery disease is infrequent in asymptomatic persons. Exercise testing would be more efficient if screening were done only in patients at relatively high risk for the disease. Two studies have adopted this approach.

Bruce and colleagues (40) increased the yield of screening by two strategies. First, they used clinical risk factors to raise the pretest risk of coronary artery disease. Second, they reduced the false-positive rate of the exercise ECG by requiring that each of several abnormal exercise test findings be present. They did an exercise ECG in 2365 healthy men and monitored them for a mean of 5.6 years. They found that four risk factors (family history of coronary artery disease, cigarette smoking, systolic blood pressure greater than 140 mm Hg, and hypercholesterolemia) predicted primary cardiac events. Four outcome measures for exercise ECG (ST-segment depression, inability to complete 6 minutes of the exercise protocol, a maximal heart rate less than 90% of that predicted, and chest pain at maximal exertion) also predicted subsequent cardiac events. There were 47 primary cardiac events in 5.6 years, an annual event rate of 3.6 per 1000 men. In men with no clinical risk factors (41% of the subjects), the annual incidence of cardiac events was 1.7 per 1000. In those with one or more clinical risk factors, and less than two risk factors for exercise testing, the annual incidence of cardiac events was 3.6 per 1000. In subjects with at least one clinical risk factor and at least two exercise risk factors, however, the annual incidence of cardiac events was 82 per 1000. Thus, Bruce and colleagues increased the pretest risk for coronary artery disease by requiring one clinical risk factor and reduced the false-positive rate of the exercise ECG by requiring two abnormalities on exercise testing. By so doing, they defined a very small group (1% of all those tested) in which more than 8% of the patients had a primary cardiac event each year. In men aged 60 to 64 years, 4.3% were in the high-risk group (41).

Most patients who had a primary cardiac event were not in the high-risk group defined by cardiovascular risk factors and exercise responses. Only 9% of those who had myocardial infarction, 19% of those who had coronary bypass surgery, and none of those who developed angina were in the high-risk group

(41). However, 25% of those who died suddenly were in the high risk group.

Uhl and colleagues (21) used a high ratio of total cholesterol to high-density lipoprotein (HDL) cholesterol to identify subjects at high risk. In their study of asymptomatic airmen referred for coronary arteriography because of an abnormal exercise test (86%) or other findings suggesting cardiac disease, only 12% of 132 patients had significant coronary artery disease. The total cholesterol:HDL ratio exceeded 6.0 in 9.6% of all subjects. The prevalence of disease was 0.64 in those with a positive exercise test and a cholesterol:HDL ratio greater than 6.0. The prevalence of disease was only 0.02 in those who had an abnormal exercise test and a cholesterol:HDL ratio less than 6.0. Thus, exercise testing has an extremely low yield when the cholesterol:HDL ratio is less than 6.0.

The results of these two studies suggest a selective strategy for screening: do an exercise ECG only in patients with at least one clinical risk factor or a cholesterol:HDL ratio of more than 6.0. Even with this selective approach, however, the yield of patients at high risk is very small. In the study by Bruce and colleagues, only 1% of the healthy persons were in the high risk group, and most of the primary disease events occurred in the other groups.

In our analysis, the cost-effectiveness of exercise testing in asymptomatic persons with risk factors for coronary artery disease compares favorably with accepted practices, such as treating mild hypertension. This result should be interpreted with caution until experimental evidence shows that asymptomatic persons with high-risk coronary artery disease live longer after early surgery or angioplasty. The Task Force on Assessment of Cardiovascular Procedures of the American College of Cardiology and American Heart Association called exercise testing in men with risk factors a class II indication (a condition in which exercise testing is frequently used but in which there is a divergence of opinion about its value) (2).

Exercise Testing before Exercise Training

Many physicians do exercise testing to screen patients who are about to undertake a program of physical conditioning. Patients who die during or after running often are found to have coronary artery disease at autopsy, although few were known to have coronary artery disease during life (42). Cardiac arrest is more likely to occur during vigorous exercise than at rest.

Among sedentary men, cardiac arrest is 56 times more likely to occur during exercise than at rest. Among those who are habitually very active, cardiac arrest is 5.0 times more likely to occur while they are exercising than while they are at rest (43). Thus, when a person is just beginning an exercise program, there appears to be a vulnerable period during which the risk of cardiac arrest during exercise is increased. By simulating the conditions experienced by a person just beginning physical conditioning, an exercise test might identify persons who are likely to die suddenly during this period of vulnerability.

Although a person's *relative* risk for death appears to be increased when starting an exercise program, his or her *absolute* risk for sudden death during running is very low. In 6 years, Thompson (44) identified 11 residents of Rhode Island who died suddenly while jogging. Assuming 1 hour of jogging per week, he calculated the incidence of sudden death during jogging to be 1 per 7620 joggers per year, or 1 death per 396 000 man-hours of jogging per year. This study did not relate a runner's risk for death while running at his or her age or fitness level.

The rationale for screening persons before they start an exercise program is to deter those who may have coronary artery disease from starting an imprudent exercise program. The argument against screening is that sudden death is a very uncommon event among runners, that exercise testing leads to many false-positive results in asymptomatic persons, and that deterring people from running may lead to a net increase in mortality from coronary artery disease. Because these conflicting views have not been resolved, it is difficult to argue that screening middle-aged men before physical training should be considered mandatory. There is insufficient evidence to make a strong recommendation for or against screening in this population. The Task Force on Assessment of Cardiovascular Procedures called this reason for exercise testing a class II indication (as defined in the preceding section) (2).

Occupations in Which a Worker's Sudden Death Would Endanger Others

Some persons, such as bus drivers and airline pilots, may deserve to be screened because their sudden death while at work could endanger people entrusted to their care. The goal of screening is not treatment of coronary artery disease but removing a person from a potentially hazardous situation. This problem has not, to our knowledge, been carefully analyzed, and there is insufficient evidence to make a strong conclusion for or against screening. This reason for exercise testing was a class II indication, according to the Task Force on Assessment of Cardiovascular Procedures (2).

Will Advancing Technology Change the Case against Screening?

The recommendations in this report pertain to the current state of knowledge. As better, less costly tests or treatments are shown to have an impact on clinical outcomes, this analysis should be updated. The decision model can be modified when new tests or treatments are shown to be superior to current technology. The main reason that screening is inefficient, however, is not inadequate technology but the nature of coronary artery disease in asymptomatic persons, as discussed below.

One of the main purposes of screening for coronary artery disease is to prevent sudden death. Most victims of sudden cardiac death have three-vessel disease or left main stenosis. These types of coronary artery disease are very uncommon in asymptomatic persons, and may become still less common if secular trends toward a reduced incidence of coronary artery disease continue. According to this argument, screening for an uncommon disease will be costly, even with improved technology, because so many people must be screened to detect so few who benefit. Strengthening the case for screening will require better tests, use of clinical risk factors to identify high-risk groups to be screened, and inexpensive interventions that alter prognosis. Three developments could make screening more worthwhile.

Percutaneous Transluminal Angioplasty
Percutaneous transluminal angioplasty is somewhat less costly than bypass surgery and is more likely to be acceptable to asymptomatic persons. However, the cost of surgery has little effect on the cost-effectiveness of screening (Table 7). This intervention will improve the case for screening only if it is more effective than bypass surgery at prolonging life in asymptomatic persons with coronary artery disease.

Silent Myocardial Ischemia
Ambulatory ECG monitoring of patients with angina pectoris has shown that 75% of episodes of ST-segment depression are asymptomatic (45). Because

these silent ischemic episodes occur without an increase in heart rate, ischemia may be due to a decrease in oxygen supply rather than an increase in oxygen demand. Episodes of silent ischemia are more frequent in patients with poor exercise tolerance and marked ST-segment depression on conventional exercise electrocardiograms; this finding suggests that silent ischemia is a marker for a poor prognosis.

Ambulatory monitoring and conventional exercise testing appear to be redundant, because the two procedures are in concordance 96% of the time, according to the results of one study (46). Furthermore, the two procedures have identical true-positive and false-positive rates in the subset of patients with angina who have coronary arteriography. As yet, little is known of the prevalence or prognosis of silent ischemia in totally asymptomatic persons.

Prevention of Myocardial Infarction by Aspirin

Aspirin is a low-cost intervention that appears to reduce the incidence of myocardial infarction in apparently healthy men. In the preliminary report of the Physicians' Health Study (47), 325 mg of aspirin taken every other day reduced the occurrence of all myocardial infarctions from 17 per 1000 to 9.5 per 1000 in 57 months. However, the total number of cardiovascular deaths was the same in aspirin and placebo groups, and the total stroke rate was unaffected by aspirin. Thus, the favorable effect of aspirin appears to be limited to myocardial infarction and may be negated by unfavorable effects on other outcomes, such as hemorrhagic stroke.

How should the decision to use the exercise ECG to screen for coronary artery disease be affected by the newly discovered effects of aspirin in apparently healthy men? The case for screening would be strengthened if most of the persons who benefited from aspirin had an abnormal exercise test. There is no evidence that the benefit of aspirin is concentrated in persons with abnormal exercise tests. Most patients destined to develop coronary artery disease are not in the high-risk group defined by clinical and exercise risk factors (41). Unless the benefit of aspirin is concentrated among those with an abnormal exercise test, the newly discovered effects of aspirin do not strengthen the case for mass screening with an exercise test.

Future Directions

Detrano and Froelicher (8) have suggested that the

goal of screening should be to detect minimal coronary artery disease, because such persons are more likely to die from the disease than persons with normal coronary arteries. These persons, rather than those with more advanced disease, may benefit most from preventive measures. Physiologically insignificant but prognostically significant coronary artery disease will probably be more difficult to detect than physiologically significant disease.

Bruce and colleagues (48) have presented preliminary evidence that persons with functional aerobic impairment on an exercise test comply better with efforts at risk factor reduction than those with no impairment. The findings are, however, based on self-reported behavior, and neither the degree of actual risk reduction nor its impact on mortality is known. No one has studied how disease outcome is affected by screening with an exercise test.

Recommendations

1. Exercise testing is not recommended as a routine screening procedure in adults with no evidence of coronary heart disease. This recommendation applies to exercise electrocardiography whether or not it is used in conjunction with thallium scintigraphy.

2. Some persons may have particular reasons to consider screening for coronary artery disease. Some persons are especially likely to have the disease because of increased age, male gender, and at least one other risk factor. Other persons have an occupation that puts others at risk (for example, bus drivers or airline pilots) or are sedentary and about to begin a program of physical conditioning. There is insufficient evidence to make a strong recommendation for or against screening in these groups.

3. An asymptomatic person who has already had a negative exercise ECG has an excellent prognosis and does not require further testing.

4. If exercise testing is to be used to screen for coronary artery disease, we recommend doing an exercise ECG and then thallium scintigraphy if the exercise ECG is abnormal. We recommend doing coronary arteriography only if the results of both noninvasive tests are abnormal. This approach detects most patients who have serious coronary artery disease and is considerably more cost-effective than doing only an exercise ECG.

Appendix

Calculating Life Expectancy from Fractional Survival Data

Life expectancy (the average length of life) is the measure of clinical outcome in this article. Life expectancy may be calculated from fractional survival by using the declining exponential approximation of life expectancy (DEALE) (18). The two principal assumptions are that the average annual mortality rate is a constant over the lifespan of the individual and that the mortality rates from different diseases are additive. The DEALE is quite accurate for persons aged 50 years or more (18).

In the example below, the life expectancy of a 60-year-old man with medically treated stable angina due to two-vessel disease is obtained from the total mortality. The total mortality is the sum of death from coronary artery disease and death from other causes.

Death from Coronary Artery Disease
The average annual mortality (m) can be calculated using the following equation: $m = (1/t) \times \ln(S/S_0)$, where t is the period of followup, ln is the natural logarithm, and S/S_0 is the fraction of surviving patients at time t. For patients with two-vessel disease, S/S_0 at five years is 0.95. Therefore, $m = (1/5) \times \ln(0.95) = (-0.2) \times (-0.0513) = 0.0103$. In CASS, essentially all deaths were due to coronary artery disease. Therefore, total mortality in the trial is equivalent to mortality from coronary artery disease.

Death from Other Causes
The life expectancy in 60-year-old men in the general population is 17.1 years (in 1980). To calculate the average annual mortality use: $m = 1/$life expectancy $= 1/17.1 = 0.0585$ per year.

Death from All Causes in 60-year-old Man with Two-Vessel Disease
The total mortality can be calculated by the following equation: mortality of coronary artery disease + mortality of other conditions $= 0.0103 + 0.0585 = 0.0688$.

The life expectancy in a 60-year-old man with two-vessel disease is $1/$total mortality $= 1/0.0688 = 14.5$ years.

Calculating the False-Positive Rate of a Screening Exercise Electrocardiogram

If possible, always use information about test performance that has been derived from a study population similar to one's own. Most studies of the accuracy of the exercise ECG used patients referred for coronary arteriography after an exercise ECG. These data probably do not apply to a screening population, in which most patients are healthy. The frequency of abnormal exercise tests in studies of the exercise ECG in persons with no symptoms of coronary artery disease can be used to estimate the false-positive rate of the exercise ECG in a screening population.

The probability (p) of a positive $(+)$ test is the probability of a positive result in a patient with coronary artery disease (CAD) plus the probability of a positive result in a patient that does not have the disease:

$$p(+) = p(+ \text{ test and CAD}) + p(+ \text{ test and no CAD})$$

When substituting from the definition of conditional probability, use the following equation:

$$p(+ \mid \text{CAD}) = \frac{p(+ \text{ and CAD})}{p(\text{CAD})}$$

$$p(+) = p(\text{CAD}) \times p(+ \mid \text{CAD}) + p(\text{no CAD}) \times p(+ \mid \text{no CAD})$$

The true-positive rate of the test (TPR) is $p[+ \mid \text{CAD}]$, and the false-positive rate of the test (FPR) is $p[+ \mid \text{no CAD}]$. Thus, $p(+) = p(\text{CAD}) \times \text{TPR} + p(\text{no CAD}) \times \text{FPR}$:

$$\text{FPR} = \frac{p(+) - p(\text{CAD}) \times \text{TPR}}{p(\text{no CAD})}$$

In a screening population, $p(\text{CAD})$ is quite small, and an imprecise estimate of the TPR will have little effect on the estimate of the FPR. The TPR derived from the CASS study $(\text{TPR} = 0.46)$ (26) is undoubtedly an overestimate of the TPR in a screening population, but any error will be small because the TPR is multiplied by a small prevalence of coronary artery disease $(p[\text{CAD}])$. To estimate $p(\text{positive exercise ECG})$, we pooled four studies (40, 49, 50, 53) that used a maximal exercise protocol in a population with a mean age of 44 years. The pooled frequency of a positive test in these four studies was 0.104. The prevalence of coronary artery disease in a population with a mean age of 41 years is 0.04 (20). The FPR is calculated as follows:

$$\text{FPR} = \frac{p(+) - p(\text{CAD}) \times \text{TPR}}{p(\text{no CAD})} = \frac{0.104 - (0.04) \times 0.46}{0.96} = 0.089$$

References

1. **Gordon T, Kannel WB.** Premature mortality from coronary heart disease: The Framingham Study. *JAMA.* 1971;**215:**1617-25.
2. **The American College of Cardiology, American Heart Association Task Force on Assessment of Cardiovascular Procedures (Subcommittee on Exercise Testing).** Guidelines for exercise testing. *J Am Coll Cardiol.* 1986;**8:**725-38.
3. **Frame PS.** A critical review of adult health maintenance: Part 1: Prevention of atherosclerotic diseases. *J Fam Pract.* 1986;**22:**341-6.
4. **Breslow L, Somers AR.** Lifetime health-monitoring: a practical approach to preventive medicine. *N Engl J Med.* 1977;**296:**601-8.
5. The periodic health examination: 2. 1984 update. Canadian Task Force on the Periodic Health Examination. *Can Med Assoc J.* 1984;**130:**1278-85.
6. **Stason WB, Fineberg HV.** Implications of alternative strategies to diagnose coronary artery disease. *Circulation.* 1982;**66**(5 pt 2):II180-6.
7. **Uhl GS, Froelicher V.** Screening for asymptomatic coronary artery disease. *J Am Coll Cardiol.* 1983;**3:**946-55.
8. **Detrano R, Froelicher V.** A logical approach to screening for coronary artery disease. *Ann Intern Med.* 1987;**106:**846-52.
9. **Bruce RA, Hornsten TR.** Exercise testing in evaluation of patients with ischemic heart disease. *Prog Cardiovasc Dis.* 1969;**11:**371-90.
10. **Bartel AG, Behar VS, Peter RH, Orgain ES, Kong Y.** Graded exercise stress tests in angiographically documented coronary artery disease. *Circulation.* 1974;**44:**348-56.
11. **McNeer JF, Margolis JR, Lee KL, et al.** The role of the exercise

test in the evaluation of patients for ischemic heart disease. *Circulation.* 1978;**57**:64-70.

12. **Stuart RJ Jr, Ellestad MH.** National survey of exercise stress testing facilities. *Chest.* 1980;**77**:94-7.

13. **Gordon DJ, Ekelund LG, Karon JM, et al.** Predictive value of the exercise tolerance test for mortality in North American men: the Lipid Research Clinics Mortality Follow-up Study. *Circulation.* 1986;**74**:252-61.

14. **Rautaharju PM, Prineas RJ, Eifler WJ, et al.** Prognostic value of exercise electrocardiogram in men at high risk of future coronary artery disease: Multiple Risk Factor Intervention Trial experience. *J Am Coll Cardiol.* 1986;**8**:1-10.

15. **Bruce RA, Hossack KF, DeRouen TA, Hofer V.** Enhanced risk assessment for primary coronary heart disease events by maximal exercise testing: 10 years' experience of Seattle Heart Watch. *J Am Coll Cardiol.* 1983;**2**:565-73.

16. Coronary artery surgery study (CASS): survival data. *Circulation.* 1983;**68**:939-50.

17. **Chaitman BR, Bourassa MG, Davis K, et al.** Angiographic prevalence of high-risk coronary artery disease in patients subsets (CASS). *Circulation.* 1981;**64**:360-7.

18. **Beck JR, Kassirer JP, Pauker SG.** A convenient approximation of life expectancy (The "DEALE"): I. Validation of the method. *Am J Med.* 1982;**73**:883-8.

19. **Killip T, Passamani E, Davis K, and the CASS Investigators and their Associates.** Coronary artery surgery study (CASS): a randomized trial of coronary bypass surgery. Eight years follow-up and survival in patients with reduced ejection fraction. *Circulation.* 1985;**72**(suppl 5):V-102.

20. **Diamond GA, Forrester JS.** Analysis of probability as an aid in the clinical diagnosis of coronary artery disease. *N Engl J Med.* 1979;**300**:1350-8.

21. **Uhl GS, Troxler RG, Heckman JR, Clark D.** Relation between high density lipoprotein cholesterol and coronary artery disease in asymptomatic men. *Am J Cardiol.* 1981;**48**:903-10.

22. **Roland ML, Fulwood R.** Coronary heart disease risk factor trends in blacks between the first and second National Health and Nutrition Examination Surveys, United States, 1971-1980. *Am Heart J.* 1984;**108**:771-9.

23. **Gensini GG, Kelly AE.** Incidence and progression of coronary artery disease: an angiographic correlation in 1,263 patients. *Arch Intern Med.* 1972;**129**:814-27.

24. **Froelicher VF Jr, Thompson AJ, Wolthuis R, et al.** Angiographic findings in asymptomatic aircrewmen with electrocardiographic abnormalities. *Am J Cardiol.* 1977;**39**:32-8.

25. **Weiner DA, McCabe CH, Ryan TJ.** Identification of patients with left main and three vessel coronary disease with clinical and exercise test variables. *Am J Cardiol.* 1980;**46**:21-7.

26. **Weiner DA, Ryan TJ, McCabe CH, et al.** Exercise stress testing: correlation among history of angina, ST-segment response and prevalence of coronary-artery disease in the coronary artery surgery study (CASS). *N Engl J Med.* 1979;**301**:230-5.

27. **Manca C, Dei Cas L, Albertini D, Baldi G, Visioli O.** Different prognostic value of exercise electrocardiogram in men and women. *Cardiology.* 1978;**63**:312-9.

28. **Erikssen J, Thaulow E.** Follow-up of patients with asymptomatic myocardial ischemia. In: Rutishauser W, Roskamm H, eds. *Silent Myocardial Ischemia.* Berlin: Springer-Verlag; 1984:154-64.

29. **Erikssen J.** Silent ischemia. *Herz.* 1987;**12**:359-68.

30. **Cohn PF.** Prognosis and treatment of asymptomatic coronary artery disease. *J Am Coll Cardiol.* 1983;**1**:959-64.

31. **Hammermeister KE, DeRouen TA, Dodge HT.** Effect of coronary surgery on survival in asymptomatic and minimally symptomatic patients. *Circulation.* 1980;**62**(2 pt 1):I98-102.

32. Long-term results of prospective randomised study of coronary artery bypass surgery in stable angina pectoris. European Coronary Surgery Study Group. *Lancet.* 1980;**2**:1173-80.

33. **Chaitman BR, Davis KB, Kaiser GC, et al.** The role of coronary bypass surgery for "left main equivalent" coronary disease: The Cor-

onary Artery Surgery Study registry. *Circulation.* 1986;**74**(suppl 3):III17-25.

34. **Fisher LD, Davis KB.** Design and study similarities and contrasts: the Veterans Administration, European, and CASS randomized trials of coronary artery bypass graft surgery. *Circulation.* 1985;**72** (suppl 5):V-110.

35. **Rahimtoola SH.** A perspective on the three large multicenter randomized trials of coronary bypass surgery for chronic stable angina. *Circulation.* 1985;**72**(suppl 5):V-123.

36. **Davis K, Kennedy JW, Kemp HG Jr, Judkins MP, Gosselin AU, Killip T.** Complications of coronary arteriography from the collaborative study of coronary artery surgery (CASS). *Circulation.* 1979;**59**:1105-12.

37. **Kennedy JW, Kaiser GC, Fisher LD, et al.** Clinical and angiographic predictors of operative mortality from the collaborative study in coronary artery surgery (CASS). *Circulation.* 1981;**63**:793-802.

38. **Showstack JA, Rosenfeld KE, Garnick DW.** Coronary artery bypass graft surgery in California, 1983: outcomes and charges. *Discussion Paper Series, Institute for Health Policy Studies.* San Francisco: University of California; April 1986.

39. **Sox HC Jr.** Exercise testing in suspected coronary artery disease. *Dis Mon.* 1985;**31**(12):1-93.

40. **Bruce RA, DeRouen TA, Hossack KF.** Value of maximal exercise tests in risk assessment of primary coronary heart disease events in healthy men: five years' experience of the Seattle heart watch study. *Am J Cardiol.* 1980;**46**:371-8.

41. **Bruce RA, Fisher LD.** Exercise-enhanced risk factors for coronary heart disease vs. age as criteria for mandatory retirement of healthy pilots. *Aviat Space Environ Med.* 1987;**58**:792-8.

42. **Thompson PD, Stern MP, Williams P, Duncan K, Haskell WL, Wood PD.** Death during jogging or running: a study of 18 cases. *JAMA.* 1979;**242**:1265-7.

43. **Siscovick DS, Weiss NS, Fletcher RH, Lasky T.** The incidence of primary cardiac arrest during vigorous exercise. *N Engl J Med.* 1984;**311**:874-7.

44. **Thompson PD, Funk EJ, Carleton RA, Sturner WQ.** Incidence of death during jogging in Rhode Island from 1975 through 1980. *JAMA.* 1982;**247**:2535-8.

45. **Nabel EG, Rocco MB, Barry J, Campbell S, Selwyn AP.** Asymptomatic ischemia in patients with coronary artery disease. *JAMA.* 1987;**257**:1923-8.

46. **Tzivoni D, Benhorn J, Gavish A, Stern S.** Holter recording during treadmill testing in assessing myocardial ischemic changes. *Am J Cardiol.* 1985;**55**:1200-3.

47. **Steering Committee of the Physicians' Health Study Research Group.** Preliminary report: findings from the aspirin component of the ongoing Physicians' Health Study. *N Engl J Med.* 1988; **318**:262-4.

48. **Bruce RA, DeRouen TA, Hossack KF.** Pilot study examining the motivational effects of maximal exercise testing to modify risk factors and health habits. *Cardiology.* 1980;**66**:111-9.

49. **Froelicher VF Jr, Thomas MM, Pillow C, Lancaster MC.** Epidemiologic study of asymptomatic men screened by maximal treadmill testing for latent coronary artery disease. *Am J Cardiol.* 1974; **34**:770-6.

50. **Cumming GR, Samm J, Borysyk L, Kich L.** Electrocardiographic changes during exercise in asymptomatic men: 3-year follow-up. *Can Med Assoc J.* 1975;**112**:578-81.

51. **Allen WH, Aronow WS, Goodman P, Stinson P.** Five-year follow-up of maximal treadmill stress test in asymptomatic men and women. *Circulation.* 1980;**62**:522-7.

52. **Giagnoni E, Secchi MB, Wu SC, et al.** Prognostic value of exercise EKG testing in asymptomatic normotensive subjects: a prospective matched study. *N Engl J Med.* 1983;**309**:1085-9.

53. **Hollenberg M, Zoltick JM, Go M, et al.** Comparison of a quantitative treadmill exercise score with standard electrocardiographic criteria in screening asymptomatic young men for coronary artery disease. *N Engl J Med.* 1985;**313**:600-6.

54. **Stason WB, Weinstein MC.** Allocation of resources to manage hypertension. *N Engl J Med.* 1977;**296**:732-9.

Screening Asymptomatic Adults for Cardiac Risk Factors:

The Serum Cholesterol Level

ALAN M. GARBER, MD, PhD; HAROLD C. SOX, Jr., MD; and BENJAMIN LITTENBERG, MD

Heart disease is the leading cause of death in the industrialized world. Physicians have long recognized that modifiable risk factors, such as hypertension, smoking, and hypercholesterolemia, contribute to the high prevalence of coronary heart disease. The ongoing development and testing of cholesterol-lowering diets and drugs have focused attention on strategies to prevent coronary heart disease by lowering patients' serum cholesterol levels. Because hypercholesterolemia usually does not cause symptoms until blood vessels have become damaged, early detection of the condition is best accomplished by screening symptom-free persons. We review evidence supporting the use of the serum cholesterol level and related screening tests for identifying asymptomatic adults at high risk for coronary heart disease. *The screening population considered here comprises men and women whose history and physical examination show no evidence of hypercholesterolemia, coronary heart disease, or hypertension.* Although we do not specifically discuss cigarette smokers and other persons whose diets or lifestyles put them at risk, they are included in the screening population. We do not address the use of these tests for other purposes, such as behavioral reinforcement or education, nor do we discuss their role in monitoring patients predisposed to lipid disorders because of coexisting medical conditions, such as diabetes, hypothyroidism, or the nephrotic syndrome, or because they have a strong family history of hyperlipoproteinemia.

By several criteria, serum lipid assays are excellent screening tests. For example, the tests themselves are safe and inexpensive. Also, they can identify persons at high risk for a serious and common condition—cardiovascular disease. Because hyperlipoproteinemia can

---

▶ This chapter was originally published in *Annals of Internal Medicine*. 1989;**110**:622-39.

be treated, lipid screening is a key component of strategies to prevent cardiovascular disease. Ultimately, though, the usefulness of any screening test depends on its ability to improve patient outcomes by expediting effective therapy. Some treatments for hypercholesterolemia have been found to reduce coronary heart disease incidence and mortality. After considering the most important links in this chain of evidence, we provide recommendations for using lipid tests for screening.

The first section summarizes the evidence connecting the most important of these tests, the serum cholesterol level, to morbidity and mortality from coronary heart disease, and to mortality from all causes. Much of this evidence is from epidemiologic studies. The characteristics of the tests used to measure total cholesterol in routine clinical practice may be different from the tests that have been used to establish the relation between the risk for coronary heart disease and the cholesterol level, as we discuss in the second section. Related tests for triglyceride levels and lipoprotein fractions are discussed in the third section. In the fourth section, we review evidence supporting the most important reason to screen for hypercholesterolemia, namely, that treating patients with elevated cholesterol levels prolongs their lives and improves other aspects of their health. Specific recommendations for using these tests to screen for coronary heart disease appear in the fifth section.

Serum Cholesterol as a Risk Factor for Coronary Heart Disease and Early Death

Epidemiologic studies that included thousands of apparently healthy patients have established that the serum cholesterol level is a powerful predictor of morbidity and mortality from coronary disease. Diverse evidence justifies this claim. Important sources include international comparisons of the rates of death from coronary heart disease in countries whose population groups have different cholesterol levels (1), and numerous prospective and retrospective studies of factors that influence mortality from coronary heart disease and other causes. Their chief findings are discussed below.

For adults whose cholesterol level exceeds the 10th or 20th percentile, the risk for symptomatic coronary heart disease or for death from coronary heart disease rises in a curvilinear fashion with the cholesterol level. The relation is approximately exponential, with the

Table 1. *Rates of Death from Coronary Heart Disease in Persons Screened for the Multiple Risk Factor Intervention Trial**

Quintile	Cholesterol	Relative Risk[†]
	mmol/L (mg/dL)	
I	< 4.69(< 181)	1.0
II	4.70-5.24(182-202)	1.3
III	5.25-5.74(203-221)	1.7
IV	5.75-6.34(222-245)	2.2
V	> 6.35(> 246)	3.4

* Data are adapted from Martin and colleagues (2).
† Relative risk is the rate of death from coronary heart disease in quintile divided by the rate in the lowest quintile.

same increment in cholesterol having a much more pronounced effect at higher levels than at lower levels of serum cholesterol. Table 1, from Martin and colleagues (2), shows how the relative risk for death from coronary heart disease varies by quintile of cholesterol level for the 361 662 men screened for the Multiple Risk Factor Intervention Trial (MRFIT). Persons whose cholesterol level exceeded 6.80 mmol/L (263 mg/dL), placing them at or above the 90th percentile, had four times the risk for death from coronary disease of those in the bottom 20%, whose cholesterol level was less than 4.71 mmol/L (182 mg/ dL).

Similar results have been obtained in the other major prospective epidemiologic studies. In the Whitehall study, the 10-year mortality from coronary heart disease rose from 2.85% in the lowest quintile to 3.44% in the next lowest quintile, and to 5.37% in the highest quintile of cholesterol levels (3). The Framingham study (4), which used the incidence of coronary heart disease as an endpoint, and a prospective study of Israeli civil servants (5), which examined death from coronary heart disease, also showed a pattern of slowly rising risk for coronary heart disease in patients with lower cholesterol levels and one of rapidly rising risk in patients with higher levels.

Total mortality is a J-shaped function of cholesterol level. Mortality rises as the cholesterol level falls, for persons whose cholesterol level is below the 10th or 20th percentile; at higher cholesterol levels, further increases in cholesterol are associated with rising mortality (6) (Figure 1). Men whose cholesterol levels were in the bottom decile had a significantly increased rate of cancer death early in MRFIT (7). Similarly, in

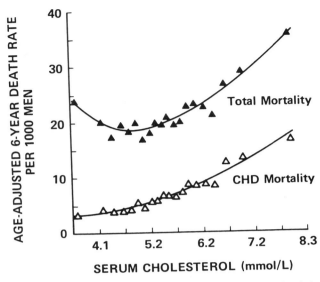

Figure 1. Age-adjusted coronary heart disease (*CHD, open triangles*) and total (*closed triangles*) mortality per 1000 men screened for the Multiple Risk Factor Intervention Trial, according to serum cholesterol level. Data are based on a cohort of 361 662 men. From Martin and colleagues (2); reproduced with the permission of *The Lancet*.

the study of Israeli civil servants, the age-adjusted overall mortality at 15 years was lowest for persons in the third decile, corresponding to a serum cholesterol level of 4.58 to 4.84 mmol/L (177 to 187 mg/dL). All-cause mortality in the bottom decile, corresponding to a cholesterol level of less than 4.16 mmol/L (161 mg/dL), was about the same as mortality in the seventh decile, corresponding to a cholesterol level of 5.61 to 5.87 mmol/L (217 to 227 mg/dL).

Most experts argue that mortality is higher in patients with low cholesterol levels because cancer and other serious underlying diseases may lower the cholesterol level before they cause symptoms. Excess cancer mortality occurred very early in MRFIT, before the intervention could have been responsible for an increased risk for cancer. Furthermore, when adjusted for age, smoking status, and randomization group, the MRFIT participants who died from cancer had much greater falls in the serum cholesterol levels after enrollment than did survivors. Finally, the drop in cholesterol was greatest among the men who died from cancer early in the trial; this finding has been interpreted to mean that cancer causes the serum cholesterol level to fall, rather than that a fall in the cholesterol level causes cancer (7). Other investigators have argued that a low cholesterol level may be more than a preclinical marker of disease and may bear a causal relation to cancer mortality (8). Although the interpretation of the negative association between the cholesterol level and all-cause mortality is controversial, the association raises doubts that further reduction of an already low cholesterol level is beneficial.

Cholesterol interacts in a synergistic fashion with other risk factors to increase patients' risk for coronary disease. Cigarette smoking and hypertension, in particular, produce greater increases in mortality from coronary heart disease when combined with hypercholesterolemia than would be predicted on the basis of each risk factor alone (9, 10). For example, if smoking and hypercholesterolemia were additive risks, the 5-year age-adjusted death rate among normotensive white hypercholesterolemic men in MRFIT who smoked would have been 9.21 per 1000 (*see* Appendix), whereas the actual death rate was 10.78 (10).

The association between elevated cholesterol levels and the incidence of and mortality from coronary heart disease has not been studied as thoroughly in elderly persons. In a Danish study (11), the cholesterol level of 70-year-old patients was not an independent predictor of the incidence of or mortality from cardiovascular disease in men or women. In this study, cardiovascular disease included cerebrovascular disease and intermittent claudication as well as coronary heart disease. In the 9-year follow-up of the Stockholm Prospective study, the serum cholesterol level did not predict the development of coronary heart disease among men age 60 and older (12). Other investigators (13, 14) have also found that the relation between cholesterol and subsequent risk for cardiac disease diminished with age.

These findings are consistent with analyses from the Framingham study suggesting that cholesterol was not a significant risk factor for coronary heart disease in elderly persons (15). With several additional years of observation, however, the Framingham investigators (16, 17) found that cholesterol was a risk factor in elderly women. They reported, on the basis of 30 years of follow-up, that the association between the cholesterol level and the incidence and mortality of coronary heart disease was significant in women, but not men, 65 years of age and older. Compared with women who had a "desirable" cholesterol level of less than 5.17 mmol/L (200 mg/dL), elderly women whose cholesterol level exceeded 7.91 mmol/L (306 mg/dL) had a significantly elevated risk for disease; the association between relative risk for disease and the cholesterol level in men was not statistically significant (17). The cholesterol level had a statistically significant negative association with overall mortality in men and women 65 years of age and older (16). Barrett-Connor and associates (18) found that the serum cholesterol was an independent predictor of death rates, but not all-cause mortality, among elderly men and women 65 to 79 years of age.

Why the relation between cholesterol level and cardiac risk changes with age is unclear. Persons with hypercholesterolemia who survive to old age without evidence of coronary disease may somehow resist the cardiac effects of hypercholesterolemia, or they may have elevated levels of high-density lipoprotein (HDL). The results of the Framingham study showed that HDL and low-density lipoprotein (LDL) levels were predictive of the risk for coronary heart disease in elderly men and women (15), and that the HDL level was a particularly strong predictor of myocardial infarction in women and the elderly (19).

Among women younger than 65 years of age, the associations between cholesterol level and coronary heart disease and overall mortality are also uncertain. Women have not been studied as extensively as men; most of the large epidemiologic studies—MRFIT, the Whitehall study, the Normative Aging study (20), the U.S. Railroad Workers study (21), and most of the studies that were part of the Pooling Project (22)—included only men. In the Stockholm Prospective study (23), the total cholesterol level in women was not a statistically significant predictor of the endpoint for coronary heart disease studied—mortality from myocardial infarction. The results of some studies may have shown that the association between cholesterol and coronary heart disease mortality was weaker in women because women tend to have higher HDL cholesterol levels than men, for a given total cholesterol level (15), and because age-adjusted rates of death from coronary heart disease are substantially lower among women (15, 24).

Characteristics of Serum Cholesterol Measurement as a Screening Test

The desirable characteristics of a screening test include low cost, convenience, safety, and accuracy. Serum cholesterol assays are inexpensive and widely available. Desktop units that measure the total serum cholesterol level in blood capillary samples obtained in a finger-stick are available, and cholesterol measurements are included in many automated blood chemistry analyzers. Lipid determinations are safe and convenient. Although it is widely believed that patients do not need to fast before blood samples are drawn for total cholesterol and HDL measurements (25-27), HDL levels vary with recent fat intake (28), and triglyceride determinations are sensitive to recent food intake. Thus, an overnight fast should precede triglyceride and HDL measurements but is unnecessary for total cholesterol measurements. Because both the cholesterol assay and further lipid tests require only blood samples, immediate risks are limited to those of venipuncture. The risks that result from screening for hyperlipoproteinemia are those of treatment and labeling (the adverse social, economic, and psychologic consequences a person might have as a result of being identified as diseased) (29, 30).

The accuracy of many screening tests can be measured by their ability to assess correctly the presence of disease. Sensitivity, specificity, and predictive value are appropriate measures of accuracy for these tests. These measures are less useful for evaluating serum cholesterol, because cholesterol assays do not detect the presence of disease. Instead, they place persons along a continuum of risk. There is no discrete threshold above which the incidence of or mortality from coronary heart disease abruptly rises. Furthermore, the distribution of serum cholesterol values among persons who later develop coronary heart disease overlaps substantially with the values for the disease-free population. Among men who were 30 to 49 years of age when they enrolled in the Framingham study, the mean cholesterol level of those who later developed coronary heart disease within 16 years was 6.31 mmol/L (244 mg/dL), whereas the mean cholesterol level for those who remained free of coronary heart disease was 5.66 mmol/L (219 mg/dL) (9). Most coronary heart disease occurs in persons who have only mild or moderate elevations in cholesterol levels.

The ability of a single cholesterol measurement to predict the risk for coronary heart disease is limited by transient variation in a person's cholesterol level. Weight loss, pregnancy, myocardial infarction, and acute illness can transiently alter cholesterol levels (27). Seasonal variation can also be responsible for temporary changes (31); in the placebo group of the Lipid Research Clinics–Coronary Primary Prevention Trial (LRC-CPPT), the measured cholesterol level averaged 0.19 mmol/L (7.4 mg/dL) higher on 30 December than on 30 June (32). The results of other studies (reviewed by Hegsted and Nicolosi [33]) have shown that even when a person adheres to a strictly controlled diet, his or her measured cholesterol levels vary substantially over short periods.

Long-term changes in a person's cholesterol level are important because they have implications for the frequency of testing. A person's cholesterol level changes as he or she ages, but this source of variation in the cholesterol level is fairly predictable. Although the mean cholesterol level for a cohort increases until patients are about 50 or 60 years old, the relative position of a person within the cohort changes slowly. After analyzing data from the Framingham study, Berwick and colleagues (34) concluded that the correlation coefficient for cholesterol levels drawn 1 year apart is 0.98. In the Muscatine study (35), the correlation between cholesterol levels measured as many as 6 years apart in children was 0.61. In young men 16 to 25 years old, the correlation coefficient between cholesterol levels measured at baseline and those measured 19 years later is 0.59; the correlation coefficient between the cholesterol levels measured at baseline and those measured 30 years later is 0.61 (36). These figures suggest that current cholesterol levels are reliable predictors of future levels, as long as diet or medications are not altered; thus, a person whose cholesterol level is well below a cutoff value for treatment is unlikely to have a level above the cutoff value for several years.

Despite both long-term and transient variation in a person's cholesterol levels, the results of epidemiologic studies have shown that the cholesterol level predicts the risk for coronary heart disease risk accurately among men. Most of these studies, however, were able to minimize variability arising from clinical laboratory practices. The cholesterol assays used in the major epidemiologic studies and randomized trials, which have served as the basis for assessments of risk and recommendations for treatment, were carefully standardized to ensure comparability over time and across sites. In contrast, the interpretation of routine measurements of serum cholesterol levels is complicated by substantial variation in the cholesterol assay among laboratories. The differences are partially due to the varied methods used to test cholesterol, but substantial variation occurs even among laboratories using the same method. The College of American Pathologists sent to 5000 clinical laboratories a sample specimen whose

directly measured the impact of triglyceride reduction on the incidence of coronary disease or death rates in asymptomatic persons. However, randomized trials (61, 62) of clofibrate, a drug that lowers both cholesterol and triglyceride levels, did not show a reduction in coronary or overall mortality rates. The Helsinki Heart study (63) assessed the effect on these outcomes of gemfibrozil, a drug that markedly lowers triglyceride levels. All of the enrollees in this trial had hypercholesterolemia, and many had hypertriglyceridemia. Although reductions in the incidence of and mortality from coronary disease correlated with the degree of cholesterol lowering, changes in the coronary endpoints did not correlate with changes in triglyceride levels.

In summary, although the results of some epidemiologic studies have shown that hypertriglyceridemia is an independent risk factor for coronary heart disease, others have shown that it is not. Persons with a type of familial hyperlipoproteinemia associated with an increased risk for coronary heart disease may have hypertriglyceridemia without hypercholesterolemia, but this condition is unlikely in the absence of a family history of hyperlipoproteinemia. The results of randomized trials do not suggest that triglyceride reduction in an asymptomatic person has an effect on coronary disease endpoints. Hypertriglyceridemia in an asymptomatic person who does not have a strong family history of coronary heart disease or a personal history of hypercholesterolemia is not a definite risk factor for coronary heart disease.

The Benefits of Cholesterol Screening

The most important reason for using the serum cholesterol as a screening test is that it detects a modifiable risk factor for premature death from coronary heart disease. This premise is a valid reason for screening if three conditions hold. First, a delay in instituting treatment must be detrimental to health outcomes or it must increase costs. If treatment at the presymptomatic stages of a disease is no cheaper, safer, or more effective than treatment initiated later, screening will impose costs on patients without providing any improvement in health or future monetary savings. Second, the test must distinguish the patients who should receive a treatment or other intervention from those who should not. If the benefits of cholesterol-lowering diets or medications were independent of the cholesterol level, the test would only offer prognostic information, because an individual patient's cholesterol level would not influence the decision to undertake treatment. Third, there must be an effective intervention. To identify a person at risk for disease will be considerably less valuable if nothing can be done to avert the disease or its consequences, or if available interventions are so costly that the same expenditure spent in other ways could improve health more. Little is known about the first of these conditions. No clinical studies have directly assessed the consequences of delays in instituting treatment for hypercholesterolemia. Because symptoms of coronary heart disease, however, develop only when the disease process is far advanced, there is widespread agreement that treatment instituted before symptoms develop has the greatest chance for success.

The epidemiologic data indicate that the second of these conditions is met. The curvilinear relation between cardiac risk and cholesterol level suggests that the benefits of cholesterol reduction are much greater at high initial levels of cholesterol than at low ones (Figure 2). Consequently, the cholesterol level identifies persons likely to benefit from therapy.

Several kinds of evidence bear on the third of these conditions. The results of studies in animals (64) and humans (65, 66) have shown that cholesterol reduction can slow or even reverse the progression of atherosclerosis. Of more direct relevance are the clinical trials that assessed the effects of cholesterol reduction on clinical outcomes. At least two of these trials found that reducing cholesterol levels that start above 6.72 mmol/L (260 mg/dL) can diminish cardiovascular mortality, and one study has shown that cholesterol-lowering interventions reduce 15-year all-cause mortality among survivors of myocardial infarction. Below, we summarize data regarding the efficacy and cost-effectiveness of interventions to lower cholesterol.

Evidence from Randomized Trials of Cholesterol Reduction

Table 2 shows the findings from several major studies of interventions to reduce mortality by lowering cholesterol (42, 53, 61, 62, 67-71). Asymptomatic hypercholesterolemic men, such as those who would be identified in a screening program, were the subjects of several primary prevention trials. These trials have shown that cholesterol reduction lowers both the incidence of and mortality from coronary heart disease among persons who have no clinical evidence of coro-

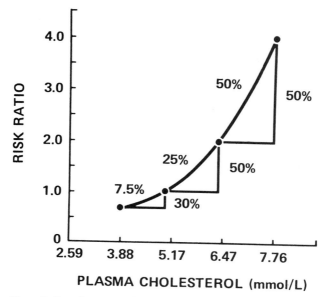

Figure 2. Hypothetical effects of the reduction of cholesterol levels on mortality from coronary heart disease among participants from the Multiple Risk Factor Intervention Trial. On the left is the percentage reduction of coronary risk resulting from a 1.29 mmol/L (50 mg/dL) decrease in plasma cholesterol level. On the right is the relative reduction in coronary risk resulting from 1.29 mmol/L (50 mg/dL) decrease in plasma cholesterol level as a function of cholesterol level at time of identification. From Grundy (6). Reproduced with the permission of the American Medical Association.

nary heart disease. However, the interventions caused only modest reductions in cholesterol and did not significantly affect all-cause mortality.

The LRC-CPPT, which was a large and well-designed randomized trial, is the most widely cited of these studies. The medication it tested, cholestyramine, is viewed by many as the best pharmacologic therapy for hypercholesterolemia. The trial included 3806 men, 35 to 59 years old, whose serum cholesterol, after an attempt at dietary management, was at least 6.85 mmol/L (265 mg/dL), and whose LDL-cholesterol level was at least 4.91 mmol/L (190 mg/dL). Both the intervention and control groups continued to receive a dietary intervention after the start of the trial. At an average of 7 years of follow-up, the cholestyramine-treated group had less morbidity and mortality from ischemic heart disease than the control group. There was a statistically significant ($P < 0.01$) reduction in the incidence of angina, which was experienced by 15% of the control group and 12% of the treatment group. Mortality from coronary heart dis-

Table 2. *Randomized, Controlled Trials of Cholesterol Reduction and Mortality in Men*

Study (Reference)	Patients	Age	Cholesterol Level	Other Characteristics
	n	*y*	*mmol/L*	
Lipid Research Clinics (42)	1906	35-59	Plasma, $\geq$ 6.85 (mean, 7.21)	. . .
Helsinki Heart Study (53)	2051	40-55	Non-HDL, > 5.17 (mean total, 7.47)	. . .
Coronary Drug Project				
1975 study (67)	1119	30-64	Mean, 6.54	Survivors of MI
1986 study (68)	. . .	. . .	. . .	. . .
World Health Organization				
1978 study (61)	5331	30-59	Mean, 6.44	Upper one third of cholesterol distribution
1984 study (62)	. . .	. . .	. . .	. . .
MRFIT (69)	6428	35-37	Mean, 6.57	High-risk
Wadsworth (70)	424	55-89	Mean, 6.03	In Veterans domicile
Oslo Study (71)	604	40-49	7.50-9.83; (mean, 8.35)	High-risk

* Difference between intervention group and control group cholesterol levels, expressed as percentage of original cholesterol level.

† Cumulative number of deaths per 100 subjects during the follow-up, with the exception of the World Health Organization trial, where deaths per 100 subjects per year are reported.

ease was also reduced by the intervention; 2.0% of the control group died from definite coronary heart disease, as compared with 1.6% of the cholestyramine group. However, all-cause mortality was 3.7% and 3.6% in the control and cholestyramine-treated groups, respectively, a difference that was not statistically significant (42). Analysis of the cholestyramine-treated patients showed that a 19% reduction in the incidence of coronary heart disease was associated with an 8% reduction in serum total cholesterol, and that the magnitude of the reduction in the incidence of coronary heart disease corresponded to the degree of reduction in total cholesterol levels. The persons who closely adhered to the pharmacologic intervention tended to have larger declines in cholesterol and a lower incidence of coronary heart disease (72). However, the incidence of coronary heart disease in the control group did not show a statistically significant

Table 2. *(Continued)*

Intervention	Mean Follow-up	Mean Change*	Deaths†			
			Coronary Heart Disease		All Causes	
			Intervention	Control	Intervention	Control
	y	*%*				
Cholestyramine	7.4	8.5	1.6	2.0	3.6	3.7
Gemfibrozil	5	11	0.7	0.9	2.2	2.1
Niacin	6	10.1	18.8	18.9	21.2	20.9
. . .	15	. . .	36.5	41.3	52.0	58.2
Clofibrate	5.3	9	0.13	0.12	0.62	0.52
. . .	13.2	. . .	0.36	0.35	0.86	0.79
Diet, smoking reduction, blood pressure control	7	2	1.8	1.9	4.1	4.0
Diet	8‡	12.7	9.6	14.2	41.0	41.9
Diet, smoking reduction	5	13	1.0	2.2	2.6	3.8

‡ Value is for the entire follow-up; the mean is not reported.

relation to the degree of cholesterol lowering due to diet (73). The LRC-CPPT showed that cholestyramine given to hypercholesterolemic, asymptomatic men diminishes morbidity and mortality from coronary heart disease, but does not reduce the overall 7-year mortality.

A more recent primary prevention trial, the Helsinki Heart Study (53), obtained similar results in 4081 asymptomatic, hypercholesterolemic men 40 to 55 years of age, who were randomly assigned to receive either a placebo or gemfibrozil. Beyond 2 years of follow-up, gemfibrozil decreased total and LDL cholesterol levels by about 9% each and raised HDL cholesterol levels by 9%. At 5 years of follow-up, the gemfibrozil group had significantly fewer cardiac events but the same overall mortality rate as the control group. Most of the excess noncardiac deaths in the treatment groups of both the LRC-CPPT and the Helsinki Heart Study were due to accidents and violence.

The Oslo study (71) enrolled more than 1200 men who reported that they had high-cholesterol, high-fat diets and whose cholesterol levels ranged from 7.50 to 9.83 mmol/L (290 to 380 mg/dL; average value, 8.51, or 328.9 mg/dL). A combined diet and smoking intervention in this population resulted in a large but statistically insignificant fall in all-cause mortality. By the end of the trial (averaging 5 years of observation), 2.6% of the intervention group died, compared with 3.8% of the control group ($P = 0.246$). Nearly 80% of the men smoked cigarettes at the time of enrollment, and the combined intervention decreased tobacco consumption by 45%. In a follow-up study conducted after the termination of the trial, or between 8.5 and 10 years after enrollment, the difference in overall mortality approached statistical significance. By that time, 3.15% of the intervention group and 4.94% of the control group had died; these values corresponded to a one-sided P value of approximately 0.05, not adjusted for multiple comparisons (74). Because the intervention substantially reduced cigarette smoking during the trial, the trend toward a significant decline in overall mortality might not have been due to cholesterol reduction alone. This trial enrolled men whose cholesterol levels were higher than in the populations included in the LRC-CPPT and Helsinki studies, and its small sample size limited its power to detect clinically significant differences in outcomes. In MRFIT, a larger trial, a multifaceted intervention did not lower coronary heart disease incidence or all-cause mortality. Because the cholesterol level in the experimental group fell by only 2% more than in the control group, this trial does not provide much information about the impact of cholesterol reduction on outcomes. However, it may affirm the difficulties of using a dietary intervention to lower cholesterol, particularly in a population that is already highly health-conscious.

Because secondary prevention trials are targeted toward persons who have clinical evidence of coronary heart disease, they do not directly apply to the screening population considered here. Nevertheless, the secondary prevention trials provide important clues to the likely effects of cholesterol reduction in asymptomatic persons. Because the subjects of these trials have advanced coronary heart disease, they might seem to be unpromising candidates for preventive efforts. They are at such a high risk of morbidity and death from (recurrent) coronary heart disease that secondary prevention might show a benefit from cholesterol reduction in this population despite a relatively short period of observation. Indeed, a well-designed secondary prevention trial has provided evidence that cholesterol reduction leads to lower all-cause mortality. The Coronary Drug Project found that niacin, when given to male survivors of myocardial infarction whose ages ranged from 30 to 64 years, reduced cholesterol levels by about 10% (68). It had no effect on mortality at a follow-up period averaging 6 years. At an average of 15 years after the inception of the trial, however, the men treated with niacin had an all-cause mortality rate that was 11% lower than the placebo group ($P = 0.0004$), even though the Coronary Drug Project regimen only lasted for about 6 years. The mortality reduction was primarily due to a fall in the coronary heart disease mortality rate. Larger benefits were reported in another secondary prevention trial, the Stockholm Ischemic Heart Disease study (75), which found a 29% reduction in 5-year all-cause mortality among survivors of myocardial infarction treated with a combination of clofibrate and niacin. However, only limited conclusions can be drawn from this trial. It was small and not double-blinded; the authors did not report whether the all-cause mortality difference was statistically significant; and 24% of the intervention group withdrew from the trial (compared with only 10% of the control group).

These trials have established that cholesterol reduction can lower the incidence of and mortality from coronary heart disease in both asymptomatic patients and in persons who have clinical evidence of coronary heart disease. Patients and physicians, however, must weigh several other aspects of treatment before embarking on a cholesterol reduction program. The interventions impose costs on patients—in the form of inconvenience, expenditures for medications, and unwanted lifestyle and dietary changes. Particularly for patients who do not have symptoms, these costs loom large in relation to the disease prevented. In undertaking cholesterol reduction, they can expect to lessen their risk for developing coronary heart disease. For many persons, a reduction in mortality will be the most important goal of cholesterol reduction, and coronary heart disease is only one of many potential causes of death.

For these persons, the key question is: "How much longer can I expect to live if I reduce my cholesterol"? Berwick and colleagues (34), and Taylor and colleagues (76), have addressed the effect of cholesterol reduction on life expectancy. These authors used similar strategies to deal with uncertainties in the relation between cholesterol reduction and mortality, and they made assumptions favorable to cholesterol-lowering interventions whenever the data were uncertain. Thus, their estimates can be viewed as the upper bounds for the effectiveness of treatment in prolonging life. The cost-effectiveness of cholesterol intervention, and its impact on the costs of care, have been addressed by Berwick and colleagues (34), by Oster and Epstein (77, 78), and most recently by Kinosian and Eisenberg (79).

Effects of Cholesterol Treatment on Life Expectancy

Berwick and colleagues (34) attempted a comprehensive cost-effectiveness analysis of cholesterol screening and treatment. Their model focused on the effect of cholesterol reduction on life expectancy. Results from the LRC-CPPT, MRFIT, and the 15-year Coronary Drug Project follow-up were not available. Drawing from data and methods of the Framingham study (80), they related the age-specific annual mortality rate to the cholesterol level and other risk factors. The formula they used to relate annual mortality to these factors is known as the Framingham logistic risk function. From this function, they were able to predict the risk for coronary heart disease as a function of cholesterol level. They applied this estimated risk to U.S. national life-table figures for annual mortality by age and sex, and they assumed that there was no effect on the risk for death from other causes. The resulting adjusted life-table figures enabled them to produce estimates of the effects of changes in cholesterol on life expectancy.

These authors assumed that the survival of persons with a specific cholesterol level was the same for untreated persons as for those whose cholesterol had been reduced to the same level by dietary or pharmacologic intervention. Their analysis, based on their "central assumption," implied that a screening program for hypercholesterolemia followed by a dietary intervention for men whose cholesterol was at or above the 95th percentile cost about $11 000 (in 1975 dollars) per year of life saved. This figure compares favorably with the cost-effectiveness of hypertension treatment, which ranges from $4000 to $20 000 per life-year saved (in 1975 dollars) (81).

Taylor and colleagues (76) also used a logistic risk function from the Framingham study to assess the change in life expectancy that results from a cholesterol-lowering diet. This function was then applied to U.S. life-table data to construct annual mortality rates be-

Table 3. *Months Added to Life Expectancy from Changes in Risk Factors among Persons at High Risk for Coronary Heart Disease**

Patients	Cholesterol Reduction		Quit Smoking	Reduction in Blood Pressure by 14.3%
	By 6.7%	By 20%		
	←————————————————— *mo* —————————————————→			
Women, age (y)				
20	4	13	37	19
40	9	24	37	26
60	13	36	23	22
Men, age (y)				
20	4	11	70	24
40	7	18	63	34
60	2	5	32	24

* Data are adapted from Taylor and colleagues (76). These figures assume a 0% discount rate and a lag period of 3 years for the achievement of full benefit. These figures are for persons whose systolic blood pressure, cigarette smoking habit, and total cholesterol are each at the 90th percentile, and whose high-density lipoprotein cholesterol level is at the 10th percentile of the age- and sex-specific population distribution.

fore and after cholesterol reduction. Taylor and co-workers also assumed that the risk for coronary heart disease associated with a given level of cholesterol was the same for untreated persons as for those who achieved the cholesterol level by dietary restrictions. They assumed, however, that a delay occurred before this full reduction in mortality could be achieved, with a base-case estimate of 3 years. Their central estimate for the cholesterol reduction achievable with diet was 6.7%, the value obtained by the intervention group in MRFIT. They did not discount future health benefits, an assumption favorable to the cholesterol-lowering intervention.

The key results from the study by Taylor and colleagues (76) are shown in Table 3. The impact of cholesterol reduction varies greatly, depending on the risk group and degree of reduction. These results apply to hypertensive smokers with hypercholesterolemia; in most cases, smoking cessation and a 14.3% reduction in blood pressure would produce greater increases in life span than would even a 20% reduction in serum cholesterol. These calculations are based on the assumption that cholesterol reduction only affects the risk from coronary heart disease, whereas smoking cessation and blood pressure control also reduce the risk from other diseases. In the absence of other risk factors, hypercholesterolemia has a small effect on life expectancy. For nonsmokers whose systolic blood pressure is at the 10th percentile and whose HDL levels are at the 90th percentile, the gains from reducing even a serum cholesterol of 7.76 mmol/L (300 mg/dL) are less than 2 months for men and 3 months for women. At lower initial levels of cholesterol, the benefits of cholesterol reduction are smaller. Thus, for most of the low-risk screening population that we consider, cholesterol reduction would not markedly prolong life.

Investigators (82) associated with the Framingham Heart Study have claimed that the effects of cholesterol reduction may be substantially larger than these calculations suggest. In their rebuttal, Taylor and colleagues (83) claimed that several of the assumptions made in the original paper that were attacked by the Framingham investigators exaggerate the effect of cholesterol on life expectancy. Although these calculations remain controversial, it is clear that most of the uncertain assumptions adopted by the authors favor cholesterol reduction. For example, Taylor and colleagues assume that diet imposes no adverse effects. If their approach were used to predict the effects of pharmacologic therapy, it would exaggerate the survival benefits of treatment.

Cholesterol Reduction and Costs of Illness

Oster and Epstein (77) assessed the effects of cholesterol reduction on the future costs of medical care and on the earnings gained by preventing premature death. Their analysis, which did not incorporate the costs of treating a patient with an elevated cholesterol level, considered the effects of cholesterol reduction on morbidity as well as mortality. They also used a logistic risk function from the Framingham study to estimate mortality from coronary heart disease, including age, cholesterol level, systolic blood pressure, cigarette smoking, and the presence of left ventricular hypertrophy as risk factors. Oster and Epstein did not assume that cholesterol reduction would always achieve "full benefit." Instead, they recognized that the mortality rate for untreated persons whose cholesterol level was 4.65 mmol/L (180 mg/dL) need not be the same as the mortality rate for persons who lowered their cholesterol levels to 4.65 mmol/L with the help of medications or diet.

Even if cholesterol reduction is assumed to be highly efficacious, the savings in the costs of medical care appear to be small. With a 5% discount rate, the fall in lifetime medical expenditures would be at most $321 (in 1980 dollars) for 45 to 49-year-old men who can reduce a cholesterol level of 8.79 mmol/L (340 mg/dL) by 25%. Savings in indirect costs—earnings lost because of early death—range from a few dollars for elderly persons to about $13 000 in 1980 dollars ($8491 in 1975 dollars) for 35 to 39-year-old men. The savings are somewhat greater for men who are hypertensive, smoke cigarettes, and have diabetes, but even in this category the maximum savings in indirect costs is $16 611 (in 1980 dollars, or $10 850 in 1975 dollars) for 35 to 39-year-old men whose initial cholesterol is 8.79 mmol/L (340 mg/dL), if their cholesterol is reduced by 15%. This method of evaluating the costs of illness can be misleading (84), but the analysis suggests that the reduction in medical expenditures would be small, even when the costs of treating hypercholesterolemia are ignored.

In a second study, Oster and Epstein (78) use similar methodology to assess the cost-effectiveness of cholestyramine therapy in treating men with hypercholesterolemia. They express the cost of the increase in life expectancy attributable to the cholestyramine treatment in a measure called "cost per year of life saved." This measure of cost decreases as the cholesterol level rises and is a U-shaped function of the age of initiating therapy. The cost per life-year saved ranges from about $56 000 for a 35 to 39-year-old man with a pretreatment cholesterol level of 8.15 mmol/L (315 mg/dL) to more than $1 million for a 70 to 74-year-old man at a cholesterol level of 8.15 mmol/L (315 mg/dL) or less, if treatment is continued throughout life. After the decline in the price of cholestyramine is taken into account, the results of this study are roughly consistent with those of an earlier study of the cost-effectiveness of cholestyramine therapy (85).

A cost-effectiveness analysis by Kinosian and Eisenberg (79) compared oat bran, cholestyramine, and colestipol as cholesterol-lowering interventions in men whose cholesterol levels averaged 7.25 mmol/L (280 mg/dL). Their methods for analyzing the impact of cholesterol reduction on health outcomes were similar to those of the other cost-effectiveness studies. Kinosian and Eisenberg used data from the LRC-CPPT to estimate the impact of cholesterol reduction on the likelihood of myocardial infarction, angina, coronary artery bypass surgery, and death from coronary disease in patients. In particular, they estimated the change in life expectancy from each therapy by assuming that the change in rates of death from coronary disease corresponding to a given reduction in cholesterol would be equal to the reduction observed in the LRC-CPPT, but that the rates of death from other causes would not be affected (Kinosian B. Personal communication). The estimates of the cost per year of life saved by the interventions varied with alternative assumptions about the costs of the drugs, the costs of treating the nonfatal cardiac events, the rate of discount applied to future health events, and the effectiveness of the interventions. Under their central assumptions, cholesterol reduction using 90 g/d (1.5 cups dry) of oat bran costs as little as $17 800 per year of life saved for a 55-year-old man. The most expensive of the three therapies considered, cholestyramine sold in packets, costs $117 400 per year of life saved. The costs per year of life saved are lower if the medications are purchased in bulk form, if the costs associated with future health events are not discounted, and if the interventions are targeted toward smokers. The costs are higher if a higher rate of discount is used or if retail medication prices are used rather than wholesale prices. As the authors note, the cost per year of life saved for therapy with oat bran compares favorably with other interventions to reduce cardiac risk, and cholestyramine and colestipol purchased in bulk form are also cost-effective, particularly if targeted toward smokers.

Additional Comments on the Efficacy of Cholesterol Reduction

The evidence that cholesterol reduction is a cost-effective approach to health improvement is incomplete. The first requirement for cost-effectiveness is therapeutic efficacy, and clinical trials have shown that cholesterol-lowering interventions improve some, but not all, important aspects of health in hypercholesterolemic men. The primary endpoints of these studies have been incidence of coronary heart disease, serious morbidity from coronary heart disease, and death from coronary heart disease. By focusing on these endpoints, we may exaggerate the advantages of treatment. These cardiovascular outcomes reflect the expected benefits of therapy, but not all of the adverse effects. The side effects of the interventions are expressed in many organ systems and in many forms; cholesterol-lowering medications produce liver abnormalities, glucose intolerance, gallbladder disease, and multiple gastrointestinal disorders. They may also be associated with cancer and impaired absorption of some medications and nutrients (86). Although many clinical trials record the incidence of noncardiovascular side effects, none of them use comprehensive measures of morbidity, such as days of work lost, measures of health care utilization, or activity limitations. Thus, a full accounting of the effects of cholesterol reduction on morbidity is unavailable. Although the results of primary and secondary prevention trials have shown that cholesterol reduction diminishes the incidence of coronary heart disease endpoints, they have indicated little or no improvement in the more global outcome measure, overall survival.

Because the randomized trials studied treatment of moderate to severe hypercholesterolemia in middle-aged men, conclusions about the effects of treatment on the young, the old, and women are speculative. The benefits of treatment in otherwise low-risk hypercholesterolemic men are probably small. During a period of 5 to 10 years, treatment for moderate hypercholesterolemia would be unlikely to reduce the already low incidence of coronary heart disease in children and women. For an entirely different reason, the treatment of hypercholesterolemia would not substantially prolong the lives of elderly men: Even though coronary heart disease is common in this group, the serum cholesterol level does not reliably predict the risk for or mortality from coronary heart disease in asymptomatic elderly persons.

Estimates of the health effects of cholesterol reduction based on the Framingham logistic risk function complement the results of the clinical trials. This approach assumes that cholesterol reduction lowers the risk for coronary heart disease without increasing mortality from other causes. The reduction in coronary heart disease incidence predicted by the Framingham logistic risk model is consistent with the results of the LRC-CPPT (72), which found that a 1% reduction in the cholesterol level was associated with a 2% reduction in coronary heart disease. The implied reduction in total mortality, however, as calculated by the authors of the cost-effectiveness studies and by Taylor and colleagues (76), exceeds the mortality reduction observed in the LRC-CPPT and the Helsinki Heart Study. These primary prevention trials did not find that treatment reduced overall mortality. By assuming that treatment can reduce the mortality of a hypercholesterolemic patient to that of an untreated patient with a lower cholesterol level, studies based on the logistic risk model estimate larger gains in life expectancy than could be inferred from the clinical trials.

Although the studies that used the Framingham risk model made assumptions favoring cholesterol-lowering interventions, they found that treating asymptomatic, low-risk persons with hypercholesterolemia results in small savings in health expenditures (77), small improvements in life expectancy (76), and large costs per year of life saved (78), unless the treatment is inexpensive (79). Other persons gain more from treatment. According to these and other (34) studies, the benefits are substantially greater among high-risk populations, such as persons who smoke, are hypertensive, or have marked hypercholesterolemia.

Recommendations

The following recommendations for screening apply only to asymptomatic persons who do not have a family history of hypercholesterolemia, who are not being treated with lipid-altering medications, and who are not known to have hypertension, coronary heart disease, or a cause of secondary hyperlipoproteinemia, such as diabetes. Despite the lack of definite evidence that treatment would diminish mortality in this population, we recommend screening because treatment reduces morbidity from coronary heart disease. Furthermore, clinical trials may have underestimated the benefits of treating patients with hypercholesterolemia.

Clinical trials may have underestimated reductions in overall mortality, because the interventions did not produce large, sustained reductions in serum cholesterol levels, and the studies may not have been in progress long enough to detect the full effect of cholesterol reduction. In some trials, such as the Helsinki Heart Study (53), there was a trend toward greater reduction in cardiac events as the duration of treatment increased. The strongest evidence for delayed benefit comes from the Coronary Drug Project, in which niacin reduced 15-year (9 years after the end of the trial) but not 6-year mortality. The evidence of delayed mortality effects suggests that even a decade-long study will underestimate the long-term benefits of cholesterol reduction.

Individualizing Screening and Treatment
Recommendations

The purpose of screening, in this context, is the detection of hypercholesterolemia. Yet no natural cutoff value separates normal from elevated serum cholesterol levels; above the 20th percentile, total mortality increases at an accelerating rate with each additional increment in the serum cholesterol level. It is most useful to define hypercholesterolemia as a cholesterol level that is high enough to warrant a specific action— further testing, a dietary recommendation, or pharmacologic therapy. Because this cholesterol level is a threshold for treatment or further testing that might lead to treatment, it represents a balance between the risks and benefits of treatment and need not be uniform. The treatment threshold differs from one person to another for at least three reasons. First, other cardiovascular risk factors, such as smoking and hypertention, modify the risk associated with a given cholesterol level. Second, the risks of treatment differ among patients. For example, niacin and lovastatin, which cause liver function abnormalities, may be especially hazardous in patients with preexisting liver disease. Third, the values that persons attach to the consequences of hypercholesterolemia or its treatment differ. Dietary modification, other lifestyle changes, and treatment with drugs that cause troublesome side effects are acceptable to some, but not all, hypercholesterolemic patients.

Recommended thresholds for the treatment of hypercholesterolemia differ. For example, the American Heart Association (87) recommended that patients whose cholesterol levels exceed the 95th percentile be treated with diet and, if they fail to respond adequately, with lipid-lowering medications. The Consensus Conference (88) of the National Institutes of Health (NIH) recommends that all adults whose cholesterol levels exceed the 75th percentile be treated by dietary means; they further recommended pharmacologic therapy to diminish very high cholesterol values (90th percentile and above) that do not fall with dietary modification. The latest in this series of recommendations from expert groups is from the Adult Treatment Panel of the National Cholesterol Education Program (27). They advise lipoprotein analysis for patients with hypercholesterolemia, and base their suggested treatment thresholds on the (calculated) LDL level. The National Cholesterol Education Program recommends cholesterol-lowering treatment for all patients whose LDL-cholesterol levels are 4.14 mmol/L (160 mg/dL) or higher, and for persons with coronary heart disease or two risk factors for cardiac disease who have LDL-cholesterol levels from 3.36 to 4.11 mmol/L (130 to 159 mg/dL).

If treatment thresholds differ among patients, screening recommendations should also be individualized. For an otherwise low-risk person who is reluctant to modify his or her lifestyle or to take cholesterol-lowering medications, there is little reason to screen for hypercholesterolemia at all. Persons whose risk for coronary heart disease is high because of other risk factors, such as cigarette smoking, are at especially high risk if they are also hypercholesterolemic. If these persons are willing to receive treatment for hypercholesterolemia and cannot modify the other risk factors, they should be screened and treated aggressively. They should be informed, however, that other risk factors are at least as harmful as hypercholesterolemia. A patient can add more to his or her life expectancy by eliminating cigarette smoking or by undergoing treatment for moderate or severe hypertension than by effecting modest reductions in his or her cholesterol level (76, 79, 89). Finally, as we note below, the interval between screening tests should vary with the treatment threshold.

The Role of Serum Triglyceride Measurements in Healthy Persons

A serum triglyceride level need not be measured from healthy persons unless they have an elevated cholesterol level or a family history suggestive of familial hyperlipidemia. In the absence of hypercholesterolemia, men with moderate elevations of triglyceride levels (6.47 to 12.90 mmol/L [250-499 mg/dL]) do not appear to have an excess risk for all-cause or cardiovascular death, according to at least one large population-based study (90). In general, the serum triglyceride level is not a consistent independent predictor of cardiac risk. Furthermore, no major study has shown that triglyceride reduction leads to lower mortality from coronary heart disease. Therefore, the serum triglyceride level is not recommended as a screening test for coronary disease.

Measurement of the triglyceride level may be useful in settings not considered here. In a person with an elevated serum cholesterol level, the triglyceride level may have prognostic significance or may influence the choice of lipid-lowering medications. Hypertriglyceridemia is sometimes the first sign that a person with a compatible family history is affected with familial combined hyperlipidemia; in this case, a person might benefit from relatively frequent cholesterol testing and early treatment of hypercholesterolemia. It may also be valuable to measure the triglyceride level in persons at risk for secondary hypertriglyceridemia from such risk factors as diabetes mellitus or obesity, because extreme elevations are associated with noncardiac complications, such as pancreatitis.

The Total Serum Cholesterol Level as a Screening Test for Men and Women

Among men, the serum total cholesterol should be measured once in early adulthood. Among women, the screening cholesterol test is optional. Only well-standardized assays should be used. For young men found to have moderate elevations of cholesterol, epidemiologic evidence and the results of clinical trials in older men suggest that treatment would reduce the likelihood of developing coronary heart disease; however, even if young men were untreated, they would have little morbidity from coronary heart disease until many years later. Young men whose cholesterol levels exceed the 95th or 97th percentile are at very high risk for developing coronary heart disease. Because these marked cholesterol elevations are infrequent, few such persons of any age have been studied in randomized, controlled trials. Mortality rises rapidly with further increases in high cholesterol levels, even among relatively young men; the results of many studies have confirmed the high prevalence of ischemic heart disease and high overall rates of mortality associated with extreme elevations of cholesterol, as is seen in familial hypercholesterolemia (91-93). These extreme elevations can be reduced by aggressive therapy (94-97). If side effects of therapy are independent of cholesterol level while benefits are greater at higher cholesterol levels, there is a strong rationale for treating persons with severe hypercholesterolemia. Therefore, although few of them have been enrolled in clinical studies of cholesterol reduction, young and middle-aged men with severe hypercholesterolemia (for example, levels above 7.76 mmol/L [300 mg/dL]) are more likely than the subjects of randomized trials to benefit from lipid-lowering therapy. Cholesterol screening can identify these persons.

Because few epidemiologic studies have included women, less is known about the association between hypercholesterolemia and the risk for coronary heart disease in women. Women have less morbidity from coronary heart disease than men, and they tend to be older when they develop symptoms. The results of the Framingham study showed that serum cholesterol is a statistically significant predictor of the incidence of and the mortality from coronary heart disease, but the risk for coronary heart disease is lower in women than in men, and the health effects of cholesterol-lowering treatment among women are unknown. The paucity of relevant information leads us to conclude that cholesterol screening should be considered optional for women. Although we feel that current evidence does not support screening in most cases, cholesterol testing would be suitable for some women. For example, those women who are at high risk because of other risk factors might benefit from screening and treatment of hypercholesterolemia. A decision to screen should be made on an individual basis, and the lack of data on the effects of treatment should be recognized.

The measured cholesterol level can vary transiently, so if the test result is near a threshold for further diagnostic investigation or for treatment, the test should be repeated on another blood sample. Even if the test is repeated, though, failure to standardize the assay and report the results in units that are equivalent to a reference method, such as the reference standard method of the Centers for Disease Control, will vitiate its value. The Laboratory Standardization Panel of the National Cholesterol Education Program has recommended that clinical laboratories take concrete steps to improve the accuracy and precision of their cholesterol assays (39). Until these steps have been taken, physicians should request evidence of standardization from the laboratories that do cholesterol assays for them.

Serum High-Density and Low-Density Cholesterol Levels as Initial Screening Tests for Lipoprotein Disorders

These assays should not be used as the initial screening tests for lipoprotein disorders. Epidemiologic studies and randomized, controlled trials have shown that the HDL level, the HDL/total cholesterol ratio, and the HDL/LDL ratios appear to be better predictors of coronary heart disease risk than the total cholesterol. There are several reasons, however, for doing lipoprotein fractionations only in patients who are hypercholesterolemic. First, few patients whose total cholesterol is low have an elevated LDL-cholesterol level. Second, although a few persons who have a low HDL-cholesterol level in the setting of a normal total cholesterol level would not be detected if only the total cholesterol were measured, the significance of this finding is unknown. Third, the HDL assays (and calculated LDL) in routine use are unreliable. Thus, only limited additional information is obtained from direct measurement of the HDL and calculated LDL in a screening population. Finally, these tests are more expensive than total cholesterol measurements. If the costs of these tests change and standardization improves, the HDL and LDL levels may become first-choice screening tests for hyperlipoproteinemia.

Measurement of the serum HDL level is indicated when the HDL level or the calculated LDL level will be used to decide whether to administer therapy, such as those occasions when the total cholesterol is near a treatment threshold. Then these lipoprotein levels can help the patient and physician assess the likely benefits of therapy by providing a more accurate estimate of the risk for coronary heart disease.

The Screening Cholesterol Test in Elderly Persons

The test is optional in men or women 70 years of age and older. The precise age limit that defines "elderly" for any analysis of cardiac risk factors is arbitrary, and investigators from different studies have used various age divisions. In virtually every study reviewed here, though, persons 70 years of age and older would be considered elderly. In the absence of data on treatment efficacy in this age group, the rationale for treating hypercholesterolemia depends heavily on the association between cholesterol level and risk for coronary heart disease. At least for men, that association weakens with age; the total cholesterol level does not consistently predict coronary heart disease risk in elderly men and may bear a negative relation to overall mortality in men and women 65 years of age and older. Because the relation between the cholesterol level and the risk for disease in elderly persons is less clearly defined than it is for middle-aged men, and because mortality from other causes increases with age, this population is likely to gain smaller benefits from lowering cholesterol than did the men who were enrolled in the clinical trials. Until there is stronger evidence that the cholesterol level is associated with risk in asymptomatic elderly persons, and that cholesterol-lowering interventions are likely to benefit elderly persons, physicians should not feel compelled to screen all elderly persons for hypercholesterolemia.

To clarify the role of screening for hypercholesterolemia in elderly persons, three areas need further study. First, increasing life expectancy may mean that people will develop coronary heart disease at older ages in the future. Then the total cholesterol may prove to be a more accurate predictor of cardiovascular risk in future cohorts of elderly persons than in the cohorts who have already been studied. Second, the effects of cholesterol treatment should be measured in elderly persons. Both the health benefits and the adverse effects of therapy may be different in this population than in the middle-aged subjects of most clinical trials. Third, the role of the HDL and LDL levels in screening for cardiovascular disease in elderly persons needs further study. The results of some studies have shown that HDL and LDL levels are independent predictors of the risk for coronary heart disease in elderly persons, although it is not known whether these lipoproteins also predict overall mortality. If HDL or LDL levels identify groups of elderly persons who benefit from cholesterol reduction, they may prove to be useful screening tests. Until data supporting these applications of the tests become available, and until these tests are better standardized, their use in screening elderly persons is not recommended.

Frequency of Screening in Healthy Persons

The serum cholesterol need not be measured more frequently than every 5 years in healthy adults, unless the cholesterol level is near a treatment threshold. We cannot recommend a precise screening interval because data needed to determine the consequences of delaying the diagnosis of hypercholesterolemia are unavailable. Furthermore, just as the treatment threshold differs from one person to another, the screening interval needs to be individualized. The screening test is aimed at finding persons whose cholesterol levels exceed the treatment threshold. In a given interval between tests, the yield—the percentage of test results that exceed the threshold for the first time—is smaller when the treatment threshold is higher. The likelihood of a positive test result is also small for persons whose previous cholesterol levels were well below the threshold. Thus, a patient whose serum cholesterol falls short of a treatment threshold by 0.26 mmol/L (10 mg/dL) should be reassessed sooner than another person whose cholesterol level is 2.59 mmol/L (100 mg/dL) less than the treatment threshold. A 5-year interval between screening tests should be sufficient for a person whose cholesterol level falls well below his or her treatment threshold, because the cholesterol level rises slowly and predictably with age unless illness, dietary change, or medications intervene.

More frequent screening may become desirable if new therapies for hypercholesterolemia are found to be effective. Several new cholesterol-lowering drugs are likely to become available soon, and other promising drugs have become available recently. For example, lovastatin, which was recently approved by the Food and Drug Administration, is one of several medications that lower serum cholesterol by inhibiting cholesterol synthesis. These drugs appear to be tolerated better and have a greater impact on cholesterol levels than previously available therapy, particularly when combined with bile acid sequestrants (98-102). Although lovastatin raises HDL levels and reduces LDL and total cholesterol levels, no reported clinical trial has measured its effectiveness in lowering coronary heart disease or overall mortality. If these or other new medications, such as the newer fibric acid derivatives (103), prove to be safe and more effective than older therapies, frequent screening might lead to the early detection and treatment of hypercholesterolemia and result in less morbidity and longer survival. A more effective treatment, however, need not mandate more frequent screening. For example, consider a hypothetical drug so effective that mortality and morbidity throughout life are the same if therapy is initiated when patients are 35 years of age as when they are 30. Then the screening test might safely be deferred until they are 35 years of age. The screening interval should be based, in part, on an assessment of the consequences of delays in initiating treatment, so the recommended interval may be modified as new treatments become available and are proved to be effective.

Recommendations of Other Authors

Although their screening recommendations differ, most authorities suggest measuring cholesterol infrequently and omitting measurement of triglycerides or HDL levels in asymptomatic persons. None of the studies cited below offers a firm justification for the recommended screening interval.

Breslow and Somers (104) recommend measurement of the serum cholesterol and triglyceride levels in persons 18 years old and then every 5 years in persons 25 to 70 years old. According to the Institute of Medicine (105) serum cholesterol levels should be screened once in persons 12 to 17 years old, and once in persons

40 to 59 years old. The Institute did not include triglyceride measurements among its recommended screening tests. Its recommendations came from an ad-hoc advisory group on preventive services that met in 1978. Although the group did not offer a specific explanation for the inclusion of the cholesterol level in screening programs, its general criteria for recommending a preventive measure were: The disease prevented was important, either by afflicting a large number of people or by causing severe illness; evidence supported the efficacy of an intervention aimed at the disease; and the preventive measure was feasible.

The Canadian Task Force (106) considered but did not recommend routine screening of serum cholesterol or triglyceride levels. Lipid screening was given a level C evaluation, meaning that "there is poor evidence regarding the inclusion of the condition in a periodic health examination, and recommendations may be made on other grounds."

The Consensus Conference (88) of the National Institutes of Health recommended measuring the blood cholesterol level in every adult patient on the first visit to a physician. The conference stated, without documentation, that a cholesterol determination at annual visits to the physician's office would be cost-effective for adults. According to Frame (107) cholesterol levels, but not triglyceride levels, should be screened every 4 years in adults younger than 70 years old. Frame argued that use of the screening cholesterol is supported by recent evidence that lowering cholesterol reduces mortality.

The American Heart Association (60) recommended measuring plasma cholesterol and triglyceride levels every 5 years in persons 20 to 60 years old. In persons older than 60 years of age, measurement of lipid levels is optional, on the basis of the results of previous examinations. Recommendations for further testing and management are essentially those of the National Cholesterol Education Program. This program (27) recommended measuring the total serum cholesterol level at least once every 5 years for all adults 20 years of age and older and advised repeating the test for any persons whose serum cholesterol level exceeds 5.17 mmol/L (200 mg/dL). The program also recommended measuring the HDL and triglyceride levels, and calculating the LDL level for all persons with high cholesterol (whose two cholesterol measurements average 6.21 mmol/L [240 mg/dL] or more), and for persons with borderline to high cholesterol levels (cholesterol measurements averaging 5.17

to 6.18 mmol/L [200 to 239 mg/dL]) who also have either coronary heart disease or two of the following risk factors: hypertension, cigarette smoking, male sex, diabetes mellitus, severe obesity, a history of definite cerebrovascular or occlusive peripheral vascular disease, and a family history of premature coronary heart disease (myocardial infarction or sudden death in a parent or sibling younger than 55 years of age).

Conclusions

The serum cholesterol level safely and inexpensively identifies persons at high risk for a serious and common disease. Randomized trials have proved that lipid-lowering medications and diet can diminish morbidity and mortality from coronary heart disease among asymptomatic men whose cholesterol levels are elevated. Its value as a screening test, however, is limited by four sources of uncertainty. First, its role as a predictor of risk in elderly persons is not well defined. Second, because many clinical laboratories produce inaccurate cholesterol measurements, the relation between the reported cholesterol value and the reference standard is unknown. Third, there is little direct evidence about the efficacy of cholesterol reduction in women, young persons, or elderly persons. Finally, clinical trials in patients with established coronary heart disease suggest that overall survival benefits may be observed many years after the initiation of therapy, but this finding has yet to be confirmed in asymptomatic, nonsmoking persons with hypercholesterolemia.

We recommend screening primarily for the purpose of detecting and treating severe hypercholesterolemia. Improvements in therapy would expand the population that benefits from cholesterol reduction and would strengthen the case for screening.

Appendix

Detecting Synergism in Risk Factors

For very small risks, independent competing risks are approximately additive. The exact calculation of competing risks for the 5-year mortality from coronary disease results in the Multiple Risk Factor Intervention Trial is as follows: Letting P_b represent the probability of (coronary) death for nonsmoking white men whose cholesterol levels are less than 250, and letting P_s represent the independent mortality risk from smoking, and P_c represent the independent mortality risk from a higher cholesterol, the probability of survival in a white man wth hypercholesterolemia who smokes would be $S = (1 - P_b)(1 - P_s)(1 - P_c)$. The probabilities of survival are $(1 - P_b)$ for a person who has neither risk factor, $(1 - P_b)(1 - P_s)$ for a smoker whose cholesterol is less than 6.46 mmol/L (250 mg/dL), and $(1 - P_b)$ $(1 - P_c)$ for a nonsmoking hypercholesterolemic person. On the basis of data reported by Neaton and colleagues (10) for white men, P_c is 0.038 and P_s is 0.033. This finding implies that the coronary death rate for a person with both risk factors would be 9.21 if the risks were "additive." The two risk factors appear to be synergistic because the actual rate of death for coronary disease for smokers with hypercholesterolemia was 17% higher than would have been predicted if the two risk factors did not have synergistic effects on coronary mortality.

References

1. **Keys A.** *Seven Countries: A Multivariate Analysis of Death and Coronary Heart Disease.* Cambridge, Massachusetts: Harvard University Press; 1980.
2. **Martin MJ, Hulley SB, Browner WS, Kuller LH, Wentworth D.** Serum cholesterol, blood pressure, and mortality: implications from a cohort of 361,662 men. *Lancet.* 1986;2:933-6.
3. **Rose G, Shipley M.** Plasma cholesterol concentration and death from coronary heart disease: 10 year results of the Whitehall study. *Br Med J [Clin Res].* 1986;293:306-7.
4. **Kannel WB, Castelli W, Gordon T, McNamara PM.** Serum cholesterol, lipoproteins, and risk of coronary heart disease: the Framingham Study. *Ann Intern Med.* 1971;74:1-12.
5. **Goldbourt U, Holtzman E, Neufeld HN.** Total and high density lipoprotein cholesterol in the serum and risk of mortality: evidence of a threshold effect. *Br Med J [Clin Res].* 1985;290:1239-43.
6. **Grundy SM.** Cholesterol and coronary heart disease: a new era. *JAMA.* 1986;256:2849-58.
7. **Sherwin RW, Wentworth DN, Cutler JA, Hulley SB, Kuller LH, Stamler J.** Serum cholesterol levels and cancer mortality in 361,662 men screened for the Multiple Risk Factor Intervention Trial. *JAMA.* 1987;257:943-8.
8. **Schatzkin A, Hoover RN, Taylor PR, et al.** Serum cholesterol and cancer in the NHANES I epidemiologic followup study: National Health and Nutrition Examination Survey. *Lancet.* 1987;2:298-301.
9. **Kannel WB, Castelli WP, Gordon T.** Cholesterol in the prediction of atherosclerotic disease: new perspectives based on the Framingham study. *Ann Intern Med.* 1979;90:85-91.
10. **Neaton JD, Kuller LH, Wentworth D, Borhani NO.** Total and cardiovascular mortality in relation to cigarette smoking, serum cholesterol concentration, and diastolic blood pressure among black and white males followed up for five years. *Am Heart J.* 1984;108:759-69.
11. **Agner E, Hansen PF.** Fasting serum cholesterol and triglycerides in a ten-year prospective study in old age. *Acta Med Scand.* 1983;214:33-41.
12. **Carlson LA, Böttiger LE.** Ischaemic heart-disease in relation to fasting values of plasma triglycerides and cholesterol: the Stockholm Prospective Study. *Lancet.* 1972;1:865-8.
13. **Gofman JW, Young W, Tandy R.** Ischemic heart disease, atherosclerosis, and longevity. *Circulation.* 1966;34:679-97.
14. **Mariotti S, Capocaccia R, Farchi G, Menotti A, Verdecchia A, Keys A.** Age, period, cohort and geographical area effects on the relationship between risk factors and coronary heart disease mortality: 15-year follow-up of the European cohorts of the Seven Countries study. *J Chronic Dis.* 1986;39:229-42.
15. **Gordon T, Castelli WP, Hjortland MC, Kannel WB, Dawber TR.** High density lipoprotein as a protective factor against coronary heart disease: the Framingham Study. *Am J Med.* 1977;62:707-14.

16. **Cupples LA, D'Agostino RB.** Some risk factors related to the annual incidence of cardiovascular disease and death using pooled repeated biennial measurements: Framingham Heart Study, 30 year followup. In: Kannel WB, Wolf PA, Garrison RJ, eds. *The Framingham Study: An Epidemiological Investigation of Cardiovascular Disease: Section 34.* Washington, DC: U.S. Department of Health and Human Services, National Institutes of Health; #1987; NIH publication no. 87-2703, pp 31, 221, 448.

17. **Harris T, Cook EF, Kannel WB, Goldman L.** Proportional hazards analysis of risk factors for coronary heart disease in individuals aged 65 or older: the Framingham Heart Study. *J Am Geriatr Soc.* 1988;**36:**1023-8.

18. **Barrett-Connor E, Suarez L, Khaw K, Criqui MH, Wingard DL.** Ischemic heart disease risk factors after age 50. *J Chronic Dis.* 1984;**37:**903-8.

19. **Abbott RD, Wilson PF, Kannel WB, Castelli WP.** High density lipoprotein cholesterol, total cholesterol screening, and myocardial infarction: the Framingham Study. *Arteriosclerosis.* 1988;**8:**207-11.

20. **Glynn RJ, Rosner B, Silbert JE.** Changes in cholesterol and triglyceride as predictors of ischemic heart disease in men. *Circulation.* 1982;**66:**724-31.

21. **Keys A, Aravanis C, Blackburn H, et al.** Probability of middleaged men developing coronary heart disease in five years. *Circulation.* 1972;**45:**815-28.

22. **Pooling Project Research Group.** Relationship of blood pressure, serum cholesterol, smoking habit, relative weight and ECG abnormalities to the incidence of major coronary events: final report of the Pooling Project. *J Chronic Dis.* 1978;**31:**201-306.

23. **Carlson LA, Böttiger LE.** Risk factors for ischaemic heart disease in men and women: results of the 19-year follow-up of the Stockholm Prospective Study. *Acta Med Scand.* 1985;**218:**207-11.

24. **Brunner D, Weisbort J, Meshulam N, et al.** Relation of serum total cholesterol and high-density lipoprotein cholesterol percentage to the incidence of definite coronary events: twenty-year follow-up of the Donolo-Tel Aviv Prospective Coronary Artery Disease Study. *Am J Cardiol.* 1987;**59:**1271-6.

25. **Hulley SB, Lo B.** Choice and use of blood lipid tests: an epidemiologic perspective. *Arch Intern Med.* 1983;**143:**667-73.

26. **National Institutes of Health Consensus Conference.** Treatment of hypertriglyceridemia. *JAMA.* 1984;**251:**1196-200.

27. Report of the National Cholesterol Education Program Expert Panel on detection, evaluation, and treatment of high blood cholesterol in adults. *Arch Intern Med.* 1988;**148:**36-69.

28. **Cohn JS, McNamara JR, Schaefer EJ.** Lipoprotein cholesterol concentrations in the plasma of human subjects as measured in the fed and fasted states. *Clin Chem.* 1988;**34:**2456-9.

29. **MacDonald LA, Sackett DL, Haynes RB, Taylor DW.** Labelling in hypertension: a review of the behavioral and psychological consequences. *J Chronic Dis.* 1984;**37:**933-42.

30. **Lefebvre RC, Hursey KG, Carleton RA.** Labeling of participants in high blood pressure screening programs: implications for blood cholesterol screenings. *Arch Intern Med.* 1988;**148:**1993-7.

31. **Thomas CB, Holljes HWD, Eisenberg FF.** Observations on seasonal variations in total serum cholesterol level among healthy young prisoners. *Ann Intern Med.* 1961;**54:**413-30.

32. **Gordon DJ, Trost DC, Hyde J, et al.** Seasonal cholesterol cycles: the Lipid Research Clinics Coronary Primary Prevention Trial placebo group. *Circulation.* 1987;**76:**1224-31.

33. **Hegsted DM, Nicolosi RJ.** Individual variation in serum cholesterol levels. *Proc Natl Acad Sci USA.* 1987;**84:**6259-61.

34. **Berwick DM, Cretin S, Keeler EB.** *Cholesterol, Children, and Heart Disease: An Analysis of Alternatives.* New York: Oxford University Press; 1980.

35. **Clarke WR, Schrott HG, Leaverton PE, Conner WE, Lauer RM.** Tracking of blood lipids and blood pressures in school age children: the Muscatine study. *Circulation.* 1978;**58:**626-34.

36. **Gillum RF, Taylor HL, Brozek J, et al.** Blood lipids in young men followed 32 years. *J Chronic Dis.* 1982;**35:**635-41.

37. Choice of cholesterol-lowering drugs. *Med Lett Drugs Ther.*

1988;**30:**81-4.

38. **Duncan IW, Mather A, Cooper GS.** *The Procedure for the Proposed Cholesterol Reference Method.* Atlanta: Centers for Disease Control; 1982.

39. **National Cholesterol Education Program.** Current status of blood cholesterol measurement in clinical laboratories in the United States: a report from the Laboratory Standardization Panel of the National Cholesterol Education Program. *Clin Chem.* 1988;**34:**193-201.

40. **Abell LL, Levy BB, Brodie BB, Kendall FE.** A simplified method for the estimation of total cholesterol in serum and demonstration of is specificity. *J Biol Chem.* 1952;**95:**357-66.

41. **National Center for Health Statistics—National Heart, Lung and Blood Institute Collaborative Lipid Group.** Trends in serum cholesterol levels among U.S. adults aged 20 to 74 years: Data from the National Health and Nutrition Examination Surveys, 1960 to 1980. *JAMA.* 1987;**257:**937-42.

42. **Lipid Research Clinics Program.** The Lipid Research Clinics Coronary Primary Prevention Trial results. I. Reduction in the incidence of coronary heart disease. *JAMA.* 1984;**251:**351-64.

43. **Kroll MH, Lindsey H, Greene J, Silva C, Hainline A Jr, Elin RJ.** Bias between enzymatic methods and the reference method for cholesterol. *Clin Chem.* 1988;**34:**131-5.

44. **Koch DD, Hassemer DJ, Wiebe DA, Laessig RH.** Testing cholesterol accuracy: performance of several common laboratory instruments. *JAMA.* 1988;**260:**2552-7.

45. **Burke JJ 2d, Fischer PM.** A clinician's guide to the office measurement of cholesterol. *JAMA.* 1988;**259:**3444-8.

46. **Friedewald WT, Levy RI, Frederickson DS.** Estimation of plasma low-density lipoprotein cholesterol concentration without use of the preparative ultracentrifuge. *Clin Chem.* 1972;**18:**499-502.

47. **Yaari S, Goldbourt U, Even-Zohar S, Neufeld HN.** Associations of serum high density lipoprotein and total cholesterol with total, cardiovascular, and cancer mortality in a 7-year prospective study of 10,000 men. *Lancet.* 1981;**1:**1011-5.

48. **Kannel WB.** High-density lipoproteins: epidemiologic profile and risks of coronary artery disease. *Am J Cardiol.* 1983;**52:**9B-12B.

49. **Davis CE, Gordon D, LaRosa J, Wood PD, Halperin M.** Correlations of plasma high-density lipoprotein cholesterol levels with other plasma lipid and lipoprotein concentrations. *Circulation.* 1980;**62**(4 pt 2):IV24-30.

50. **Heiss G, Johnson NJ, Reiland S, Davis CE, Tyroler HA.** The epidemiology of plasma high-density lipoprotein cholesterol levels: The Lipid Research Clinics Program Prevalence Study Summary. *Circulation.* 1980;**62**(4 pt 2):IV116-36.

51. **Havel RJ.** High-density lipoproteins, cholesterol transport and coronary heart disease [Editorial]. *Circulation.* 1979;**60:**1-3.

52. **LaRosa JC, Chambless LE, Criqui MH, et al.** Patterns of dyslipoproteinemia in selected North American populations: the Lipid Research Clinics Program Prevalence Study. *Circulation.* 1986;**73**(1 pt 2):II2-29.

53. **Frick MH, Elo O, Haapa K, et al.** Helsinki Heart Study: primary-prevention trial with gemfibrozil in middle-aged men with dyslipidemia: Safety of treatment, changes in risk factors, and incidence of coronary heart disease. *N Engl J Med.* 1987;**317:**1237-45.

54. **College of American Pathologists.** *Comprehensive Chemistry 1987 Survey.* Skokie, Illinois: College of American Pathologists; 1987.

55. **Cowan LD, Wilcosky T, Criqui MH, et al.** Demographic, behavioral, biochemical, and dietary correlates of plasma triglycerides: Lipid Research Clinics Program Prevalence Study. *Arteriosclerosis.* 1985;**5:**466-80.

56. **Brunzell JD, Schrott HG, Motulsky AG, Bierman EL.** Myocardial infarction in the familial forms of hypertriglyceridemia. *Metabolism.* 1976;**25:**313-20.

57. **Goldstein JL, Schrott HG, Hazzard WR, Bierman EL, Motulsky AG.** Hyperlipidemia in coronary heart disease: II. Genetic analysis of lipid levels in 176 families and delineation of a new inherited disorder, combined hyperlipidemia. *J Clin Invest.* 1973;**52:**1544-68.

58. **Goldstein JL, Hazzard WR, Schrott HG, Bierman EL, Motulsky AG.** Hyperlipidemia in coronary heart disease: I Lipid levels in 500 survivors of myocardial infarction. *J Clin Invest.* 1973;**52**:1533-43.
59. **Hulley SB, Rosenman RH, Bawol RD, Brand RJ.** Epidemiology as a guide to clinical decisions: the association between triglyceride and coronary heart disease. *N Engl J Med.* 1980;**302**:1383-9.
60. **Grundy SM, Greenland P, Herd A, et al.** Cardiovascular and risk factor evaluation of healthy American adults: a statement for physicians by an Ad Hoc Committee appointed by the Steering Committee, American Heart Association. *Circulation.* 1987;**75**:1340A-62A.
61. **Committee of Principal Investigators.** A cooperative trial in the primary prevention of ischaemic heart disease using clofibrate: report from the Committee of Principal Investigators. *Br Heart J.* 1978;**40**:1069-118.
62. **Committee of Principal Investigators.** WHO Cooperative Trial on primary prevention of ischaemic heart disease with clofibrate to lower serum cholesterol: final mortality follow-up. *Lancet.* 1984;**2**:600-4.
63. **Manninen V, Elo MO, Frick MH, et al.** Lipid alterations and decline in the incidence of coronary heart disease in the Helsinki Heart Study. *JAMA.* 1988;**260**:641-51.
64. **Malinow MR, Blaton V.** Regression of atherosclerotic lesions. *Arteriosclerosis.* 1984;**4**:292-5.
65. **Levy RI, Brensike JF, Epstein SE, et al.** The influence of changes in lipid values induced by cholestyramine and diet on progression of coronary artery disease: results of the NHLBI Type II Coronary Intervention Study. *Circulation.* 1984;**69**:325-37.
66. **Blankenhorn DH, Nessim SA, Johnson RL, Sanmarco ME, Azen SP, Cashin-Hemphill L.** Beneficial effects of combined colestipol-niacin therapy on coronary atherosclerosis and coronary venous bypass grafts. *JAMA.* 1987;**257**:3233-40.
67. **Coronary Drug Project Research Group.** Clofibrate and niacin in coronary heart disease. *JAMA.* 1975;**231**:360-81.
68. **Canner PL, Berge KG, Wenger NK, et al.** Fifteen year mortality in Coronary Drug Project patients: long-term benefit with niacin. *J Am Coll Cardiol.* 1986;**8**:1245-55.
69. **Multiple Risk Factor Intervention Trial Research Group.** Multiple risk factor intervention trial: risk factor changes and mortality results. *JAMA.* 1982;**248**:1465-77.
70. **Dayton S, Pearce ML, Hashimoto S, Dixon WJ, Tomiyasu U.** A controlled clinical trial of a diet high in unsaturated fat in preventing complications of atherosclerosis. *Circulation.* 1969;**40**(Suppl II):II1-63.
71. **Hjermann I, Velve Byre K, Holme I, Leren P.** Effect of diet and smoking intervention on the incidence of coronary heart disease: report from the Oslo Study Group of a randomized trial in healthy men. *Lancet.* 1981;**2**:1303-10.
72. **Lipid Research Clinics Program.** The Lipid Research Clinics Coronary Primary Prevention Trial results. II. The relation of reduction in incidence of coronary heart disease to cholesterol lowering. *JAMA.* 1984;**251**:365-74.
73. **Kronmal RA.** Commentary on the published results of the Lipid Research Clinics Coronary Primary Prevention Trial. *JAMA.* 1985;**253**:2091-3.
74. **Holme I, Hjermann I, Helgeland A, Leren P.** The Oslo study: diet and antismoking advice. Additional results from a 5-year primary preventive trial in middle-aged men. *Prev Med.* 1985;**14**:279-92.
75. **Rosenhamer G, Carlson LA.** Effect of combined clofibrate-nicotinic acid treatment in ischemic heart disease. *Atherosclerosis.* 1980;**37**:129-42.
76. **Taylor WC, Pass TM, Shepard DS, Komaroff AL.** Cholesterol reduction and life expectancy: a model incorporating multiple risk factors. *Ann Intern Med.* 1987;**106**:605-14.
77. **Oster G, Epstein AM.** Primary prevention and coronary heart disease: the economic benefits of lowering serum cholesterol. *Am J Public Health.* 1986;**76**:647-56.
78. **Oster G, Epstein AM.** The cost-effectiveness of antihyperlipemic

therapy in the prevention of coronary heart disease: the case of cholestyramine. *JAMA*. 1987;**258**:2381-7.

79. **Kinosian BP, Eisenberg JM.** Cutting into cholesterol: cost-effective alternatives for treating hypercholesterolemia. *JAMA*. 1988;**259**:2249-54.

80. **Shurtleff D.** Some characteristics related to the incidence of cardiovascular disease and death: Framingham Study, 18 year follow-up. In: Kannel WB, Gordon T, eds. *The Framingham Study: An Epidemiological Investigation of Cardiovascular Disease: Section 30*. Washington, D.C.: U.S. Department of Health, Education, and Welfare (DHEW Publication no. [NIH] 74-599); 1974.

81. **Weinstein MC, Stason WB, Blumenthal D.** *Hypertension: A Policy Perspective*. Cambridge, Massachusetts: Harvard University Press; 1976.

82. **Frommer PL, Verter J, Witters J, Castelli W.** Cholesterol reduction and life expectancy [Letter]. *Ann Intern Med*. 1988;**108**:313-4.

83. **Taylor WC, Pass TM, Shepard DS, Komaroff AL.** Cholesterol reduction and life expectancy [Letter]. *Ann Intern Med*. 1988;**108**:313-4.

84. **Thompson MS.** Willingness to pay and accept risks to cure chronic disease. *Am J Public Health*. 1986;**76**:392-6.

85. **Weinstein MC, Stason WB.** Cost-effectiveness of interventions to prevent or treat coronary heart disease. *Annu Rev of Public Health*. 1985;**6**:41-63.

86. **Tikkanen MJ, Nikkilá EA.** Current pharmacologic treatment of elevated serum cholesterol. *Circulation*. 1987;**76**:529-33.

87. **Grundy SM, Gotto AM Jr, Bierman EL, Conner WE.** Recommendations for treatment of hyperlipidemia in adults: a joint statement of the Nutrition Committee and the Council on Arteriosclerosis. *Circulation*. 1984;**69**:1065A-90A.

88. **National Institutes of Health Consensus Conference.** Lowering blood cholesterol to prevent heart disease. *JAMA*. 1985;**253**:2080-90.

89. **Winkelstein W Jr.** Some ecological studies of lung cancer and ischaemic heart disease in mortality in the United States. *Int J Epidemiol*. 1985;**14**:39-57.

90. **Barrett-Connor E, Khaw KT.** Borderline fasting hypertriglyceridemia: absence of excess risk of all-cause and cardiovascular disease mortality in healthy men without hypercholesterolemia. *Prev Med*. 1987;**16**:1-8.

91. **Jensen J, Blankenhorn DH, Kornerup V.** Coronary disease in familial hypercholesterolemia. *Circulation*. 1967;**36**:77-82.

92. **Stone NJ, Levy RI, Frederickson DS, Verter J.** Coronary artery disease in 116 kindred with familial type II hyperlipoproteinemia. *Circulation*. 1974;**49**:476-82.

93. **Gagné C, Moorjani S, Brun D, Toussaint M, Lupien PJ.** Heterozygous familial hypercholesterolemia: relationship between plasma lipids, lipoproteins, clinical manifestations and ischaemic heart disease in men and women. *Atherosclerosis*. 1979;**34**:13-24.

94. **Kane JP, Malloy MJ, Tun P, et al.** Normalization of low-density-lipoprotein levels in heterozygous familial hypercholesterolemia with a combined drug regimen. *N Engl J Med*. 1981;**304**:251-8.

95. **Mabuchi H, Haba T, Tatami R, et al.** Effects of an inhibitor of 3-hydroxy-3-methylglutaryl coenzyme A reductase on serum lipoproteins and ubiquinone-10-levels in patients with familial hypercholesterolemia. *N Engl J Med*. 1981;**305**:478-82.

96. **Bilheimer DW, Grundy SM, Brown MS, Goldstein JL.** Mevinolin and colestipol stimulate receptor-mediated clearance of low-density lipoprotein from plasma in familial hypercholesterolemia heterozygotes. *Proc Natl Acad Sci USA*. 1983;**80**:4124-8.

97. **Illingworth DR.** Mevinolin plus colestipol in therapy for severe heterozygous familial hypercholesterolemia. *Ann Intern Med*. 1984;**101**:598-604.

98. **Mabuchi H, Sakai T, Sakai Y, et al.** Reduction of serum cholesterol in heterozygous patients with familial hypercholesterolemia: additive effects of compactin and cholestyramine. *N Engl J Med*. 1983;**308**:609-13.

99. **Lovastatin Study Group II.** Therapeutic response to lovastatin (mevinolin) in nonfamilial hypercholesterolemia: a multicenter study. *JAMA.* 1986;**256**:2829-34.
100. **Vega GL, Grundy SM.** Treatment of primary moderate hypercholesterolemia with lovastatin (mevinolin) and colestipol. *JAMA.* 1987;**257**:33-8.
101. **Tobert JA.** New developments in lipid-lowering therapy: the role of inhibitors of hydroxymethylglutaryl-coenzyme A reductase. *Circulation.* 1987;**76**:534-9.
102. **Lovastatin Study Group II.** A multicenter comparison of lovastatin and cholestyramine therapy for severe primary hypercholesterolemia. *JAMA.* 1988;**260**:359-66.
103. **Knopp RH, Brown WV, Dujovne CA, et al.** Effect of fenofibrate on plasma lipoproteins in hypercholesterolemia and combined hyperlipidemia. *Am J Med.* 1987;**83**(suppl 5B):50-9.
104. **Breslow L, Somers AR.** The lifetime health-monitoring program: a practical approach to preventive medicine. *N Engl J Med.* 1977;**296**:601-8.
105. **Fielding JE.** Preventive services for the well population. In: The Institute of Medicine of the National Academy of Sciences. *Healthy People: The Surgeon General's Report on Health Promotion and Disease Prevention. Background Papers.* Washington, DC: U.S. Government Printing Office DHEW (PHS) Pub. No. 70-55071A;**1979**:277-304.
106. **Canadian Task Force on the Periodic Health Examination.** The periodic health examination. *Can Med Assoc J.* 1979;**121**:1194-254.
107. **Frame PS.** A critical review of adult health maintenance. Part 1: Prevention of atherosclerotic diseases. *J Fam Pract.* 1986;**22**:341-6.

Screening for Diabetes Mellitus

DANIEL E. SINGER, MD; JEFFREY H. SAMET, MD;
CHRISTOPHER M. COLEY, MD; and
DAVID M. NATHAN, MD

We have analyzed the clinical and epidemiologic studies bearing on screening for type I, type II, and gestational diabetes. We stress that screening is justified only when it results in net therapeutic benefit; increased detection of disease is an insufficient justification. From this perspective, our analyses suggest that screening for gestational diabetes is reasonable, whereas screening for type I or type II diabetes is not. Such recommendations necessarily depend on the current body of evidence. We indicate what future findings would alter our conclusions.

The Diagnosis of Diabetes

Diabetes mellitus is a common heterogeneous group of disorders characterized by elevated plasma glucose concentrations resulting from insufficient insulin or insulin resistance. In developed societies diabetes can be usefully subdivided into the following categories (1): *Insulin-dependent,* or *type I diabetes,* appears to result from immunologically mediated destruction of the insulin-secreting islet cells producing absolute insulin deficiency (2, 3). The resulting extreme abnormalities in glucose metabolism allow clear-cut diagnosis. *Non-insulin dependent,* or *type II diabetes,* is associated with insulin resistance and relative insulin deficiency (3). Obesity is prominent in most patients. Glucose abnormalities may be mild, and thereby pose a problem in diagnosis. Type II diabetes accounts for 90% of diabetes prevalence. *Gestational diabetes* is a disorder of carbohydrate metabolism with onset or first recognition during pregnancy (1). It results from the distinctive hormonal environment and metabolic demands of pregnancy (4). The diabetes usually remits after parturition. However, it is a risk factor for development of nongestational diabetes (usually type II) in succeeding decades *(see below). Secondary diabetes* occurs rarely. Some adults with diabetes have identifi-

▶ This chapter was originally published in *Annals of Internal Medicine.* 1988;**109**:639-49.

able underlying illnesses producing the diabetes, fc. example, chronic pancreatitis, hemochromatosis, or acromegaly (1). In these patients the diabetes is considered secondary.

Disordered glucose metabolism is common to all forms of diabetes, and the resultant hyperglycemia the source of many distinctive symptoms in diabetic patients. In addition to metabolic abnormalities, diabetes is also characterized by a greatly increased risk for subsequent vascular and neuropathic disease. Epidemiologic studies have focused primarily on vascular lesions. Retinopathy and nephropathy are the results of microvascular disease highly specific for diabetes mellitus. The risk for such lesions is strongly dependent on the duration of diabetes and perhaps dependent on the level of hyperglycemia (5-8). Microvascular lesions are found in patients with all nongestational forms of diabetes and across many ethnic groups (9). Macrovascular disease manifested as coronary, peripheral vascular, or cerebrovascular disease is also significantly associated with diabetes, but is a much less specific outcome of diabetes than microvascular disease. Macrovascular disease is not clearly related to duration of diabetes or severity of hyperglycemia, and is not frequently found among diabetic patients from societies with low rates of atherosclerosis (10, 11).

Persistent controversy surrounds the question of what extent the achievement of near-normal glucose levels will alter the development or progression of microvascular and neuropathic complications of diabetes mellitus (12-18). The one condition where strong evidence linking "tight" glucose control and improved (fetal and neonatal) outcome has emerged is in pregnant women with type I diabetes (19-24). Such pregnancies have historically been associated with substantial rates of intrauterine and neonatal mortality, macrosomia, congenital malformation, and postpartum metabolic derangements in the infant (25, 26). With the exception of fetal malformations (27, 28), these complications have been clearly reduced by maintaining strict glycemic control after pregnancy is discovered.

A relatively mild form of diabetes may develop during pregnancy and disappear after delivery. Such gestational diabetes generally develops in the third trimester. Early experience (29, 30) with gestational diabetes suggested infant perinatal mortality rates of 7% to 10%. Today, this risk approaches that for nondiabetic patients (2%) (31, 32). Macrosomia and neonatal complications in patients with gestational diabetes are reported (32-36) to occur at substantially higher rates than for nondiabetic patients. As with pregnant patients with type I diabetes, tight control of maternal glycemia has been associated with improved perinatal outcome (35, 37, 38). However, with gestational diabetes it is less certain that glucose control itself provides benefits beyond those provided by the other features of modern obstetrical management.

Prevention and amelioration of the vascular and neuropathic sequelae of diabetes mellitus in nonpregnant adults and the reduction of adverse effects on pregnancy outcome are the primary motivations for screening and early intervention in asymptomatic persons.

Criteria for Diagnosing Diabetes Mellitus

A diagnosis of diabetes should identify persons with abnormal glucose levels and accurately convey an increased risk for developing vascular complications. For many diabetic patients treated in clinical practice the diagnosis is straightforward, characterized by typical symptoms of hyperglycemia (for example, polyuria and polydipsia) and clearly abnormal glucose levels (fasting plasma glucose, greater than 140 mg/dL; or any plasma glucose, greater than 200 mg/dL) (39). However, population surveys have shown many persons with abnormal glucose metabolism who are undiagnosed and often asymptomatic (40, 41). These persons are the proper focus of screening programs. For this group the diagnosis depends on the oral glucose tolerance test, a nonphysiologic challenge to insulin secretion and tissue responsiveness. In recent years consensus standards have emerged for both the administration and the interpretation of the oral glucose tolerance test. The most important feature of these new standards is the considerably higher glycemic thresholds used for diagnosis. The epidemiologic basis for these new standards includes the following. First, most persons with mild abnormalities of glucose tolerance do not progress to frank diabetes (42-45). Second, the risk for developing the specific microvascular lesions of diabetes appear to be limited to patients with marked hyperglycemia (fasting plasma glucose, greater than 140 mg/dL, or 2-hour postglucose plasma glucose, greater than 200 mg/dL) (46-49). Third, in ethnic groups where diabetes is particularly prevalent, the Pimas (50) and Nauruans (51), population blood glucose distributions are bimodal with the optimal separation of diabetic and nondiabetic persons occurring at relatively high glucose levels, that is, a 2-hour plasma glucose level of greater than 200 mg/dL. Finally, earlier standards using lower glycemic thresholds resulted in large proportions of older persons being classified as asymptomatic diabetic patients (52), an unappealing nosologic consequence of the progressive glucose intolerance of aging.

The National Diabetes Data Group standards are presented in Appendix 1 (1). They constitute the current gold standard for the diagnosis of diabetes in the United States. The World Health Organization (WHO) standards (39), which are similar, are also widely cited. The National Diabetes Data Group standards reserve the diagnosis of diabetes for persons with considerable elevations in glucose levels. They also identify an intermediate category of impaired glucose tolerance where the risk for deterioration into frank diabetes is heightened but not absolute. In earlier classifications impaired glucose tolerance would have been considered "chemical" diabetes.

The diagnosis of gestational diabetes mellitus is particularly important from the perspective of screening for disease. The criteria for the diagnosis of gestational diabetes mellitus have been kept separate from criteria for nonpregnant diabetes. These criteria essentially perpetuate the standards of O'Sullivan and Mahan (53) that were developed more than 20 years ago. These investigators administered 100-g oral glucose tolerance tests to pregnant women not known to be diabetic, and identified cut-offs greater than two standard deviations above the mean. In a follow-up (53) of a separate set of pregnant women, patients above the threshold levels of blood glucose had a 22% risk for developing nonpregnant diabetes during the study period (up to 8 years), compared with a 4.3% risk for patients below the cut-off point. However, the glucose threshold criteria for subsequent nonpregnant diabetes used in these studies were considerably lower than current National Diabetes Data Group standards. Indeed it appears from later publications (54) that only about 10% of the cohort of gestational diabetic patients developed nonpregnant diabetes by the National Diabetes Data Group criteria. Currently the standards for gestational diabetes all primarily defended as indicating heightened risk for fetal and neonatal complications, thereby shifting the clinical importance of the diagnosis from maternal to fetal health.

Rationale for Screening

The primary purpose of screening programs is to identify persons with disease in asymptomatic populations

Table 1. *Recommendations for Screening for Diabetes Mellitus*

GESTATIONAL

Rationale: Has been associated with pregnancy loss and complications. Glycemic control appears to improve outcome. Gestational diabetes may be silent.

Recommendation: Screening may be beneficial and not likely to incur much risk or cost. Screening of all pregnant women seems reasonable. The screening test should be a 50-g glucose load given between weeks 24 and 28. Patients with plasma glucose values > 140 mg/dL at 1 h should have a full oral glucose tolerance test.

PREGESTATIONAL (women planning pregnancy)

Rationale: Pregnant diabetic patients face substantial risks for pregnancy loss and other complications. Careful glycemic control and obstetric management reduces risks.

Recommendation: "Silent" diabetes in women of childbearing age is probably rare. Pregnancy risk for such women and benefits of early therapy are not known. Screening of women at heightened risk for diabetes may be reasonable, but there is little evidence bearing on this issue.

TYPE I

Rationale: Early therapy may forestall complications. Immunosuppressive therapy may prevent further beta-cell destruction.

Recommendation: Prevalence of type I diabetes detectable by screening is low. Benefits of early hypoglycemic therapy are unknown. Immunosuppressive strategies are still experimental. Screening is not currently recommended.

TYPE II

Rationale: The prevalence of undiagnosed impaired glucose tolerance or type II diabetes is high. Early intervention might prevent deterioration of impaired glucose tolerance to frank diabetes, or improve glycemic control among diabetic patients and thereby prevent vascular and neurologic complications. Identification of undiagnosed diabetes might lead to early diagnosis of vision-threatening retinopathy and timely laser therapy.

Recommendation: Benefits of early diagnosis and therapy in preventing worsening glucose tolerance or diabetic complications have not been shown. Vision-threatening retinopathy rarely precedes the diagnosis of diabetes. Screening for type II diabetes is not recommended. For selected obese persons, screening for impaired glucose tolerance or diabetes may better motivate weight loss, which may prevent progression of glucose intolerance.

(Table 1). Screening makes sense only when treatment begun in the presymptomatic phase of disease is more effective than treatment begun after symptoms lead a person to seek medical care. However, even when this condition is satisfied screening may not be appropriate. Inaccurate, dangerous, or expensive screening tests and difficult treatment regimens may make screening programs more costly in health and dollar terms than they are worth (55-61). In recent decades, enthusiasm for screening for diabetes increased with the belief that many diabetic persons were undiagnosed and therefore untreated, but then diminished with disappointment over the objective benefits of early intervention (62, 63). Our analysis begins with gestational diabetes where the rationale for screening is strongest.

Screening for Gestational Diabetes Mellitus

Gestational diabetes is estimated to occur in 3% of pregnancies. There is considerable variation in its frequency across different study populations. Most patients are asymptomatic (64-66). Gestational diabetes has been associated with increased perinatal mortality; increased rates of macrosomia, serious birth trauma, and cesarian section; and neonatal hyperbilirubinemia, hypocalcemia, and hypoglycemia (36, 37). Without screening, gestational diabetes mellitus may remain undetected. As a result of these considerations the Second International Workshop-Conference on Gestational Diabetes Mellitus recommended that "all pregnant women should be screened for glucose intolerance . . . by glucose measurement in blood" (67). The conference recommended that 50 g of glucose be given orally, without regard to the time of the last meal or the time of day, between 24 and 28 weeks of gestation (the onset of the period of greatest glucose intolerance). A 1-hour plasma glucose level of 140 mg/dL would be the threshold for further evaluation with the definitive diagnostic test, the oral glucose tolerance test (53). Measurement of glycated hemoglobin (HbA1$_c$) was not recommended as a screening modality because of its inadequate sensitivity for the mild derangements in glycemia typical of gestational diabetes (68). We will consider the evidence bearing on these recommendations, and will incorporate the conference screening test with its threshold plasma glucose of 140 mg/dL in our cost-effectiveness analysis.

Screening programs can be assessed in terms of the efficiency and ease of case identification, and the net therapeutic benefit for screening-identified cases. The conference's proposed gestational diabetes screening test (1 hour after a 50-g glucose assay) is not expensive or greatly inconvenient to the patient. It appears to have a sensitivity of 83% and a specificity of 87% (69, 70) using the O'Sullivan and Mahan (53) criteria as the gold standard. If we assume a prevalence of gestational diabetes of 3% in unselected pregnant populations, then for each 10 000 women tested we can anticipate 249 true cases identified along with 1261 false-positive and 51 false-negative results.

There are four possible adverse effects of screening in general: the medical complications of the screening test; the false reassurance of a false-negative test result; the psychological stress of a false-positive test result; and the medical complications of the intervention in screen-detected cases. Here the screening test (post-glucose phlebotomy) is trivial. Patients with false-negative test results probably do no worse than if they had not been screened. The psychological trauma of false-positive results is not easily quantitated but should be minimized by rapid definitive classification by full glucose tolerance testing. The intervention might lead to important toxic sequelae such as hypoglycemia, but this risk must be small because diet is the primary therapy for gestational diabetes. Moreover, studies of pregnant type I diabetic patients, where insulin use is universal, have not strongly linked maternal hypoglycemic reactions with adverse effects on the child (71). The diagnosis of gestational diabetes may, by itself, lead to unnecessary monitoring and operative deliveries. This effect may be important, but the potential induced costs and risks are currently unmeasured.

The prevalance of asymptomatic gestational diabetes and the relative ease of its detection would favor screening. But the issue can only be settled by clear evidence for the efficacy of therapy for screen-detected cases. The first trial with concurrent controls was done by O'Sullivan and associates (72) in Boston between 1954 and 1960. Treatment of 615 women with gestational diabetes was alternated between insulin (fixed dose of 10 units NPH) and diet, or treatment with ordinary antenatal care. There was a modest improvement in glycemic control (mean fasting blood glucose, 69.1 mg/dL in the insulin group compared with 74.3 mg/dL in the "ordinary" care group), and a significant reduction in macrosomia (4.3% compared with 13.1%, respectively), but no significant difference in neonatal mortality (4.3% in patients treated with insulin compared with 4.9% in controls).

In this study and other studies of gestational diabetes, macrosomia serves as an index of morbidity. Macrosomia, generally defined as a birth weight exceeding 4100 g, is a frequent consequence of maternal hyperglycemia, but occurs in nondiabetic pregnant patients as well (72). Macrosomia is not a morbid condition, but it is associated with an increased risk for birth trauma, including skull and clavicular fracture, shoulder dystocia, and peripheral nerve injury. Gabbe and colleagues (73) reported that 5 of 49 macrosomic infants of mothers with gestational diabetes had birth trauma, a rate about four times higher than nonmacrosomic infants of mothers with gestational diabetes. Cyr and coworkers (74) estimate that 6% of babies over 4500 g have birth trauma. Macrosomia may lead to cesarian section. It is also linked to subsequent obesity in the child (75).

In the second experimental trial of therapy for gestational diabetes, Coustan and Lewis (76) studied the effect of insulin and diet, compared with diet alone, compared with no therapy in 72 gestational diabetic women. The initial 20 patients in this study were assigned therapy based on their gestational age (35 weeks or less, insulin and diet; more than 35 weeks, no therapy). The remaining 52 patients were randomly assigned to one of the three treatment groups. The study analysis was based on all 72 patients. The difference in glycemic control was statistically significant (fasting blood sugar, 86.8 mg/dL, in patients treated with insulin compared with 98.9 mg/dL in untreated controls $[P < 0.01]$ and 94.7 mg/dL in patients treated with diet $[P < 0.05]$). A significant reduction in macrosomia (defined here as birth weight greater than 3.86 kg [8.5 pounds] was noted in patients treated with insulin compared with untreated patients (7% and 50%, respectively $[P < 0.005]$). There was 36% macrosomia in patients treated with diet alone. No significant difference in perinatal mortality, cesarian section rate, or forceps delivery rate was found among the three groups. There was one case of shoulder dystocia with Erb palsy in an untreated patient, and none in patients treated with diet or insulin.

These two controlled clinical trials provide useful estimates of the effect of hypoglycemic therapy in cases of gestational diabetes detected by screening. They do not address the benefit of screening itself. It is possible that early detection led to more effective care independent of hypoglycemic therapy, that is, the outcome in the control patients was better than if their gestational diabetes had not been discovered.

Other nonexperimental analyses have offered more dramatic evidence that meticulous regulation of glycemia in patients with gestational diabetes favorably influences neonatal outcome. However, each of the supporting studies is seriously weakened by one or more design limitations. These limitations include the mixing of gestational and pregnant type I diabetic patients, use of historical controls in the face of changes in general obstetrical care over the same period, and use of a patient's previous pregnancy outcome as the control for the studied pregnancy. This last practice may introduce substantial bias if patients were selected on the basis of a preceding problem pregnancy. Such selection effects are common since previous problem pregnancy has been a criterion for screening for gestational diabetes, or for referral to research-oriented clinics. Patients with a previous problem pregnancy would be expected to have a better outcome with a subsequent pregnancy regardless of medical management (such "regression to the mean" issues are discussed in reference 77). A brief review of frequently cited observational studies (73, 78-82) is provided in Appendix 2.

On the basis of these past investigations, it is difficult to determine the unbiased magnitude of improvement in the outcome of pregnancy in patients with gestational diabetes, particularly rates of perinatal death, and whether such improvement was the result of actions specific for gestational diabetes or because of significant advances in general obstetric management. Despite these considerable uncertainties, strong support (67, 83, 84) for screening for gestational diabetes exists. This support is understandable given the importance of minimizing fetal morbidity and mortality, the numerous studies reporting better outcome in patients with gestational diabetes identified through screening, and the relatively short period of therapy (the remaining 15 weeks of pregnancy). As currently recommended, insulin is reserved for the relatively rare patient for whom diet alone does not produce euglycemia (38). This method minimizes the inconvenience and potential morbidity of treatment. The assumption is that the benefits of therapy are preserved (84).

Cost-Effectiveness of Screening for Gestational Diabetes

Approaches for screening for gestational diabetes have varied. Early screening strategies (85) focused only on high-risk groups, defined by obesity, glucosuria, previous macrosomic infants, and other clinical features. Research (85) has since shown that such risk factors have little discriminating ability. Other proposed strategies have incorporated an age threshold for screening because gestational diabetes disproportionately affects the older pregnant population.

We will outline the cost-effectiveness implications of

several screening strategies. In all cases screening is done once between weeks 24 and 28 of pregnancy. We assume that identified cases would receive therapy to maintain glycemic control within the recent American Diabetes Association guidelines (fasting plasma glucose, less than 105 mg/dL, or 2-hour postprandial plasma glucose, less than 120 mg/dL) (67, 83). These levels would be achieved by nutritional counseling (67, 84) in most patients, with only a small fraction (10% to 15%) requiring insulin (38). Glycemic control would be monitored by frequent fasting and postprandial glucose tests. The detailed component assumptions of our cost-effectiveness analysis are presented in Appendix 3. The results of this analysis are shown in Table 2. Four different strategies of screening for gestational diabetes mellitus are examined on a hypothetical cohort of 10 000 pregnant women: First, screen all pregnant women with the definitive oral glucose tolerance test. Second, screen all pregnant women with the 1-hour plasma glucose after 50-g glucose load (the "glucose screening test"), and test patients with positive results further with the glucose tolerance test. Third, screen with the glucose screening test only in women over 25 years old. Fourth, screen with the glucose screening test only in women with positive risk factors.

Screening all pregnant women with full oral glucose tolerance tests (Table 2; strategy 1) will identify all 300 expected cases of gestational diabetes in the cohort of 10 000 pregnant women with no false-positive results. This approach is the most expensive but has the greatest total benefit. The strategies using an initial glucose screening test (Table 2; strategies 2, 3, and 4) have a lower cost per case detected because a cheaper screening test is substituted for the full glucose tolerance test in most women, and the screening test identifies 83% of cases with a low level of false-positive results. The true difference in costs between strategies using the initial full glucose tolerance test compared with an initial screening test is probably greater than we have estimated because full glucose tolerance tests often have to be repeated for technical reasons, for example, lack of proper fasting. Only 17% of cases are missed using an initial glucose screening test, resulting in a very small expected difference in pregnancy outcome, at a substantial savings with reduced patient inconvenience. Screening on the basis of risk factors is not useful because such risk factors are poor discriminators. By contrast, restricting screening to women over 25 years old would add efficiency with a modest reduction in total cases identified.

Table 2. *Screening for Gestational Diabetes: Cost-Effectiveness of Four Screening Strategies*

Strategy	Effectiveness per 10 000 Women, *n*			
	Cases Detected	Cases Missed (%)	Estimated Neonatal Deaths Prevented* (range)	Estimated Macrosomic Infants Prevented*
Screen all patients with oral glucose tolerance test	300	0 (0)	0 (0-77)	26
Screen all patients with glucose screening test;*§ glucose tolerance test for all patients with positive results	249	51 (17)	0 (0-64)	22
Screen all patients over 25 with glucose screening test; glucose tolerance test for all positives	212	88 (29)	0 (0-54)	19
Screen all patients with risk factors with glucose screening test; glucose tolerance test for all positives	119	181 (60)	0 (0-31)	10

* Estimate of effect found in controlled trial (72).
† Includes $300 per case treated.

We feel the most reasonable approach is to screen all pregnant women with an initial glucose screening test followed by full glucose tolerance testing in women with positive results. By our calculations this method would add an average cost of 17 dollars per pregnant woman ($9.62 for screening; the remainder for treatment), and would reduce the risk for macrosomia in each woman by 2.2 in 1000 and the risk for associated birth trauma by about 2 in 10 000. Such small estimates for expected efficacy are only part of the motivation for screening. The potential for reducing neonatal deaths, dramatically but likely unreliably estimated in the cited observational studies, influences the decision in favor of screening.

Using the initial glucose screening test in all pregnant women is the strategy supported by the Second International Workshop-Conference on Gestational Diabetes Mellitus (67) and by the American Diabetes

Table 2. *(Continued)*

Estimate of Costs, $			
Screening 10 000 Pregnant Women	Per Case Detected	Per Neonatal Death Prevented*† (*range*)	Per Macrosomic Infant Prevented*†
240 000	800	NM‡ (≥ 4286)	12 692
96 240	387	NM‡ (≥ 2671)	7770
49 896	235	NM‡ (≥ 2102)	5973
44 352	373	NM‡ (≥ 2582)	8005

‡ Not meaningful (denominator is zero).
§ Glucose screening test: 50-g oral glucose load followed by 1-hour plasma glucose determination.

Association (83). The strategy of limiting screening to older pregnant women is also reasonable, and lowers the cost of the program to $11 per pregnant woman while reducing macrosomia by 1.9 per 1000. The American College of Obstetrics and Gynecology recently recommended (86) screening all pregnant women over age 30 as well as any woman with glucosuria, hypertension, or a risk factor for gestational diabetes. Our recommendation differs from the position of the Canadian Task Force on the Periodic Health Examination (58). The Canadian Task Force recommended screening via risk factors for gestational diabetes and repeated urine glucose testing, both inadequately sensitive tests for gestational diabetes (30, 69, 85). Such differences in recommendations should not spark great controversy. It should be clear that by any strategy, screening for gestational diabetes is a low cost intervention with low expected benefit.

There are substantial uncertainties in our analysis. This field would be advanced by better and more current information about the efficacy of glucose control and other aspects of modern obstetric care in gestational diabetes. Large prospective cohort studies with uniform data collection would be helpful if randomized trials are unworkable. Further issues that might be explored include: the optimal time during gestation for screening (87); the optimal screening test—2-hours post-load plasma glucose compared with the recommended 1-hour test (88); fingerstick meter compared with laboratory venous measurements (89, 90); the true costs induced by a diagnosis of gestational diabetes ("extra" ultrasound tests, operative deliveries); and the value of screening for occult type II diabetes in high-risk (for example, both parents diabetic) women planning pregnancy or very early in their pregnancy (67, 91) (Tables 1 and 2).

Screening for Non-Insulin Dependent Diabetes Mellitus

Non-insulin dependent (type II) diabetes mellitus is a common chronic illness with a substantial frequency of severe vascular and neuropathic complications (92). Approximately 3% of the United States population have this disease; the rate is strongly dependent on age (40, 41). Lifetime rates of renal failure (93) and blindness (94) are many times that of nondiabetic patients. Cardiovascular disease manifested as coronary artery disease or congestive heart failure is two to three times commoner than that for nondiabetic patients (95, 96). The natural history of this disease often includes an asymptomatic initial phase that may persist for years. The National Health and Nutrition Examination Survey estimated that the national prevalence of undiagnosed non-insulin dependent diabetes mellitus was about the same as that for diagnosed non-insulin dependent diabetes mellitus (40, 41). Earlier studies (97) provided lower estimates for the prevalence of undiagnosed diabetes (1%). Screening fasting or post-load plasma glucose and now hemoglobin $A1_C$ (98, 99), and follow-up full glucose tolerance testing can be done relatively easily on a large scale. Such considerations prompted screening programs in the 1960s and 1970s (62, 100-103). Many of these programs were primarily research-oriented, studying the operating characteristics of screening tests, the prevalence of screen-detected disease, and the association of glucose intolerance with concurrent or future vascular disease. For the most part, these programs limited their assessment of the value of screening to the efficiency of disease detection. A notable exception was the work of Genuth and colleagues (62) of Cleveland's mass diabetes screening program. These authors observed that disease detection was merely the first step toward the therapeutic effect of screening, and that continued medical follow-up of screen-detected cases and demonstration of efficacy of treatment were needed for screening to be beneficial. Their work generally questioned the value of mass screening, highlighting problems with medical follow-up and patient compliance as well as the negative effect of misdiagnosis. Several recent reviews (57, 58) of screening policy have concluded that screening for diabetes in the non-pregnant adult is not justified.

Once again, the crux of the issue is whether treatment in the asymptomatic phase yields a clinical outcome superior to treatment first begun after symptoms lead to a diagnosis. If early treatment is beneficial, then the pragmatic issues of efficient detection of cases and patient compliance become important. The question of therapeutic efficacy involves at least two issues. First, is there evidence that therapy can ameliorate or prevent chronic complications? Second, is therapy begun in the asymptomatic phase more effective than therapy begun after symptomatic discovery of diabetes?

Although there are observational data linking diabetic microvascular complications to hyperglycemia (5-8, 47, 48), there is little evidence that therapy can forestall such complications. Of course, techniques have only recently become available to effect and monitor near-normal blood glucose control. Currently there is a great deal of investigation of the effect of modern therapeutic approaches on vascular complications, particularly in type I diabetes (16), but the issue is not settled (104). For type II diabetes, the largest controlled clinical trial to date, the University Group Diabetes Program study (105), showed no benefit of improved glycemic control. Despite a mean fasting glucose level of 122 mg/dL in patients randomly assigned to the variable-dose insulin regimen compared with 165 mg/dL in all other treatment groups (including the notorious tolbutamide group), no corresponding significant decreases in retinopathy or cardiovascular mortality or morbidity were found. No recent work clearly contradicts these findings. Although treatment begun in the presymptomatic phase might be more effective, the evidence to substantiate such a view is meager.

The reader should appreciate the nature of the epidemiologic argument. There is evidence linking hyperglycemia and microvascular complications, but there is little evidence that standard diabetic therapy prevents such complications. There is evidence that aggressive hypoglycemic therapy can acutely improve some of the defects in insulin physiology found in type II diabetes (106), but the long-term impact of such measures is unknown. Tighter glycemic control might be effective, but the proof is pending. The data are simply not sufficient to justify population screening to improve glycemic control among undetected diabetics.

Disease detection would be more efficient if the search were restricted to high-risk populations. Such populations would include first-degree relatives of type II diabetic patients, obese persons, women who formerly had gestational diabetes (1), and ethnic groups with a particularly high prevalence of diabetes, including Mexican-Americans (107) and Pima Indians (50). However, the efficiency of disease detection is a moot issue so long as the net therapeutic benefit is unproved.

We should consider other possible beneficial effects of screening for type II diabetes. First, persons who have not sought medical care may have symptoms due to hyperglycemia, and these symptoms may be explained and successfully treated as a result of a screening program. This finding has been reported in previous screening programs (97). However, such undiagnosed symptomatic persons are not the usual focus of screening (asymptomatic persons are). The same benefit might accrue from other potentially less costly programs, for example, community education, as from screening.

Second, persons with diabetes or impaired glucose tolerance are at heightened risk for atherosclerotic disease to a large extent because of other risk factors that are associated with diabetes mellitus (95, 108). Such persons identified by a screening program might benefit greatly by reduction in concurrent risk factors such as obesity, hypertension, elevated serum cholesterol, and smoking even if the risk from diabetes itself is immutable. But this fact seems more of an argument for screening for the associated risk factors rather than for diabetes itself.

Third, persons with impaired glucose tolerance identified by a screening program might be treated so as to prevent progression to frank diabetes. Trials of hypoglycemic therapy for impaired glucose tolerance have generally been disappointing (109, 110), although one trial (111) provided suggestive positive findings. Degree of obesity is strongly associated with progression from impaired glucose tolerance to frank diabetes (112-114), and weight loss in the established type II obese diabetic patient can greatly improve glycemia (115). Weight loss in obese patients with impaired glucose tolerance certainly seems prudent. Although broad population screening for diabetes may provide little net health benefit, screening in targeted populations, especially obese persons, might be more valuable. More effective weight-loss techniques would stimulate study of such screening programs. Forestalling progression of impaired glucose tolerance is an important issue and merits large-scale investigation.

Finally, there is an established preventative therapy for one diabetic complication. Progression of diabetic retinopathy can be slowed by laser therapy (116). Screening could uncover diabetic patients whose vision might be saved. However, several studies have shown that vision-threatening retinopathy rarely develops early in type II diabetes (117, 118). Severe retinopathy is an unusual presentation of diabetes. Screening for diabetic retinopathy is most efficient when done on populations of known diabetic patients. (This conclusion assumes a "usual" level of medical care. Among groups of patients with reduced access to care, the prevalence of advanced retinopathy would be greater, the value of screening increased [119].)

The Canadian Task Force on the Periodic Health Examination reached similar conclusions, stating that because treatment of asymptomatic persons has not been shown to be effective in ameliorating complications there was "fair evidence" to recommend that screening for type II diabetes not be routinely done by physicians (58).

Screening for Insulin-Dependent Diabetes Mellitus

Screening for insulin-dependent diabetes mellitus (type I) has generally not been considered, much less recommended, by policy studies (57, 58). The disease is rarer than type II diabetes (1.6 cases of type I diabetes per 1000 school-age children) (120) and seems to have a briefer presymptomatic phase. Recent prospective studies (121, 122) have shown a longer presymptomatic phase than previously estimated. Nevertheless, the prevalence of type I diabetes detectable by screening is small. The benefit of early presymptomatic therapy with insulin in preventing later complications is not shown or widely anticipated. Unlike type II diabetes, type I diabetes often presents with a life-threatening metabolic disorder, for example, ketoacidosis. Early diagnosis and therapy might prevent this initial episode of ketoacidosis. This theoretical benefit of screening is made unlikely by the low probability of detecting a patient at such a point in the illness. As such, standard glycemic screening for type I diabetes is not justified.

Recent insight into the immunopathologic basis of type I diabetes has raised the possibility of screening for immunologic markers and abnormal glucose metabolism to identify persons at high risk for type I diabetes. These patients might have their diabetes prevented by immunosuppressive therapy (2). These approaches are still too new to fall within the scope of this paper, but we recognize their potential for completely changing our notion of screening for type I diabetes.

References

1. **National Diabetes Data Group.** Classification and diagnosis of diabetes mellitus and other categories of glucose intolerance. *Diabetes.* 1979;**28**:1039-57.
2. **Eisenbarth GS.** Type I diabetes mellitus: a chronic autoimmune disease. *N Engl J Med.* 1986;**314**:1360-8.
3. **Fajans SS, Cloutier MC, Gorother RL.** Clinical and etiologic heterogeneity of idiopathic diabetes mellitus. *Diabetes.* 1978;**27**:1112-25.
4. **Freinkel N, Metzger BE, Potter JM.** Pregnancy in diabetes. In: **Ellenberg M, Rifkin H,** eds. *Diabetes Mellitus: Theory and Practice.* 3rd edition. New Hyde Park, New York: Medical Examination Publishing Company; 1983:689-714.
5. **Burditt AGF, Caird FI, Draper GJ.** The natural history of diabetic retinopathy. *Q J Med.* 1968;**37**:303-17.
6. **Nathan DM, Singer DE, Godine JE, Harrington CH, Perlmuter LC.** Retinopathy in older type II diabetics: association with glucose control. *Diabetes.* 1986;**35**:797-801.
7. **Davidson MB.** The case for control in diabetes mellitus. *West J Med.* 1978;**129**:193-200.
8. **West KM, Erdreich LJ, Stober JA.** A detailed study of risk factors for retinopathy and nephropathy in diabetes. *Diabetes.* 1980;**29**:501-8.
9. **West KM.** *Epidemiology of Diabetes and its Vascular Complications.* New York:Elsevier North-Holland;1978:351-402.
10. **International Collaboration Group.** Joint Discussion. *J Chronic Dis.* 1979;**32**:829-37.
11. **Prosnitz LR, Mandell GL.** Diabetes mellitus among Navajo and Hopi Indians: the lack of vascular complications. *Am J Med Sci.* 1967;**253**:700-5.
12. **Pirart J.** Diabetes mellitus and its degenerative complications: a prospective study of 4400 patients observed between 1947 and 1973. *Diabetes Care.* 1978;**1**:168-88.
13. **The Kroc Collaborative Study Group.** Blood glucose control and the evaluation of diabetic retinopathy and albuminuria: a preliminary multi-center trial. *New Engl J Med.* 1984;**311**:365-72.
14. **Lauritzen T, Frost-Larsen K, Larsen HW, Deckert T.** Effect of 1 year of near-normal blood glucose levels on retinopathy in insulin-dependent diabetics. *Lancet.* 1983;**1**:200-4.

15. **Raskin P, Rosenstock J.** Blood glucose control and diabetic complications. *Ann Intern Med.* 1986;**105**:254-63.
16. **The DCCT Research Group.** Diabetes Control and Complications Trial (DCCT): results of feasibility study. *Diabetes Care.* 1987;**10**:1-19.
17. **Knatterud GL, Klimt CR, Levin ME, Jacobson ME, Goldner MG.** Effects of hypoglycemic agents on vascular complications in patients with adult onset diabetes. VII. Mortality and selected nonfatal events with insulin treatment. *JAMA.* 1978;**240**:37-42.
18. **Kilo C, Williamson JR, Choi SC, Miller JP.** Refuting the UGDP conclusion that insulin treatment does not prevent vascular complications in diabetes. *Adv Exp Med Biol.* 1979;**119**:307-11.
19. **Freinkel N, Dooley SL, Metzger BE.** Care of the pregnant woman with insulin-dependent diabetes mellitus. *New Engl J Med.* 1985;**313**:96-101.
20. **Jovanovic L, Peterson CM.** Management of the pregnant, insulin-dependent diabetic woman. *Diabetes Care.* 1980;**3**:63-8.
21. **Gabbe SG.** Management of diabetes mellitus in pregnancy. *Amer J Obstet Gynecol.* 1985;**153**:824-8.
22. **Coustan D, Berkowitz R, Hobbins JC.** Tight metabolic control of overt diabetes in pregnancy. *Am J Med.* 1980;**68**:845-52.
23. **Schade DS, Santiago JU, Skyler JS, Rizza RA.** *Intensive Insulin Therapy.* New York:Medical Examination Publishing Company; 1983;241-63.
24. **Jovanovic L, Druzin M, Peterson CM.** Effect of euglycemia on the outcome of pregnancy in insulin-dependent diabetic women as compared with normal control subjects. *Am J Med.* 1981;**71**:921-27.
25. **Freinkel N.** Banting Lecture 1980: of pregnancy and progeny. *Diabetes.* 1980;**29**:1023-35.
26. **Miller E, Hare JW, Cloherty JP, et al.** Elevated maternal hemoglobin A1c in early pregnancy and major congenital anomalies in infants of diabetic mothers. *New Engl J Med.* 1981;**304**:1331-4.
27. **Fuhrmann K, Reiher H, Semmler K, Fischer F, Fischer M, Glöckner E.** Prevention of congenital malformation in infants of insulin-dependent mothers. *Diabetes Care.* 1983;**6**:219-23.
28. **Mills JL, Knopp RH, Simpson JL, et al.** Lack of relation of increased malformation rates in infants of diabetic mothers to glycemic control during organogenesis. *N Engl J Med.* 1988;**318**:671-6.
29. **O'Sullivan JB, Charles D, Mahan CM, Dandrow RV.** Gestational diabetes and perinatal mortality rate. *Am J Obstet Gynecol.* 1973;**116**:901-4.
30. **Pettitt DJ, Knowler WC, Baird HR, Bennett PH.** Gestational diabetes: infant and maternal complications of pregnancy in relation to third-trimester glucose tolerance in the Pima Indians. *Diabetes Care.* 1980;**3**:458-64.
31. **Gabbe SG.** Effects of identifying a high risk population. *Diabetes Care.* 1980;**3**:486-8.
32. **Gabbe SG.** Application of scientific rationale in the management of the pregnant diabetic. *Seminar Perinatol.* 1978;**2**:361-71.
33. **Widness JA, Cowett RM, Coustan DR, Carpenter MW, Oh W.** Neonatal morbidities in infants of mothers with glucose intolerance in pregnancy. *Diabetes.* 1985;**34**(Suppl 2):61-5.
34. **Kalkhoff RK.** Therapeutic results of insulin therapy in gestational diabetes mellitus. *Diabetes.* 1985;**34**(Suppl 2):97-100.
35. **Roversi GD, Gargiulo M, Nicolini V, et al.** Maximal tolerated insulin therapy in gestational diabetes. *Diabetes Care.* 1980;**3**:489-94.
36. **Gyves MT, Schulman PK, Merkatz IR.** Results of individualized intervention in gestational diabetes. *Diabetes Care.* 1980;**3**:495-6.
37. **Beard RW, Hoet JJ.** Is gestational diabetes a clinical entity? *Diabetologia.* 1982;**23**:307-10.
38. **Gabbe SG.** Gestational diabetes mellitus [Editorial]. *N Engl J Med.* 1986;**315**:1025-6.
39. **Expert Committee on Diabetes Mellitus, World Health Organization.** *WHO Technical Report Series 646.* Geneva: World Health Organization; 1980:1-80.
40. **Harris MI.** Prevalence of non-insulin-dependent diabetes and im-

paired glucose tolerance. In: **National Diabetes Data Group.** *Diabetes In America: Diabetes Data Compiled 1984.* Washington, DC: U.S. Department of Health and Human Services; 1985. (NIH Publication No. 85-1468, August 1985:VI-1 through VI-31).

41. **Harris MI, Hadden WC, Knowler WC, Bennett PH.** Prevalence of diabetes and impaired glucose tolerance and plasma glucose levels in U.S. population aged 20-74 yr. *Diabetes.* 1987;**36**:523-34.

42. **O'Sullivan JB, Mahan CM.** Prospective study of 352 young patients with chemical diabetes. *N Engl J Med.* 1968;**278**:1038-41.

43. **Keen H, Jarrett RJ, McCartney P.** The ten-year follow-up of the Bedford survey (1962-1972): glucose tolerance and diabetes. *Diabetologia.* 1982;**22**:73-8.

44. **Sasaki A, Suzuki J, Horiuchi N.** Development of diabetes in Japanese subjects with impaired glucose tolerance: a seven year follow-up study. *Diabetologia.* 1982;**22**:154-7.

45. **King H, Zimmet P, Raper LR, Balkau B.** The natural history of impaired glucose tolerance in the Micronesian population of Nauru: a six-year follow-up study. *Diabetologia.*1984;**26**:39-43.

46. **Knowler WC, Bennett PH, Hamman RF, Miller M.** Diabetes incidence and prevalence in Pima Indians: a 19-fold greater incidence than in Rochester, Minnesota. *Am J Epidemiol.* 1978;**108**:497-505.

47. **Pettitt DJ, Knowler WC, Lisse JR, Bennett PH.** Development of retinopathy and proteinuria in relation to plasma glucose concentrations in Pima Indians. *Lancet.* 1980;**2**:1050-2.

48. **Sayegh HA, Jarrett RJ.** Oral glucose tolerance tests and the diagnosis of diabetes: results of a prospective study based on the Whitehall survey. *Lancet.* 1979;**2**:431-3.

49. **Jarrett RJ, Keen H.** Hyperglycemia and diabetes mellitus. *Lancet.* 1976;**2**:1009-12.

50. **Bennett PH, Rushforth NB, Miller M, LeCompte PM.** Epidemiologic studies in diabetes in the Pima Indians. *Recent Prog Horm Res.* 1976;**32**:333-76.

51. **Zimmet P, Whitehouse S.** Bimodality of fasting and two-hour glucose tolerance distributions in a Micronesian population. *Diabetes.* 1978;**27**:793-800.

52. **Hayner NS, Kjelsberg MO, Epstein FH, Francis T.** Carbohydrate tolerance and diabetes in a total community, Tecumseh, Michigan: 1. effects of age, sex, and test conditions on one-hour glucose tolerance in adults. *Diabetes.* 1965;**14**:413-23.

53. **O'Sullivan JB, Mahan CM.** Criteria for the oral glucose tolerance test in pregnancy. *Diabetes.* 1964;**13**:278-85.

54. **O'Sullivan JB, Charles D, Dandrow RV.** Treatment of verified prediabetics in pregnancy. *J Reprod Med.* 1971;**7**:21-4.

55. **Browder AA.** Screening for diabetes. *Prev Med.* 1974;**3**:220-4.

56. **Frame PS, Carlson SJ.** A critical review of periodic health screening using specific screening criteria. Part 2: selected endocrine, metabolic and gastrointestinal diseases. *J Fam Prac.* 1975;**2**:123-9.

57. **Frame PS.** A critical review of adult health maintenance: Part 4. Prevention of metabolic, behavioral, and miscellaneous conditions. *J Fam Pract.* 1986;**23**:29-39.

58. **Canadian Task Force on the Periodic Health Examination.** The periodic health examination. *Can Med Assoc J.* 1979;**121**:1193-254.

59. **Breslow L, Somers AR.** The lifetime health-monitoring program: a practical approach to preventive medicine. *N Engl J Med.* 1977;**296**:601-8.

60. **Eddy DM.** *Screening for Cancer: Theory, Analysis, and Design.* Englewood Cliffs, New Jersey: Prentice-Hall;1980.

61. **Morrison AS.** *Screening in Chronic Disease.* New York: Oxford University Press; 1985.

62. **Genuth SM, Houser HB, Carter JR Jr, et al.** Observations on the value of mass indiscriminate screeni for diabetes mellitus based on a five-year follow-up. *Diabetes.* 1978;**27**:377-83.

63. **Bennett PH, Knowler WC.** Early detection and intervention in diabetes mellitus: is it effective? *J Chronic Dis.* 1984;**37**:653-66.

64. **Merkatz IR, Duchon MA, Yamashita TS, Houser HB.** A pilot community-based screening program for gestational diabetes. *Diabetes Care.* 1980;**3**:453-7.

65. **Amankwah KS, Prentice RL, Fleury FJ.** The incidence of gestational diabetes. *Obstet Gynecol.* 1977;**49**:497-8.

66. **Mestman JH.** Outcome of diabetes screening in pregnancy and perinatal morbidity in infants of mothers with mild impairment in glucose tolerance. *Diabetes Care.* 1980;**3**:447-52.
67. **Summary and recommendations of the Second International Workshop-Conference on Gestational Diabetes Mellitus.** *Diabetes.* 1985;**34**:123-6.
68. **Cousins L, Dattel BJ, Hollingsworth DR, Zettner A.** Glycosylated hemoglobin as a screening test for carbohydrate intolerance in pregnancy. *Am J Obstet Gynecol.* 1984;**150**:455-60.
69. **O'Sullivan JB, Mahan CM, Charles D, Dandrow RV.** Screening criteria for high-risk gestational diabetic patients. *Am J Obstet Gynecol.* 1973;**116**:901-4.
70. **Carpenter MW, Coustan DR.** Criteria for screening tests for gestational diabetes. *Am J Obstet Gynecol.* 1982;**144**:768-73.
71. **Churchill JA, Berendes HW.** Intelligence of children whose mothers had acetonuria during pregnancy. In: *Perinatal Factors Affecting Human Development.* Washington, DC: Pan American Health Organization; 1969. (Scientific publication No. 185: 30-35).
72. **O'Sullivan JB, Gellis SS, Dandrow RV, Tenney BO.** The potential diabetic and her treatment in pregnancy. *Obstet Gynecol.* 1966;**27**:683-9.
73. **Gabbe SG, Mestman JG, Freeman RK, Anderson GV, Lowensohn RI.** Management and outcome of class A diabetes mellitus. *Am J Obstet Gynecol.* 1977;**127**:465-9.
74. **Cyr RM, Usher RH, McLean FH.** Changing patterns of birth asphyxia and trauma over 20 years. *Am J Obstet Gynecol.* 1984;**148**:490-8.
75. **Pettitt DJ, Baird HR, Aleck KA, Bennett PH, Knowler WC.** Excessive obesity in offspring of Pima Indian women with diabetes during pregnancy. *N Engl J Med.* 1983;**308**:242-5.
76. **Coustan DR, Lewis SB.** Insulin therapy for gestational diabetes. *Obstet Gynecol.* 1978;**51**:306-10.
77. **Campbell DT, Stanley JC.** *Experimental and Quasi-Experimental Designs for Research.* Chicago: Rand McNally College Publishing Company; 1963:10-3.
78. **Gyves MT, Rodman HM, Little AB, Fanaroff AA, Merkatz IR.** A modern approach to management of pregnant diabetics: a two year analysis of perinatal outcomes. *Am J Obstet Gynecol.* 1977;**128**:606-16.
79. **Roversi GD, Gargiulo M, Nicolini U, et al.** A new approach to the treatment of diabetic pregnant women report of 479 cases seen from 1963 to 1975. *Am J Obstet Gynecol.* 1979;**135**:567-76.
80. **Adashi EY, Pinto H, Tyson JE.** Impact of maternal euglycemia on fetal outcome in diabetic pregnancy. *Am J Obstet Gynecol.* 1979;**133**:268-74.
81. **Coustan DR, Imarah J.** Prophylactic insulin treatment of gestational diabetes reduces the incidence of macrosomia, operative delivery, and birth trauma. *Am J Obstet Gynecol.* 1984;**150**:836-42.
82. **Karlsson K, Kjellmer I.** The outcome of diabetic pregnancies in relation to the mother's blood sugar level. *Am J Obstet Gynecol.* 1972;**112**:213-20.
83. **American Diabetes Association, Inc.** Gestational diabetes mellitus. *Ann Intern Med.* 1986;**105**:461.
84. **Persson B, Stangenberg M, Hansson U, Nordlander E.** Gestational diabetes mellitus (GDM): comparative evaluation of two treatment regimens, diet versus insulin and diet. *Diabetes.* 1985;**34**(suppl 2):101-5.
85. **Lavin JP, Jr.** Screening of high-risk and general populations for gestational diabetes: clinical application and cost analysis. *Diabetes.* 1985;**34**(Suppl 2):24-7.
86. **American College of Obstetrics and Gynecology.** Management of diabetes mellitus in pregnancy. *ACOG Technical Bulletin.* Chicago: 1986;No.**92**:1-5.
87. **Jovanovic L, Peterson CM.** Screening for gestational diabetes: optimum timing and criteria for retesting. *Diabetes.* 1985;**34**(Suppl 2):21-3.
88. **Weiner CP, Fraser MM, Burns JM, Schnoor D, Herrig J, Whitaker LA.** Cost efficacy of routine screening for diabetes in pregnancy: 1-h versus 2-h specimen. *Diabetes Care.* 1986;**9**:255-9.

89. **Landon MB, Cembrowski GS, Gabbe SG.** Capillary blood glucose screening for gestational diabetes: a preliminary investigation. *Am J Obstet Gynecol.* 1986;**155:**717-21.

90. **Weiner CP, Faustich MW, Burns J, Fraser M, Whitaker L, Klugman M.** Diagnosis of gestational diabetes by capillary blood samples and a portable reflectance meter: derivation of threshold values and prospective validation. *Am J Obstet Gynecol.* 1987;**156:**1085-9.

91. **Morris MA, Grandis AS, Litton JC.** Glycosylated hemoglobin concentration in early gestation associated with neonatal outcome. *Am J Obstet Gynecol.* 1985;**153:**651-4.

92. **West KM.** *The Epidemiology of Diabetes and its Vascular Lesions.* New York: Elsevier North-Holland; 1978. op.cit.

93. **Herman WH, Teutsch SM.** Kidney diseases associated with diabetes. In: **National Diabetes Data Group.** *Diabetes in America: Diabetes Data Compiled 1984.* Washington, DC: U.S. Department of Health and Human Services; 1985. (NIH Publication No. 85-1468, August 1985: XIV-1 to XIV-31).

94. **Klein R, Klein BEK.** Vision disorders in diabetes. In: **National Diabetes Data Group.** *Diabetes in America: Diabetes Data Compiled 1984* Washington, DC: U.S. Department of Health and Human Services; 1985 (NIH Publication No. 85-1468, August 1985: XIII-1 to XIII-36).

95. **Barrett-Connor E, Orchard T.** Diabetes and heart disease In: **National Diabetes Data Group. Diabetes in America; Diabetes Data Compiled 1984.** Washington, DC: U.S. Department of Health and Human Services; 1985. (NIH Publication No. 85-1468, August 1985: XVI-I to XVI-41).

96. **Kannel WB, McGee DL.** Diabetes and cardiovascular disease: the Framingham Study. *JAMA.* 1979;**241:**2035-8.

97. **Sharp CL.** Diabetes survey in Bedford in 1962. *Proc R Soc Lond [Med].* 1964;**57:**193-5.

98. **Forrest RD, Jackson CA, Yudkin JS.** The glycohaemoglobin assay as a screening test for diabetes mellitus: the Islington Diabetes Survey. *Diabetic Med.* 1987;**4:**254-9.

99. **Little RR, England JD, Wiedmeyer HM, et al.** Relationship of glycosylated hemoglobin to oral glucose tolerance: implications for diabetes screening. *Diabetes.* 1988;**37:**60-4.

100. **Orzeck EA, Mooney JH, Owen JA Jr.** Diabetes detection with a comparison of screening methods. *Diabetes.* 1971;**20:**109-16.

101. **Kent GT, Leonards JR.** Analysis of tests for diabetes in 250,000 persons screened for diabetes using finger blood after a carbohydrate load. *Diabetes.* 1968;**17:**274-80.

102. **Reid DD, Brett GZ, Hamilton PJ, Jarrett RJ, Keen H, Rose G.** Cardiorespiratory disease and diabetes among middle-aged male Civil Servants: a study of screening and intervention. *Lancet.* 1974;**1:**469-73.

103. **Medalie JH.** Risk factors other than hyperglycemia in diabetic macrovascular disease. *Diabetes Care.* 1979;**2:**77-84.

104. **The Diabetes Control and Complications Trial.** Are continuing studies of metabolic control and microvascular complications in insulin-dependent diabetes mellitus justified? *N Engl J Med.* 1988;**318:**246-50.

105. Effects of hypoglycemic agents on vascular complications in patients with adult-onset diabetes. VIII. Evaluation of insulin therapy: final report. *Diabetes.* 1982;**31:**(Suppl 5):1-81.

106. **Scarlett JA, Gray RS, Griffin J, Olefsky JM, Kolterman OG.** Insulin treatment reverses the insulin resistance of type II diabetes mellitus. *Diabetes Care* 1982;**5:**353-63.

107. **Stern MP, Rosenthal M, Haffner SM, Hazuda HP, Franco LJ.** Sex differences in the effects of sociocultural status on diabetes and cardiovascular risk factors in Mexican Americans: the San Antonio Heart Study. *Am J Epidemiol.* 1984;**120:**834-51.

108. **Wingard DL, Barrett-Connor E, Criqui MH, Suarez L.** Clustering of heart disease risk factors in diabetic compared to nondiabetic adults. *Am J Epidemiol.* 1983;**117:**19-26.

109. **Keen H, Jarrett RJ, McCartney P.** The ten-year follow-up of the Bedford survey (1962-1972): glucose tolerance and diabetes. *Diabetologia.* 1982;**22:**73-8.

110. **Jarrett RJ, Keen H, Fuller JH, McCartney M.** Treatment of bor-

derline diabetes: controlled trial using carbohydrate restriction and phenformin. *Br Med J.* 1977;2:861-5.

111. **Sartor G, Scherstén B, Carlström S, Melander A, Nordén A, Persson A.** Ten-year follow-up of subjects with impaired glucose tolerance: prevention of diabetes by tolbutamide and diet regulation. *Diabetes.* 1980;29:41-9.

112. **O'Sullivan JB, Mahan CM.** Blood sugar levels, glycosuria, and bodyweight related to development of diabetes mellitus. *JAMA.* 1965;194:587-92.

113. **Knowler WC, Pettitt DJ, Savage PJ, Bennett PH.** Diabetes incidence in Pima Indians: contributions of obesity and parental diabetes. *Am J Epidemiol.* 1981;113:144-56.

114. **Westlund K, Nicolaysen JM.** Ten-year mortality and morbidity related to serum cholesterol: a follow-up of 3751 men aged 40-49. *Scand J Clin Lab Invest.* 1972;30(Suppl 127):1-24.

115. **Hadden DR, Montgomery DA, Skelly RJ, et al.** Maturity onset diabetes mellitus: response to intensive dietary management. *Br Med J.* 1975;3:276-8.

116. **Diabetic Retinopathy Study Research Group.** Preliminary report on effects of photocoagulation therapy. *Am J Ophthalmol.* 1976;81:383-96.

117. **Dorf A, Ballantine EJ, Bennett PH, Miller M.** Retinopathy in Pima Indians: relationship to glucose level, duration of diabetes, age at diagnosis of diabetes, and age at examination in a population with a high prevalence of diabetes mellitus. *Diabetes.* 1976;25:554-60.

118. **Dwyer MS, Melton LJ 3d, Ballard DJ, Palumbo PJ, Trautmann JC, Chu CP.** Incidence of diabetic retinopathy and blindness: a population-based study in Rochester, Minnesota. *Diabetes Care.* 1985;8:316-22.

119. **Velez R, Haffner S, Stern MP, Van Heuven WAJ.** Ophthalmologist vs retinal photographs in screening for diabetic retinopathy [Abstract]. *Clin Res.* 1987;35:363A.

120. **LaPorte RE, Tajima N.** Prevalence of insulin-dependent diabetes. In: **National Diabetes Data Group.** *Diabetes in America: Diabetes Data Compiled 1984.* Washington, DC: U.S. Department of Health and Human Services; 1985. (NIH Publication No. 85-1468, August 1985: V-I).

121. **Gorsuch AN, Spencer KM, Lister J, et al.** Evidence for a long prediabetic period in type I (insulin-dependent) diabetes mellitus. *Lancet.* 1981;2:1363-5.

122. **Rosenbloom AL, Hunt SS, Rosenbloom EK, Maclaren NK.** Ten-year prognosis of impaired glucose tolerance in siblings of patients with insulin-dependent diabetes. *Diabetes.* 1982;31:385-7.

123. **Reed BD.** Screening for gestational diabetes—analysis by screening criteria. *J Fam Pract.* 1984; 19:751-5.

124. **Bochner CJ, Medearis AL, Williams J 3d, Castro L, Hobel CJ, Wade ME.** Early third-trimester ultrasound screening in gestational diabetes to determine the risk of macrosomia and labor dystocia at term. *Am J Obstet Gynecol.* 1987;157:703-8.

Appendix 1

The Diagnosis of Diabetes Mellitus

The criteria of the National Diabetes Data Group (1) for nonpregnant adults include the following. First, "unequivocal elevation of plasma glucose concentration together with the classic symptoms of diabetes" are required. Both criteria are left undefined. The World Health Organization defines unequivocal elevation of plasma glucose as 140 mg/dL or greater on a fasting specimen or any plasma glucose of 200 mg/dL or greater (39). Fasting plasma glucose less than 115 mg/dL is considered definitely normal. Second, "elevated fasting plasma glucose concentration on more than one occasion," that is, 140 mg/dL or greater, is required. Third, "elevated plasma glucose concentration after an oral glucose challenge on more than one occasion" is required. Both the 2-hour plasma or serum and some other sample before 2 hours after glucose must be 200 mg/dL or greater.

Impaired glucose tolerance is diagnosed when fasting plasma glucose is less than 140 mg/dL, the oral glucose tolerance test 2-hour plasma glucose is between 140 mg/dL and 200 mg/dL, and an oral glucose tolerance test plasma glucose before 2 hours is 200 mg/dL or greater.

Standards for the oral glucose tolerance test are as follows: The dose is 75-g oral glucose consumed over 5 minutes. The patient should remain seated throughout the test. The test should be done in the morning after a 10- to 16-hour fast that was preceded by 3 days of diet containing at least 150 g of carbohydrate and unrestricted physical activity.

Gestational diabetes (1, 53), which first appears during pregnancy, is diagnosed by two or more of the following values after a 100-g oral glucose challenge: fasting plasma glucose, 105 mg/dL or greater; 1-hour plasma glucose, 190 mg/dL or greater; 2-hour plasma glucose, 165 mg/dL or greater; or 3-hour plasma glucose, 145 mg/dL or greater. There is no official category of gestational impaired glucose tolerance.

The diagnosis of diabetes can be unambiguously assigned only when other physiologic stresses or drugs that produce hyperglycemia are not present (1).

Appendix 2

Observational Studies Bearing on Screening for Gestational Diabetes Mellitus

Gyves and colleagues (78) reported a 2-year analysis of perinatal outcomes with a "modern approach to management of pregnant diabetics" using the patient's own previous pregnancy as a historical control. In this study the 52 previously pregnant gestational diabetic patients had a history of an 8.3% perinatal mortality rate (11 deaths per 133 potential viable pregnancies) compared with no losses in the study period.

Roversi and associates (79) also used the patient's previous pregnancies as the historical control to determine the effect of "maximally tolerated dose" insulin regimen on pregnant diabetic patients from 1963 to 1975. The subset of 109 previously pregnant women with gestational diabetes mellitus (White's Class A) had a decreased perinatal mortality from a remarkable 27.5% before therapy to 1.8% with therapy.

Adashi and coworkers (80) followed 113 pregnant diabetic patients using the patient's previous pregnancies as historical controls. The cumulative past reproductive loss in 50 parous patients with gestational diabetes mellitus was 13 of 247 potentially viable pregnancies, for a rate of 52 per 1000. This historical control rate decreased to zero in the study where maternal euglycemia was pursued.

Coustan and Imarah (81) retrospectively analyzed treatment and outcome of 445 gestational diabetic patients managed between 1975 and 1980. Patients were categorized according to therapy: insulin and diet (115 patients); diet alone (184 patients); and neither insulin nor dietary manipulation (146 patients). The frequency of birth complications was significantly less in the insulin and diet treatment group compared with the diet treatment and no treatment groups, respectively: macrosomia, 7.0% compared with 18.5% and 17.8%; operative delivery (midforceps, midcavity vacuum extraction, or primary cesarean section, 16.3% compared with 30.4% and 28.5%; and birth trauma, 4.8% compared with 13.4 and 20.4%). There was no difference in perinatal mortality with all groups having rates of 1% or less. Although the treatment cohorts differed in several respects, the authors attributed the improved outcome in the first group to the combined therapy of insulin and diet.

Gabbe and associates (73) retrospectively reviewed the outcome of 261 gestational diabetic patients (White Class A with normal fasting serum glucose and abnormal glucose tolerance test) who were managed between 1970 and 1972 with a uniform protocol that included dietary supervision and close surveillance of glycemia. Although the results showed a perinatal death rate less than the general population rate (19 per 1000 compared with 32 per 1000) no concurrent control group was used.

Karlsson and Kjellmer (82) reviewed the outcome of diabetic pregnancies in relation to the mother's blood sugar level. Although significant reductions in perinatal mortality were found with lower mean blood sugars, only 11% (20 of 180) of the patients had gestational diabetics.

Appendix 3

Screening for Gestational Diabetes Mellitus: Assumptions Underlying the Cost-Effectiveness Analysis

1. The cost (hospital charges) of the glucose screening test is $6.00. (Personal communication. Billing office, Beth Israel Hospital, Boston, Massachusetts, 1987.)

2. The cost (hospital charges) of the oral glucose tolerance test is $24.00. No indirect costs to the patient are included.

3. The prevalence of gestational diabetes in the general pregnant population is 3% (64-66).

4. The sensitivity of the glucose screening test is 83% (70).

5. The specificity of the glucose screening test is 87% (70).

6. Two estimates of the reduction in neonatal mortality are used to bound the range observed by previous studies: 0 and 25.7 per 100 singleton pregnancies. The latter is the largest estimate derived from observational studies (79). The estimate of zero derives from the two controlled trials described above (72, 76).

7. Neonatal morbidity is assessed as rates of macrosomia. We use the estimate of reduction in macrosomia of 8.8% found by O'Sullivan and coworkers (72) using a more stringent definition (more than 4.09 kg [9 pounds]).

8. The rates of neonatal mortality and morbidity are constant with maternal age. This finding is supported by more recent series (73, 78, 80) but runs counter to the original observations of O'Sullivan and associates (29, 72).

9. The population aged over 25 years accounts for approximately 50% of pregnancies but 85% of gestational diabetic pregnancies (123).

10. The relative risk for gestational diabetes of patients with positive risk factors is 1.07 (85).

11. The proportion of pregnant women with risk factors for gestational diabetes is 46% (85).

12. A conservative estimate of the cost of treating identified cases is $300 per case for additional glucose tests, extra visits, and (rarely) medications. Patients with gestational diabetes may receive more ultrasound and other nonglucose testing as well as more frequent operative deliveries (67, 124) because they have been labeled as gestationally diabetic. Estimates for these induced costs are difficult to determine, and are not included in this analysis.

13. Only cases of gestational diabetes detected by screening benefit.

Screening for Thyroid Disease

MARK HELFAND, MD, MS; and
LAWRENCE M. CRAPO, MD, PhD

Elderly patients with thyrotoxicosis or hypothyroidism can present with subtle and nonspecific signs and symptoms that can be mistakenly attributed to other illnesses or to "old age." Epidemiologic surveys have shown that screening can detect unsuspected thyrotoxicosis and hypothyroidism and that some patients who are detected can benefit from therapy (1, 2). In addition, established programs to screen infants for congenital hypothyroidism show that inexpensive, non-invasive thyroid function tests can detect significant, treatable disease before clinical manifestations occur (3-5). These considerations have intensified interest in screening adults for thyroid disease.

Our goal is to make recommendations based on what is currently known about the benefits, risks, and costs of screening for thyrotoxicosis and hypothyroidism in adults. We rely primarily on a critical evaluation of studies of both screening and the benefits of detecting thyroid disease in its early stages. In addition, we examine the influence of clinical setting, target population, and choice of screening tests on effectiveness and costs of different strategies for early diagnosis of thyroid disease.

Definitions

Screening Programs

Strategies for early diagnosis can be classified into screening and case-finding (6). Screening programs invite the general public to have tests or examinations intended to find early evidence of disease. Epidemiologic studies of screening for thyroid disease attempt to recruit a population sample of a particular geographic area. Such research studies show the extent of unsuspected disease and the potential benefits of universal screening but do not represent the effectiveness of screening in practice. For example, when patients are invited to have a periodic health examination and mul-

---

▶ This chapter was originally published in *Annals of Internal Medicine.* 1990;112:840-9.

tiphasic screen, patients at high risk who have avoided regular care in the past are unlikely to participate (7, 8).

In contrast to screening, case-finding tests patients who have come to their physicians for unrelated reasons for the disease. Usually, physicians can do the thyroid screening test when blood would be drawn for other reasons. Case-finding can cover a larger proportion of the population than other strategies because most adults visit a physician at some time, even if they do not use medical care regularly or will not respond to a special invitation to be screened (6). The patient's primary physician orders and interprets the screening test and supervises follow-up tests and treatment. For these reasons, case-finding can be more effective and less costly than screening (9). Case-finding for thyroid disease has been done in general medical clinic patients; geriatric, general medical, and psychiatric hospital patients; and postpartum patients. (We discuss each of these settings for case-finding later.)

Serial testing in some groups of patients might be called surveillance rather than screening. For example, patients with a history of neck irradiation for malignancy are likely to develop nodular thyroid disease or hypothyroidism (10). Patients who have had surgery or radioiodine therapy for Graves disease are also very likely to become hypothyroid. Examination of the thyroid gland and testing for thyroid function are an important part of managing these patients, and our recommendations for screening are not meant to be applied to them.

Screening Tests

Tests that have been used to screen for thyroid disease are described in Table 1. The most commonly used initial tests for screening are the total thyroxine (TT4), free thyroxine index (FT4I), and the sensitive thyrotropin (sensitive-TSH). Tests for triiodothyronine (TT3) and antithyroid antibodies are not useful as screening tests for thyroid dysfunction, but may be used as follow-up tests in some situations.

Many factors other than choice of initial test, including choice of follow-up tests and coordination between agencies that do screening tests and physicians who follow patients with abnormal results, affect the effectiveness and costs of a screening strategy. Table 1 shows customary charges for thyroid function tests. Charges bear little relation to laboratory costs; for example, a laboratory that processes a large volume of

Table 1. *Thyroid Function Tests Used for Screening*

Test	Typical Normal Range	Charge, $*
Total thyroxine (TT4) Measures total amount of thyroxine in serum	50–142 nmol/L (4–11 µg/dL)	18 ± 9
T3 resin uptake (T3 uptake)† Estimates thyroid binding hormone capacity using T3 as a tracer	30%–40% (or 100% normalized)	16 ± 8
Free thyroxine index (FT4I) Indirectly estimates unbound thyroxine in serum (TT4 × T3 uptake)	5–12	23 ± 10
Free thyroxine (FT4) Measures or estimates unbound thyroxine in serum by dialysis, filtration, or other methods	‡	27 ± 10
Thyrotropin (TSH) Measures total thyrotropin using older radioimmunoassays	0–10 mU/L	40 ± 17
Sensitive-thyrotropin (sensitive-TSH) Measures total thyrotropin using immunoradiometric or other new assay methods	0.2–5 mU/L	55
Total triiodothyronine (TT3) Measures total amount of triiodothyronine in serum	1.2–3.4 nmol/L (75–220 ng/dL)	39 ± 17
Free triiodothyronine (FT3) Measures unbound thyroxine in serum	‡	55 ± 17

* The sources for these figures were Northern California Blue Shield reimbursements, 1987; and a survey of reference labs (Wu R. Unpublished data). Data are expressed as the mode and the approximate range.

† The T3 resin uptake is one of various methods of measuring thyroid-hormone-binding sites. Direct radioimmunoassay of thyroid-binding globulin (TBG) is an alternative method. The American Thyroid Association recommends that the term "thyroid hormone binding ratio" (THBR) replace "T3 uptake," because the latter is often confused with a measure of triiodothyronine (T3).

‡ Widely varying commercial methods are used. Different assays have different normal ranges.

tests can do a TT4 for less than $1 but will typically charge much more. Therefore, the costs of screening in organized health systems (such as HMOs or public health clinics) may be much less than the cost to patients in other settings.

Costs also depend on clinicians' responses to abnormal test results (11). Clinicians may ignore or repeat an abnormal test; refer patients unnecessarily before doing follow-up tests that can exclude false-positive results; or provide long-term follow-up for patients with early (or nonexistent) disease that is detected by one strategy but not another. The choice of initial test is less important than how abnormal test results are interpreted and acted on.

Thyroid Disease and Dysfunction

Screening is intended to find patients who have clinically unsuspected thyroid dysfunction (hypothyroidism or thyrotoxicosis). Patients with abnormal thyroid function are a small subset of all patients with anatomic or serologic evidence of thyroid disease. For example, most patients over 60 years of age who, while alive, had no evidence of thyroid disease have histologic abnormalities of the thyroid gland at autopsy (12-14). Serologic evidence of autoimmune thyroid disease is also common among euthyroid persons: Approximately 15% of elderly women and 2% of other persons have circulating antithyroid antibodies, suggesting autoimmune thyroiditis (1, 15-17). When careful physical examination is used to screen for disease, a goiter or nodule is found in 1% of men and 10% of women (1). However, most of these patients have normal thyroid function and would not be detected by screening with thyroid function tests.

Modern tests of thyroid function have led to the recognition that detectable biochemical abnormalities may precede clinical thyroid disease. The course of disease and the benefits of treatment depend on the stage at which diagnosis is made. Thyroid dysfunction is classified by severity of clinical findings, serum hormone levels (T4, T3, and TSH), the presence or absence of thyroid autoantibodies, and physiologic and biochemical evidence of deficient or excessive thyroid hormone effect in target tissues.

The terms "overt" and "subclinical" have been introduced to distinguish clinically apparent disease from earlier grades of dysfunction (18). Unfortunately, there is disagreement on the criteria for these new diagnoses. Table 2 reflects the complexity and ambiguity of current usage, showing that even such terms as "overt hypothyroidism" are used ambiguously. This term means "clinically and biochemically hypothyroid" in some studies and "biochemically hypothyroid, regardless of clinical status" in others. Such disagreement is important because the apparent prevalence of disease as well as expectations about its course differ among studies that use different definitions.

An ideal classification would distinguish subgroups of patients who need therapy or follow-up from those who do not. Few of the designations listed in Table 2 meet this criterion. In our review, we emphasize studies that use an adequate period of follow-up to distinguish patients who need treatment from those who have biochemical abnormalities but are free of thyroid disease.

Screening for Thyroid Disease in the Community

Some investigators recommend screening for thyroid disease in the general or elderly population (1, 2). There are no studies of the health benefits of screening for thyroid disease in the community. Instead, the potential benefits must be inferred from the number of cases of unsuspected disease uncovered by screening. Screening is aimed at detecting both hypothyroid and thyrotoxic patients. Studies of screening in the community are summarized in Table 3 and discussed below by diagnosis.

Overt Hypothyroidism

This condition is usually defined as the combination of clinical findings of hypothyroidism as well as low serum TT4 and elevated serum TSH levels. Screening benefits patients with this condition by reducing the length of time between onset of the disease and detection. In various studies, the prevalence of unsuspected overt hypothyroidism ranges from 0 to 18 cases per 1000 persons (1, 2, 19-24). Because patients with hypothyroidism have near-normal life spans, routine screening in the community will "detect" far more cases of known hypothyroidism than of previously unsuspected disease. Tunbridge's prospective survey (1) in a small English town used a screening history and physical examination to diagnose 28 cases of overt hypothyroidism among the 2779 persons screened. Of these 28 cases, all but 5 were already known to have the disease. All 5 were women. Thus the yield of unsuspected overt hypothyroidism was 0 per 1000 men and 3 per 1000 women. Another study (19) used a thyroid panel (T4, T3, and TSH) instead of clinical examination as the initial test; in this study, the prevalence of previously undiagnosed hypothyroidism was 6 cases per 1000 middle-aged women.

Most studies focus on older persons, especially older women (2, 20-27). In these studies, the prevalence of unsuspected overt hypothyroidism is usually from 0 to 7 per 1000 men and from 3 to 18 per 1000 women. One

Table 2. *Definitions of Thyroid Dysfunction**

Diagnosis and Clinical Findings

Overt hyperthyroidism
Definition 1: Signs or symptoms of hyperthyroidism

Definition 2: Not a criterion
T3 toxicosis: Signs and symptoms of hyperthyroidism

Subclinical hyperthyroidism
Definition 1: May have symptoms and signs

Definition 2: No signs or symptoms

Definition 3: No signs or symptoms

Euthyroidism with thyroid disease
Definition 1: Goiter, Graves ophthalmopathy, nodule
Definition 2: Goiter, Graves ophthalmopathy, nodule

Euthyroidism without thyroid disease: No evidence of thyroid disease
Subclinical hypothyroidism
Definition 1: No signs or symptoms

Definition 2: May have symptoms and signs
Mild hypothyroidism: Single or few symptoms
Overt hypothyroidism
Definition 1: Signs and symptoms of hypothyroidism

Definition 2: Not a criterion

---

* T4 = serum thyroxine; T3 = triiodothyronine; TSH = thyrotropin; TRH = thyrotropin-releasing hormone; R = raised; L = low; Sup = suppressed; N = normal; Ex = exaggerated; NA = not applicable. Studies disagree on criteria for diagnosis. Some require the presence or absence of clinical findings; others rely only on biochemical tests of thyroid function (T4 and T3) or of pituitary function (basal TSH and TSH response to TRH).

study, however, reported a much higher prevalence, 30 cases per 1000 (27). Unlike the other studies, this study did not use an independent standard or follow-up to verify diagnosis; in addition, asymptomatic patients with biochemical evidence only were classified as having "overt" disease. These features of the study design explain the unusually high prevalence of disease found.

Table 2. *(Continued)*

T4	T3	Basal TSH	TSH Response to TRH	Comments
R	R	L	Sup	Clinically and biochemically hyperthyroid
R	R	L	Sup	Only biochemical criteria
N	R	L	Sup	Some require normal FT4 instead of TT4
N	N	L	Sup	Symptomatic but biochemically euthyroid
N	N	L	Sup	Asymptomatic but abnormal TSH and TSH response to TRH
R	R	L	Sup	Asymptomatic but biochemically hyperthyroid
N	N	N	N	Clinically and biochemically euthyroid
N	N	L or N	Sup or N	May have suppressed basal TSH and TRH response
N	N	N	N	
N	NA	R	Ex	Studies differ on cutoff for elevated TSH; some studies require demonstration of antithyroid antibodies
N	NA	R	Ex	
N	NA	R	Ex	
L	NA	R	Ex	Clinical and biochemical overt hypothyroidism
L	NA	R	Ex	"Biochemical overt hypothyroidism"

Overt Thyrotoxicosis

This condition is usually defined as the combination of clinical findings of thyrotoxicosis and elevated TT4 and TT3 levels. Early detection of overt thyrotoxicosis might prevent some episodes of thyroid storm and acute cardiac decompensation, although the extent of these benefits is unknown. The prevalence of unsuspected overt thyrotoxicosis ranges from 2 to 20 cases per 1000 persons (1, 2, 19-24). Using physical examination and history as the primary screening test, Tunbridge's ex-

Table 3. *Effects of Screening for Thyroid Disease in the Community*

Study Description (Reference)	Subject Description (n)
Population surveys	
Small town, Great Britain; 4-year follow-up (1)	Men (1285)
	Women (1494)
	Women over 55 years of age (528)
Rural Sweden (2, 19)	Women over 60 years of age (1442)
	Women 39 to 60 years of age (3885)
Small town, Sweden; 6-year follow-up (20, 21)	Women 44 to 66 years of age (1283)
Town, New Zealand (22)	Residents over 80 years of age (427)
Town, Japan (23)	Men over 40 years of age (1026)
	Women over 40 years of age (1395)
Rural Norway (24)	Men over 70 years of age (86)
	Women over 70 years of age (114)
London, England (25)	Elderly residents (114)
Other designs	
Analysis of data from Framingham cohort (26)	Men over 60 years of age (892)
	Women over 60 years of age (1256)
Survey at a senior citizen's center, Boston (27)	Senior citizens (374)

* Number of new cases detected when 1000 community residents are screened. TSH = thyrotropin.

† Prevalence varies, because the studies define subclinical hypothyroidism differently. In most studies, an asymptomatic patient with a serum thyrotropin level over 6 mU/L (TSH > 6) is classified as having subclinical hypothyroidism. In other studies, a TSH level over 5, 7, or 10 mU/L is required. Some studies include only asymptomatic patients, and some require the presence of circulating antithyroid antibodies.

tensive survey found no cases among 1285 men and 7 cases among 1494 women (5 per 1000 women). Laboratory tests were also done but did not detect any additional cases. The annual incidence of thyrotoxicosis ranges from 1 to 5 cases per 10 000 persons (28, 29). If an effective screening program is repeated, far fewer cases will be detected. Studies of the prevalence of overt thyrotoxicosis in elderly persons give conflicting results. In a Swedish study of 1442 elderly women, 20 per 1000 were thyrotoxic (2, 30). In a smaller Norwegian study, however, no cases were found among 114 elderly women (24).

Subclinical Hypothyroidism

Prevalence of Disease

Subclinical hypothyroidism is usually defined as an elevated TSH level in an asymptomatic patient. Many studies define subclinical hypothyroidism as a TSH level over 6 mU/L. By this definition, the prevalence is between 25 and 104 per 1000 persons, depending on the

Table 3. *(Continued)*

Prevalence of Disease, *n/1000**			Definition of Subclinical Hypothyroidism†
Unsuspected Overt Hyperthyroidism	Unsuspected Overt Hypothyroidism	Subclinical Hypothyroidism	
0	0	28	TSH > 6
5	3	75	TSH > 6
Not given	Not given	104	TSH > 6
19	6	11	TSH > 7
6	6	Not given	Not given
6	0	12	TSH > 14
5	9	Not given	Not given
0	4	33	TSH > 4.1‡
2	6	55	TSH > 4.1‡
12	12	24	TSH > 6
0	18	35	TSH > 6
0	17	Not given	Not given
Not given	Not given	24	TSH > 10
Not given	Not given	59	TSH > 10
Not given	32	27	TSH > 10

‡ Values of the sensitive-TSH assay used in this study are lower than those of the older assays used in other studies.

sex and age of the population (Table 3), and approximately 10% of women between 40 and 60 years of age are diagnosed to have subclinical hypothyroidism.

Some studies use a stricter definition. If subclinical hypothyroidism is defined as a TSH level above 10 mU/L, the prevalence is between 11 and 60 per 1000 women over 50 years of age (*see* Table 3). The most stringent definition requires a TSH level over 10 mU/L and a positive test for circulating antithyroid antibodies; the additional criterion lowers the apparent prevalence by about 30% (1, 16).

It seems likely that, when subclinical hypothyroidism is defined as a TSH level over 6 mU/L instead of a higher value, almost all of the additional cases that are detected are actually in healthy persons. In the Tunbridge study (1, 31), 8% of patients with TSH levels over 6 mU/L developed overt hypothyroidism within 5 years; 92% remained well. However, nearly all patients who progressed to overt hypothyroidism had TSH levels over 10 mU/L and high titers of circulating antithyroid antibodies. By itself, a TSH level between 6 and 10 mU/L was not a risk factor for development of overt hypothyroidism.

Women with TSH levels over 10 mU/L and high titers of antithyroid antibodies become overtly hypothyroid at a rate of 7% per year (31, 34). Other estimates range from 1% to 20% per year (17, 20, 24, 31-34). Extreme estimates reflect more or less stringent criteria for defining an elevated TSH level or a high antibody titer, the number of patients with mild symptoms at the beginning of the study, and the inclusion in some studies of patients who have had antithyroid treatment or neck irradiation in the past. Rigid criteria increase the likelihood of progression but greatly decrease the apparent prevalence of disease. In one study, for example, only patients with TSH levels over 14 mU/L and very high titers of antithyroid antibodies were considered to have subclinical hypothyroidism. These patients progressed at a rate of 20% per year, but only 7 per 1000 women screened had subclinical hypothyroidism by this definition (20).

By the first definition, if 1000 elderly women are screened, 60 (at most) would be diagnosed to have subclinical hypothyroidism, and 12 of these women would progress to overt disease within 5 years. Even if follow-up and early treatment helped these 12, the other 48 patients would be treated unnecessarily. If the strictest criteria are used, few patients are found, but most of them will progress to overt hypothyroidism within 5 years.

Effect of Diagnosis on Patient Outcomes

Does subclinical hypothyroidism warrant early detection? Patients with subclinical hypothyroidism are said to have a higher prevalence of coronary artery disease, possibly due to a relative increase in low-density lipoprotein and decrease in high-density lipoprotein (35). The prevalence of subclinical hypothyroidism is higher among women in their 40s and 50s than among women in their 70s and 80s, a pattern that suggests selective mortality (16). In addition, some patients with subclinical hypothyroidism become overtly hypothyroid. For these reasons, some investigators have suggested that asymptomatic patients found to have elevated TSH levels and antithyroid antibodies should be treated with thyroxine to prevent the emergence of clinical disease (36, 37).

There have been six studies of the benefits of early treatment in subclinical hypothyroidism (35-40). In one of these studies, treatment with thyroxine effected a statistically significant increase in left ventricular ejection fraction with exercise but had no effect on total cholesterol, high-density lipoprotein, or triglyceride levels (38). In a randomized, placebo-controlled trial of 33 patients (37), treatment did not affect serum cholesterol level or body weight after 1 year. In the same trial, a composite score of the severity of six symptoms was significantly better in the treated group than in the controls after 1 year. The patients studied in this trial were symptomatic; some would, therefore, argue that these patients had "mild" hypothyroidism rather than subclinical hypothyroidism. In a randomized, placebo-controlled crossover study of 20 patients, four patients improved during treatment as measured by tests of short-term memory, calculation speed, and reaction time (40). Interestingly, the titer of antithyroid antibodies bore no relation to clinical improvement. Two patients felt nervous on thyroxine therapy and quit the study. Eight patients said they felt better while receiving thyroxine. Since thyroxine therapy might impart a sense of well-being in some euthyroid persons, this study should be interpreted cautiously.

Detecting subclinical hypothyroidism allows closer follow-up of patients at risk for overt hypothyroidism and, possibly, ischemic heart disease or elevations in low-density lipoprotein cholesterol level. These benefits are difficult to quantify and have not been systematically studied. Reliance on the patient's history is hazardous, because symptoms traditionally associated with hypothyroidism are common in elderly patients. One study in 79-year-old women compared those whose TSH levels were under 10 with those whose TSH levels were over 10. There were no differences in frequency of tiredness (30%), cold sensitivity (19%), constipation (25%), or other symptoms (41). On the other hand, treating asymptomatic patients with subclinical hypothyroidism when TT4 levels fall below normal has not been shown to improve outcomes.

If widely used for subclinical hypothyroidism, levothyroxine therapy might aggravate co-existing coronary artery disease and osteoporosis and impose unnecessary medication on many well persons. At present, no study has followed patients on therapy for longer than 1 year, and only 53 patients have been formally observed. Presently, the balance between the short-term benefits and potential long-term risks cannot be estimated.

Recommendations for Screening

Screening for thyroid disease in healthy persons is not useful. The studies summarized in Table 3 show that screening in the community can detect some patients with overt thyroid disease. These studies, however, were done in a research program that included meticulous population sampling, extensive testing, and thorough follow-up. An actual screening program may be less effective for many reasons and, because no demonstration has been done, there is no way to estimate the actual benefits and costs of such a program.

Screening in the community also detects early and subclinical disease. Asymptomatic patients have not been shown to benefit from screening. The evidence suggests that, among women over 40 years of age, an elevated TSH level (over 10 mU/L) is a risk factor for development of overt hypothyroidism. However, screening to detect a risk factor is only justified if a safe and effective therapy has been shown to reduce the risk for disease. If typical criteria are used, about four euthyroid patients would be followed or treated for every patient who develops overt hypothyroidism. If the strictest criteria are used, the chance of treating well patients is reduced, but only 7 per 1000 women screened would be candidates for treatment.

Thyroxine therapy in subclinical hypothyroidism has not been extensively evaluated, and the available evidence for a benefit is equivocal. In addition, even if therapy were effective, it would only benefit those patients who would later develop overt hypothyroidism and who had escaped detection by other means at that time. No study has examined the long-term risks of using thyroxine therapy for subclinical hypothyroidism, risks that might include osteoporosis. Given the evidence, screening for subclinical hypothyroidism is not recommended.

Case-Finding for Thyroid Disease

Case-Finding in General Clinics

Case-finding identifies disease in patients who visit their physicians for unrelated reasons. Why is there interest in case-finding for thyroid disease? Although patients with overt thyroid disease are symptomatic, the signs and symptoms may be subtle. Studies show that, in retrospect, patients detected by laboratory screening have clinical findings that suggest a thyroid disorder, but these findings did not lead clinicians to suspect the problem. In many patients, especially in elderly patients, symptoms may be nonspecific–mental clouding, poor appetite, constipation–and typical findings, such as a goiter, are usually absent. Thus, advocates of case-finding argue that broad indications for testing are needed because clinical findings are insensitive and not specific.

Studies of case-finding and office-based screening confirm these views (Table 4) (42-47). In one study, 2704 self-selected, healthy adults who responded to an offer for a multiphasic screening examination were screened for thyroid disease with FT4I tests (42). If a patient's FT4I level was low, a TSH was done; if high, a TT3 was done. Final diagnosis was made by a combination of clinical examination, test results, radioactive iodine uptake, response to therapy, and chart review 1 year later. In all, 25 patients (1%) had unsuspected overt thyroid disease. In retrospect, some of the 25 diagnosed patients had a nodular goiter (5) or typical symptoms, but these did not lead physicians to suspect the diagnosis.

Among women over 40 years of age in the same study, the rate of unsuspected hypothyroidism was 8 per 1000 and the rate of unsuspected hyperthyroidism was 9 per 1000. Case-finding was much less useful in other groups of patients. No cases were found among 492 men under 40 years of age. Rates for younger women and older men were intermediate. As would be expected from population studies, the prevalence of unsuspected thyroid disease and the potential benefit of case-finding are highest among women who are over 40 years of age.

Case-finding in general clinics detects patients who benefit from therapy. Nolan and colleagues (43) used the TT4 to screen for overt thyroid disease in 5002 outpatients and inpatients. If a patient's TT4 result was abnormal, a T3 resin uptake was done on the same specimen of serum. If a patient's FT4I level (TT4 × T3 resin uptake) was high, a TT3 was done; if low, a TSH was done. The prevalence of unsuspected overt disease was 6.6 per 1000 (26 patients with hypothyroidism and 7 with thyrotoxicosis). The 26 hypothyroid patients were treated with thyroxine. Of the thyrotoxic patients, 5 had goiters consistent with Graves disease, 1 had a toxic adenoma, and 1 had a self-limited subacute thyroiditis. Thus, 6 of these 7 patients also had a change in management as a result of the case-finding program. Two large prospective studies from Sweden document that patients detected in this manner obtain relief of symptoms and improved function from therapy (44, 45).

The yield of case-finding in these studies is not far below that found in patients who have thyroid function tests ordered because of mild symptoms (48). In one of these studies (42), the results of screening were compared with the yield of tests done by clinic physicians.

Table 4. *Studies of Case-Finding or Periodic Health Examination in Clinic Patients**

Study (Reference)	Number of Patients	Primary Screening Test
Health maintenance organization, Oakland, Calif. (42)	2704	FT4I
Private hospital and clinic, Mass. (43)	5002	TT4
Primary care center, Sweden (44)	2000	s-TSH
Outpatient clinic, large hospital, Sweden (45)	496	FT4
Private practice, Conn. (46)	1554	History and physical
Primary care center, Japan (47)	1114	FT4 or TT4

* FT4I = free thyroxine index; TT4 = total thyroxine; s-TSH = sensitive thyrotropin; FT4 = free thyroxine; NG = not given; and NA = not available.

† Patients with hyperthyroidism and hypothyroidism are combined to calculate the true-positive rate (sensitivity). Most studies use a specially calculated reference range to increase sensitivity.

Of 579 tests done in symptomatic patients, 13 patients (2%) had thyroid disease. By comparison, case-finding identifies disease in 0.5% to 1% of all patients and in 1% to 2% of women over 50 years of age. These data suggest that physicians have a low threshold for investigating thyroid dysfunction in clinic patients and that test performance in case-finding represents that found in actual practice.

Test Performance

When the reference range is adjusted appropriately for the patient population, the TT4, FT4I, FT4, and sensitive-TSH are highly sensitive screening tests for thyroid disease (*see* Table 4). In dos Remedios and colleagues' study (42), both the TT4 and FT4I were 100% sensitive (sensitivity defined as in Table 4). The studies of the FT4 (45) and sensitive-TSH (44) did not report sensitivity but, because both studies used a modified reference range, it is very likely that the sensitivity was close to 100%.

The four tests also have similar specificities. Specificity depends on the prevalence of conditions that cause misleading thyroid function test results. Among women attending general outpatient clinics, pregnancy, oral contraceptives, and estrogen therapy are the commonest conditions. Hypoalbuminemia and drugs, such as propranolol, phenytoin, and prednisone, are also fre-

Table 4. *(Continued)*

Test Performance		Prevalence, *n/1000*			
Sensitivity†	Specificity‡	Overtly Hyperthyroid		Overtly Hypothyroid	
		Men	Women	Men	Women
1.0	0.996	0	5	3	6
1.0§	0.906	0.5	2	5	5
NG	0.93‖	1¶	5	1	12
NG	0.92	NA	6	NA	10
NG	NG	0	8	3	5
NG	0.96	4	2	0	5

‡ Falsely elevated and falsely decreased test results are combined to calculate the false-positive rate (1 − specificity).
§ Estimated from initial study of 200 patients.
‖ Estimated after excluding patients receiving thyroxine.
¶ Assumes 1250 women and 750 men in population.

quently encountered. Familial dysalbuminemias and thyroid-binding globulin abnormalities occur in approximately 1% to 2% of the population. In dos Remedios and colleagues' study, the specificity of the TT4 was 98% and that of the FT4I was 99.6% when patients taking estrogens were excluded. Approximately 18% of women seen in their clinic took estrogens. If these women were included, the specificity of the TT4 would still be 95%. Nolan's study (43) included a higher proportion of patients who received drugs that affect thyroid function tests; in this study, the specificity of the TT4 was 91%. This figure is very close to the specificity of the FT4 and sensitive-TSH when they are used for case-finding (Table 4) (44, 45).

Cost and Efficiency

What is the best strategy for case-finding? Because the TT4, FT4I, FT4, and sensitive-TSH perform similarly as initial tests, it is reasonable to consider other factors, such as cost and convenience. The sensitive-TSH-based strategy is more expensive because of the costs of initial testing. Using the average prices listed in Table 1, the cost per case detected is $5000 for the sensitive-TSH, $3000 for the FT4I, and $2000 for the TT4 strategy.

The studies in Table 4 evaluate explicit, efficient strategies for acting on abnormal test results, including

Table 5. *Case-Finding in Patients Admitted to Geriatric Units**

Description of Patient Conditions (Reference)	Number of Patients
General disability, failure to thrive, mental slowing (49)	3417
Similar to above (50)	490
Apathy, depression, nonspecific symptoms, anemia, arthritis, and other medical problems (51)	2000
Geriatric assessment, hip fracture, rehabilitation (52)	229
Similar to above (one third of patients were transferred from acute care facility for rehabilitation) (53)	307
Geriatric assessment, some rehabilitation, medical problems (54)	125
Geriatric patients (55)	4780

* PBI = protein-bound iodine; T3 uptake = T3 resin uptake; TT4 = total thyroxine; FT4I = free thyroxine index; TT3 = total triiodothyronine; TSH = thyrotropin; and NA = not available.

careful examination and appropriate follow-up tests. For example, when the TT4 is the initial test, an abnormal result automatically prompts the laboratory to do the T3 resin uptake and additional tests when they are needed. Case-finding is less effective and more expensive when follow-up is haphazard. When a TT4 is included with a biochemical profile, physicians often ignore or repeat abnormal test results, or they order an inappropriate barrage of tests. In one study, 3606 routine biochemical profiles that included a TT4 determination were done. These tests identified 2 cases of thyrotoxicosis and 6 cases of hypothyroidism, for a total yield of 2.2 per 1000 patients tested (11). This yield is much lower than those of the studies reviewed above. When a TT4 is included in every biochemical profile, many patients with protein-binding abnormalities will be tested. Indiscriminate testing reduces the specificity of the TT4 and increases the number of follow-up tests, visits, and referrals without detecting more patients with disease.

Case-Finding in Geriatric Admissions

Case-finding has been studied among patients admitted to geriatric hospitals (49-56). The geriatric unit must be distinguished from the acute care medical ward or intensive care unit. In most geriatric units, patients are admitted for chronic disability, failure to thrive, mental

Table 5. *(Continued)*

Primary Screening Test	Response to Therapy Reported?	Prevalence, *n/1000*	
		Overtly Hyperthyroid	Overtly Hypothyroid
Clinical suspicion	Yes	5	17
PBI, T3 uptake	Yes	23	20
PBI, FT4I	Yes	NA	21
TT4, FT4I, TT3, TSH	Yes	30	26
FT4I	Yes	3	7
TSH, TT4, FT4I, TT3	No	8	94†
PBI	No	12	6

† Includes previously diagnosed patients and asymptomatic patients with elevated TSH and low FT4I levels (*see* text).

slowing or depression, psychosocial problems, or exacerbations of chronic diseases, such as rheumatoid arthritis or congestive heart failure. In most studies, from 30% to 50% of patients had suggestive symptoms of thyroid disease, and the remainder were at least sufficiently ill or debilitated to require hospital care.

The studies are summarized in Table 5. To confirm final diagnoses, most of these studies used the results of a trial of therapy (either thyroxine or antithyroid therapy). In these studies, the prevalence of overt thyroid disease was 20 to 40 cases per 1000 admissions. One study that did not report the results of treatment also appears to have a much higher prevalence of hypothyroidism than the others (54). In this study, 125 patients were screened. Hypothyroidism, defined as a TSH level over 10 mU/L with either a low FT4I level or clinical findings, was diagnosed in 11 patients. Of these, 3 patients were already receiving levothyroxine, 3 had clinical findings and isolated elevated TSH levels, and 3 had no clinical findings but had elevated TSH and low FT4I levels. If the patients with previously known hypothyroidism and no symptoms are excluded, the prevalence of unsuspected overt hypothyroidism is 4%. The results of other studies indicate that a trial of therapy would reduce this figure even further (37, 51).

Case-Finding in Acute Medical Admissions

All thyroid function tests may give misleading results in patients with acute medical illnesses (57, 58). Routine testing of medical ward admissions identifies few patients with true thyroid disease and even fewer who may benefit from treatment. Most studies identify unsuspected thyroid disease in fewer than 1% of hospitalized patients (45, 57-61). Higher estimates of the prevalence of thyroid disease among hospital admissions result from lax diagnostic criteria or from patients with suspected thyroid disease being included in the sample.

Testing hospital admissions is less efficient than case-finding in the clinic. In a direct comparison, the yield of case-finding in one medical ward was 0.8% of patients screened, whereas the yield in the general medical clinic of the same hospital was 1.8% (45). The lower yield is accompanied by added expense and confusion, because many patients have false-positive test results that mimic hypothyroidism and thyrotoxicosis. Mortality from other causes also limits the value of routine testing on admission (59, 61). In one study, for example, one case of thyrotoxicosis and nine cases of hypothyroidism were diagnosed among 425 elderly patients admitted to a county hospital (59). Three of the nine patients with hypothyroidism died during hospitalization. In another series, 10 of 945 persons admitted (1%) were diagnosed as hypothyroid; of these, 3 died within a few weeks from malignancy and another died from cancer after a few months (61).

There is no evidence that testing thyroid function on admission affects clinical management or outcomes during hospitalization. The reason is that diagnosis is not secure until acute illness has passed. Some acutely ill patients have elevated TSH and decreased FT4I or FT4 levels in the absence of thyroid disease (45, 62). Importantly, there is no way to distinguish patients with true hypothyroidism from others during hospitalization. In fact, no study has shown that patients identified by screening benefited from treatment during hospitalization.

Case-Finding in Other Groups

A recent National Institutes of Health Consensus Conference (63) recommended that thyroid tests be done in patients with a diagnosis of dementia. In the studies on which the recommendation is based, the prevalence of hypothyroidism ranged from 0% to 5% (64, 65). In all the studies combined, only 12 hypothyroid patients have been identified. We agree with a recent review that existing data on test performance, response to therapy, and the value of clinical findings are insufficient to estimate the benefits and costs of case-finding in this setting (64).

Case-finding has been studied among patients with depression (66-68), psychosis (69-74), and panic attacks (75, 76). Some depressed or psychotic patients have transient abnormalities in thyroid function tests that may be confused with thyrotoxicosis (66-74). Physicians cannot distinguish true thyroid disease from these abnormalities until such patients have been treated for some time (74). If patients taking lithium and those with clinical evidence of thyroid disease are excluded, the prevalence of thyroid dysfunction among psychiatric admissions is not clearly different from that among the general population (74). For these reasons, routine testing of all psychiatric admissions is not useful.

Case-finding has also been studied in postpartum patients (77-79) and in patients attending an obesity clinic (80). Postpartum screening reveals a 5% prevalence of symptomatic thyroid disease 6 or more months after delivery (77, 78). The prevalence may be much lower in some areas (79). In a large retrospective study, 6% of patients attending an obesity clinic had laboratory findings consistent with overt hypothyroidism (80). These applications of case-finding will not be discussed in this article.

Recommendations for Case-Finding

If tests are properly interpreted in light of the clinical findings, case-finding in women over 40 years of age can be useful. Up to 2% of these women may benefit. Since only patients with symptoms have been shown to benefit from case-finding, it is not necessary to test all patients who have no complaints and no evidence of thyroid dysfunction. The best candidates are women over 40 years of age who have one or more nonspecific complaints. Because the annual incidence of disease is much lower than the prevalence, repeated testing of the same patients is not useful. Case-finding is not useful in younger women or in men who have a very low prevalence of clinically unsuspected thyroid disease.

These recommendations are based on studies that evaluated a clinical laboratory algorithm that triggers confirmatory tests and examinations without waiting for physicians to order them (42-45). In contrast, including the TT4 in screening biochemical profiles without a specific plan for action is not useful. In practice, abnormal results are often ignored, or they prompt excessive investigations. Patients with conditions that cause misleading results are tested, reducing the efficiency of

testing. In our view, testing that is not part of an organized, laboratory-based effort is not case-finding and is
not helpful. The TT4, FT4I, FT4, or sensitive-TSH can
be used as the initial test; at current prices, the sensitive-TSH is much less cost-effective than the other
choices.

The prevalence of thyroid disease (mostly hypothyroidism) appears to be between 1% and 4% among
elderly patients admitted to specialized geriatric units.
Compared with elderly inpatients in acute medicine
wards, these patients have a higher prevalence of
vague, chronic, unexplained disability and depression or
mental clouding (49-56). Most studies of geriatric admissions were done using outdated diagnostic tests and
criteria. Nevertheless, it is reasonable to obtain a FT4I
when a patient is admitted for one of these reasons.

Screening is not indicated for patients admitted with
acute medical or psychiatric illnesses, because transient
abnormalities are indistinguishable from true thyroid
disease. In these settings, testing is only useful if there
is clinical suspicion of thyroid disease. Studies that define asymptomatic patients with biochemical abnormalities as diseased have not shown that these patients
benefit from identification and treatment.

References

1. **Tunbridge WM, Evered DC, Hall R, et al.** The spectrum of thyroid disease in a community: the Whickham survey. *Clin Endocrinol (Oxf).* 1977;**7**:481-93.
2. **Falkenberg M, Kågedal B, Norr A.** Screening of an elderly female population for hypo- and hyperthyroidism by use of a thyroid hormone panel. *Acta Med Scand.* 1983;**214**:361-5.
3. American Academy of Pediatrics, American Thyroid Association: newborn screening for congenital hypothyroidism: recommended guidelines. *Pediatrics.* 1987;**80**:745-9.
4. **Fisher DA.** Effectiveness of newborn screening programs for congenital hypothyroidism: prevalence of missed cases. *Pediatr Clin North Am.* 1987;**34**:881-90.
5. **Schoen EJ, dos Remedios LV, Backstrom M.** Heterogeneity of congenital primary hypothyroidism: the importance of thyroid scintigraphy. *J Perinat Med.* 1987;**15**:137-42.
6. Early diagnosis. In: **Sackett DL, Haynes RB, Tugwell P.** *Clinical Epidemiology: A Basic Science for Clinical Medicine.* Boston: Little, Brown and Co.; 1985;139-55.
7. **Greenlick MR, Bailey JW, Wild J, Grover J.** The characteristics of men most likely to respond to an invitation to be screened. In: Greenlick MR, Freeborn DK, Pope CR, eds. *Health Care Research in an HMO: Two Decades of Discovery.* Baltimore: Johns Hopkins University Press; 1988:131-7.
8. **Fink R, Shapiro S, Roester R.** Impact of efforts to increase participation in repetitive screenings for early breast cancer detection. *Am J Public Health.* 1972;**62**:328-36.
9. **Canadian Task Force on the Periodic Health Examination.** The periodic health examination. *Can Med Assoc J.* 1979;**121**:1193-254.
10. **Shimaoka K, Bakri K, Sciascia M, et al.** Thyroid screening program; follow-up evaluation. *N Y State J Med.* 1982;**82**:1184-7.
11. **Epstein KA, Schneiderman LJ, Bush JW, Zettner A.** The "abnor-

mal'' screening thyroxine (T4): analysis of physician response, outcome, cost and health effectiveness. *J Chronic Dis.* 1981;**34:**175-90.

12. **Bastenie PA, Bonnyns M, Neve P, Vanhaelst L, Chailly M.** Clinical and pathological significance of atrophic thyroiditis. A condition of latent hypothyroidism. *Lancet.* 1967;**1:**915-8.

13. **Goudie RB, Anderson JR, Gray KG.** Complement-fixing antithyroid antibodies in hospital patients with asymptomatic thyroid lesions. *J Path Bacteriol.* 1959;**77:**389-400.

14. **Blumenthal HT, Perlstein IB.** The aging thyroid. I. A description of lesions and an analysis of their age and sex distribution. *J Am Geriatr Soc.* 1987;**35:**843-54.

15. **Couchman KG, Wigley RD, Prior IA.** Autoantibodies in the Carterton population survey. The prevalence of thyroid and gastric antibodies, antinuclear, and rheumatoid factors in a probability based population sample. *J Chronic Dis.* 1970;**23:**45-53.

16. **Hawkins BR, Cheah PS, Dawkins RL, et al.** Diagnostic significance of thyroid microsomal antibodies in randomly selected population. *Lancet.* 1980;**2:**1057-9.

17. **Lazarus JH, Burr ML, McGregor AM, et al.** The prevalence and progression of autoimmune thyroid disease in the elderly. *Acta Endocrinol (Copenh).* 1984;**106:**199-202.

18. **Evered DC, Ormston BJ, Smith PA, Hall R, Bird T.** Grades of hypothyroidism. *Br Med J.* 1973;**1:**657-62.

19. **Kågedal B, Månson JC, Norr A, Sorbo B, Tegler L.** Screening for thyroid disorders in middle-aged women by computer-assisted evaluation of a thyroid hormone panel. *Scand J Clin Lab Invest.* 1981; **41:**403-8.

20. **Nyström E, Bengtsson C, Lindquist O, Noppa H, Lindstedt G, Lundberg PA.** Thyroid disease and high concentration of serum thyrotrophin in a population sample of women. A 4-year follow-up. *Acta Med Scand.* 1981;**210:**39-46.

21. **Nyström E, Bengtsson C, Lindquist O, Lindberg S, Lindstedt G, Lundberg PA.** Serum triiodothyronine and hyperthyroidism in a population sample of women. *Clin Endocrinol (Oxf).* 1984;**20:**31-42.

22. **Campbell AJ, Reinken J, Allan BC.** Thyroid disease in the elderly in the community. *Age Ageing.* 1981;**10:**47-52.

23. **Okamura K, Ueda K, Sone H, et al.** A sensitive thyroid stimulating hormone assay for screening of thyroid functional disorder in elderly Japanese. *J Am Geriatr Soc.* 1989;**37:**317-22.

24. **Brochmann H, Bjøro T, Gaarder PI, Hanson F, Frey HM.** Prevalence of thyroid dysfunction in elderly subjects. A randomized study in a Norwegian rural community (Naerøy). *Acta Endocrin (Copenh).* 1988;**117:**7-12.

25. **Hodkinson HM, Denham MJ.** Thyroid function tests in the elderly in the community. *Age Ageing.* 1977;**6:**67-70.

26. **Sawin CT, Castelli WP, Hershman JM, McNamara P, Bacharach P.** The aging thyroid. Thyroid deficiency in the Framingham Study. *Arch Intern Med.* 1985;**145:**1386-8.

27. **Sawin CT, Chopra D, Azizi F, Mannix J, Bacharach P.** The aging thyroid. Increased prevalence of elevated serum thyrotropin levels in the elderly. *JAMA.* 1979;**242:**247-50.

28. **Furszyfer J, Kurland LT, McConahey WM, Elveback LR.** Graves' disease in Olmsted County, Minnesota, 1935 through 1967. *Mayo Clin Proc.* 1970;**45:**636-44.

29. **Barker DP, Phillips DI.** Current incidence of thyrotoxicosis and past prevalence of goitre in 12 British towns. *Lancet.* 1984;**2:**567-70.

30. **Falkenberg M, Kågedal B.** Hyperthyroidism in elderly women. Registered and detected by screening in a primary health care district. *Scand J Prim Health Care.* 1985;**3:**11-3.

31. **Tunbridge WM, Brewis M, French JM, et al.** Natural history of autoimmune thyroiditis. *Br Med J [Clin Res].* 1981;**282:**258-62.

32. **Gordin A, Lamberg BA.** Spontaneous hypothyroidism in symptomless autoimmune thyroiditis. A long-term follow-up study. *Clin Endocrinol (Oxf).* 1981;**15:**537-43.

33. **Salabè G, Salabè HL, Urbinati G, et al.** A longitudinal study of thyroid autoimmunity and subclinical hypothyroidism in a random population of central Italy. In: Walfish PG, Wall JR, Volpe R, eds. *Autoimmunity and the Thyroid.* Orlando, Florida: Academic Press; 1985:317-8.

34. **Rosenthal MJ, Hunt WC, Garry PJ, Goodwin JS.** Thyroid failure in the elderly. Microsomal antibodies as discriminant for therapy. *JAMA.* 1987;**258**:209-13.
35. **Althaus BU, Staub JJ, Ryff-de-Lèche A, Oberhänsli A, Stähelin HB.** LDL/HDL-changes in subclinical hypothyroidism: possible risk factors for coronary heart disease. *Clin Endocrinol (Oxf).* 1988;**28**:157-63.
36. **Tibaldi J, Barzel US.** Thyroxine supplementation. Method for the prevention of clinical hypothyroidism. *Am J Med.* 1985;**79**:241-4.
37. **Cooper DS, Halpern R, Wood LC, Levin AA, Ridgway EC.** L-Thyroxine therapy in subclinical hypothyroidism. A double-blind, placebo-controlled trial. *Ann Intern Med.* 1984;**101**:18-24.
38. **Bell GM, Todd WT, Forfar JC, et al.** End-organ responses to thyroxine therapy in subclinical hypothyroidism. *Clin Endocrinol (Oxf).* 1985;**22**:83-9.
39. **Ridgway EC, Cooper DS, Walker H, Rodbard D, Maloof F.** Peripheral responses to thyroid hormone before and after L-thyroxine therapy in patients with subclinical hypothyroidism. *J Clin Endocrinol Metab.* 1981;**53**:1238-42.
40. **Nyström E, Caidahl K, Fager G, Wikkelso C, Lundberg PA, Lindstedt G.** A double-blind cross-over 12-month study of L-thyroxine treatment of women with "subclinical" hypothyroidism. *Clin Endocrinol (Oxf).* 1988;**29**:63-75.
41. **Edén S, Sundbeck G, Lindstedt G, et al.** Screening for thyroid disease in the elderly. Serum concentrations of thyrotropin and 3,5,3'-triiodothyronine in a representative population of 79-year-old women and men. *Compr Gerontol [A].* 1988;**2**:40-5.
42. **dos Remedios LV, Weber PM, Feldman R, Schurr DA, Tsoi TG.** Detecting unsuspected thyroid dysfunction by the free thyroxine index. *Arch Intern Med.* 1980;**140**:1045-9.
43. **Nolan JP, Tarsa NJ, DiBenedetto G.** Case-finding for unsuspected thyroid disease: costs and health benefits. *Am J Clin Pathol.* 1985;**83**:346-55.
44. **Eggertsen R, Peterson K, Lundberg PA, Nyström E, Lindstedt G.** Screening for thyroid disease in a primary care unit with a thyroid stimulating hormone assay with a low detection limit. *Br Med J [Clin Res].* 1988;**297**:1586-92.
45. **Nyström E, Peterson K, Lindstedt G, Lundberg PA.** Screening for thyroid disease in women greater than or equal to 50 years of age seeking hospital care: influence of common nonthyroidal illness on serum free thyroxin as determined by analog radioimmunoassay. *Clin Chem.* 1986;**32**:603-8.
46. **Baldwin DB, Rowett D.** Incidence of thyroid disorders in Connecticut. *JAMA.* 1978;**239**:742-4.
47. **Fukazawa H, Sakurada T, Yoshida K, et al.** Free thyroxine estimation for the screening of hyper- and hypothyroidism in an adult population. *Tohoku J Exp Med.* 1986;**148**:411-20.
48. **Schectman JM, Kallenberg GA, Shumacher RJ, Hirsch RP.** Yield of hypothyroidism in symptomatic primary care patients. *Arch Intern Med.* 1989;**149**:861-4.
49. **Lloyd WH, Goldberg IJ.** Incidence of hypothyroidism in the elderly. *Br Med J [Clin Res].* 1961;1256-9.
50. **Jefferys PM, Farran HE, Hoffenberg R, Fraser PM, Hodkinson HM.** Thyroid-function tests in the elderly. *Lancet.* 1972;**1**:924-7.
51. **Bahemuka M, Hodkinson HM.** Screening for hypothyroidism in elderly inpatients. *Br Med J [Clin Res].* 1975;**2**:601-3.
52. **Palmer KT.** A prospective study into thyroid disease in a geriatric unit. *N Z Med J.* 1977;**86**:323-4.
53. **Scott MA, Kidd BL, Croxson MS, Evans MC.** Admission thyroid function testing in elderly patients. *Aust N Z J Med.* 1986;**16**:699-702.
54. **Livingston EH, Hershman JM, Sawin CT, Yoshikawa TT.** Prevalence of thyroid disease and abnormal thyroid tests in older hospitalized and ambulatory persons. *J Am Geriatr Soc.* 1987;**35**:109-14.
55. **Jussila MT, Kaarela RH, Heikinheimo RJ.** Screening of thyroid disease in the hospitalized aged. *Arch Gerontol Geriatr.* 1987;**6**:117-21.
56. **Byrne E, Gilmore DH, Beringer TR.** Thyroid screening in elderly hospital patients. *Ulster Med J.* 1988;**57**:80-4.

57. **Kaplan MM, Larsen PR, Crantz FR, Dzau VJ, Rossing TH, Haddow JE.** Prevalence of abnormal thyroid function test results in patients with acute medical illnesses. *Am J Med.* 1982;**72**:9-16.
58. **Spencer C, Eigen A, Shen D, et al.** Specificity of sensitive assays of thyrotropin (TSH) used to screen for thyroid disease in hospitalized patients. *Clin Chem.* 1987;**33**:1391-6.
59. **Atkinson RL, Dahms WT, Fisher DA, Nichols AL.** Occult thyroid disease in an elderly hospitalized population. *J Gerontol.* 1978; **33**:372-6.
60. **Montoro M, Guttler RB, Spencer CA, Kaptein EM, Nicoloff JT.** Adult thyroid screening in hospitalized patients. *Clin Res.* 1981; **29**:39A.
61. **Riniker M, Tieche M, Lupi GA, Grob P, Studer H, Burgi H.** Prevalence of various degrees of hypothyroidism among patients of a general medical department. *Clin Endocrinol (Oxf).* 1981;**14**:69-74.
62. **Helfand M, Crapo LM.** Testing for suspected thyroid disease. In: Sox HC Jr., ed. *Common Diagnostic Tests.* 2d edition. Philadelphia: American College of Physicians; 1990:148-81.
63. **Consensus Conference.** Differential diagnosis of dementing diseases. *JAMA.* 1987;**258**:3411-6.
64. **Barry PP, Moskowitz MA.** The diagnosis of reversible dementia in the elderly. A critical review. *Arch Intern Med.* 1988;**148**:1914-8.
65. **Larson EB, Reifler BV, Sumi SM, Canfield CG, Chinn NM.** Diagnostic tests in the evaluation of dementia. A prospective study of 200 elderly outpatients. *Arch Intern Med.* 1986;**146**:1917-22.
66. **Gold MS, Pottash AL, Extein I.** Hypothyroidism and depression. Evidence from complete thyroid function evaluation. *JAMA.* 1981; **245**:1919-22.
67. **Kirkegaard C, Faber J.** Altered serum levels of thyroxine, triiodothyronines, and diiodothyronines in endogeneous depression. *Acta Endocrinol (Copenh).* 1981;**96**:199-207.
68. **Sweer L, Martin DC, Ladd RA, Miller JK, Karpf M.** The medical evaluation of elderly patients with major depression. *J Gerontol.* 1988;**43**:M53-8.
69. **Caplan RH, Pagliara AS, Wickus G, Goodlund LS.** Elevation of the free thyroxine index in psychiatric patients. *J Psychiatr Res.* 1983; **17**:267-74.
70. **Spratt DI, Pont A, Miller MB, McDougall IR, Bayer MF, McLaughlin WT.** Hyperthyroxinemia in patients with acute psychiatric disorders. *Am J Med.* 1982;**73**:41-8.
71. **Lambert TJ, Davidson R, McLellan GH.** Euthyroid hyperthyroxinaemia in acute psychiatric admissions. *Aust N Z J Psychiatry.* 1987;**21**:608-12.
72. **McLarty DG, Ratcliffe WA, Ratcliffe JG, Shimmins JG, Goldberg A.** A study of thyroid function in psychiatric in-patients. *Br J Psychiatry.* 1978;**133**:211-8.
73. **Checkley SA.** Thyrotoxicosis and the course of manic-depressive illness. *Br J Psychiatry.* 1978;**133**:219-23.
74. **Bannister P, Mortimer A, Shapiro L, Simms AC.** Thyroid function screening of psychiatric inpatient admissions: a worthwhile procedure? *J R Soc Med.* 1987;**80**:77-8.
75. **Fishman SM, Sheehan DV, Carr DB.** Thyroid indices in panic disorder. *J Clin Psychiatry.* 1985;**46**:432-3.
76. **Lesser IM, Rubin RT, Lydiard RB, Swinson R, Pecknold J.** Past and current thyroid function in subjects with panic disorder. *J Clin Psychiatry.* 1987;**48**:473-6.
77. **Hayslip CC, Fein HG, O'Donnell VM, Friedman DS, Klein TA, Smallridge RC.** The value of serum antimicrosomal antibody testing in screening for symptomatic postpartum thyroid dysfunction. *Am J Obstet Gynecol.* 1988;**159**:203-9.
78. **Nikolai TF, Turney SL, Roberts RC.** Postpartum lymphocytic thyroiditis. Prevalence, clinical course, and long-term follow-up. *Arch Intern Med.* 1987;**147**:221-4.
79. **Freeman R, Rosen H, Thysen B.** Incidence of thyroid dysfunction in an unselected postpartum population. *Arch Intern Med.* 1986;**146**: 1361-4.
80. **Lima N, Cavaliere H, Medeiros-Neto G.** Communications: a retrospective study of thyroid autoimmunity and hypothyroidism in a random obese population. *Medical Science Research.* 1987;**15**:31-2.

Screening for Osteoporosis

L. JOSEPH MELTON III, MD; DAVID M. EDDY, MD, PhD; and C. CONRAD JOHNSTON, Jr., MD

Osteoporosis, the commonest metabolic bone disorder, is characterized by a reduction in bone mass that compromises the biomechanical integrity of the skeleton and leads to an increased risk for fractures. Fractures of the proximal femur (hip), vertebrae (spine), and distal forearm (Colles) are often linked with osteoporosis; however, because bone is lost throughout the skeleton, osteoporosis results in fractures at other skeletal sites as well. At least 1.3 million fractures in the United States each year are attributable to osteoporosis, including roughly 250 000 hip, 250 000 wrist, and 500 000 vertebral fractures (1, 2). This large number of fractures and the disability that is often associated with fracture (3) make osteoporosis an enormous public health problem as well as a difficult patient management issue. The national cost of osteoporosis was estimated at $6.1 billion in 1984 (4) and will rise because fracture rates increase with age, and the elderly population is growing rapidly. In 30 years, there may be 350 000 hip fractures each year in the United States, at an annual cost of between $31 and $62 billion (5).

Because any substantial reduction in these costs depends on preventing fractures rather than improving the treatment of patients with fractures, virtually every assessment of the problem has concluded that the impact of osteoporosis is sufficient to justify prophylaxis if a suitable program could be defined. Preventive efforts might be directed at falls, the usual source of trauma, but no specific intervention has been widely effective (6). Consequently, interest has centered on preventing excessive bone loss. We review the evidence on the clinical utility of screening for osteoporosis to preserve bone mass and reduce the incidence of associated fractures.

Bone Loss and Fractures

Bone is removed and replaced throughout life at spe-

▶ This chapter was originally published in *Annals of Internal Medicine*. 1990;**112**:516-28.

cific foci called bone remodeling units (7). In young adults, the two processes are closely coupled: Bone resorption is matched by bone formation, and bone mass increases or at least remains constant. With aging, however, bone formation does not keep pace with resorption, and bone mass is gradually lost throughout the skeleton. Due to its greater surface area, trabecular (or cancellous) bone in the vertebrae, limb metaphyses, pelvis, and other flat bones has a higher remodeling rate. More trabecular than cortical (or compact) bone, which makes up about 80% of the skeleton, may be lost. In either type of bone, a decline in bone mass results in a disproportionately greater decrease in bone strength (8, 9). This decrease in strength is especially dramatic in trabecular bone; halving the cross-sectional area of a vertical trabecular column reduces its load-carrying capacity by 75%, as does doubling the effective length of the column through loss of horizontal support trabeculae. Thinning and loss of trabeculae both occur with aging (Figure 1).

The biomechanical effects of age-related bone loss are partially compensated for by modeling of the shafts of long bones (through endosteal resorption and periosteal apposition) to increase the diameter and, thus, increase resistance to bending and torsion (8). However, this process is less marked at the ends of limb bones and in the vertebrae, where fractures typically associated with osteoporosis occur. Strength may also be compromised by age-related impairments in bone quality, including decreased elasticity of the collagen matrix of bone, creation of local stress risers by large apatite crystals and other geometric defects, increased fragility of hypermineralized old bone, and reduced repair of microfractures (9). Although bone architecture and quality are important determinants of bone strength, neither can be accurately quantified in vivo with non-invasive techniques.

Because bone mass accounts for 75% to 85% of the variance in ultimate strength of bone tissue (9), bone mineral density should be related to fracture risk in patients; evidence supports this hypothesis. Population-based studies have shown a gradient of continuously increasing hip fracture incidence associated with declining bone mineral density in the proximal femur (10), rising Colles fracture incidence with decreasing bone mass in the radius (11, 12), and increasing vertebral fracture incidence (13) and prevalence (14) with falling bone density in the lumbar spine. Trauma is also important, of course, because falling increases the chance for fracture at any given level of bone mass

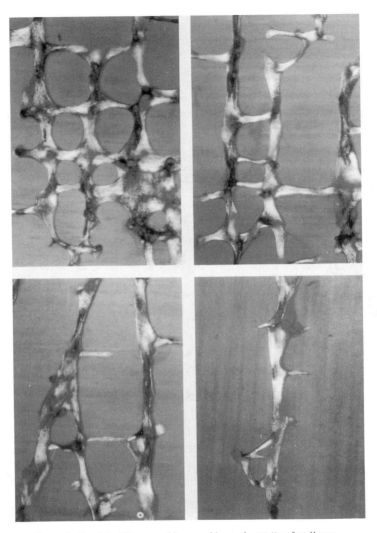

Figure 1. Top left. Fifty-year-old man with an almost "perfect," continuous trabecular network (vertical trabeculae, yellow; horizontal, blue-green). **Top right.** Fifty-eight-year-old man with discernible thinning of the horizontal trabeculae and some loss of continuity. **Bottom left.** Seventy-six-year-old man with a continued thinning of the horizontal trabeculae and a wider separation of the vertical structures. **Bottom right.** Eighty-seven-year-old woman with advanced breakdown of the whole network showing unsupported vertical trabeculae. (Reprinted with permission from *Bone* (New York), **Mosekilde LI.** Age-related changes in vertebral trabecular bone architecture—assessed by a new method. 1988;**9:**247-50. Pergamon Press.)

(15) as does inability to dissipate the kinetic energy produced by a fall (16, 17). The pathophysiology of falling is not well understood, however, and many of the risk factors that have been recognized, such as gait and balance disorders, diminished reflexes and strength, and reduced vision (18), are difficult to correct. Fortunately, only about 6% of falls result in fractures and only 1%, in hip fractures (19).

Diagnosis of Osteoporosis

Although fundamentally a histologic diagnosis (a reduced amount of normally mineralized bone), osteoporosis is manifested clinically as fractures and, on non-invasive imaging tests, as low bone mass (osteopenia). Once bone mass has decreased to the point where fractures begin to occur, however, therapeutic options are limited. Generally accepted treatments for osteoporosis (estrogen, calcium, and calcitonin) reduce bone resorption (20); these agents may maintain existing bone mass but cannot increase it substantially. As a consequence, interest has shifted from treating patients with fractures to preventing fractures by preserving bone mass. We need a test that predicts the incidence of fractures (fracture risk) in individual patients so that intervention can be initiated before irreversible bone loss has occurred.

Because the risk for fracture increases with decreasing bone mass (Figure 2), predicting fracture risk may be done with several bone mass measurement techniques. However, no sharp dividing line for bone density separates persons at high risk for fracture from others; thus, the definition of an "abnormal" bone mass for screening purposes must be based on clinical criteria such as the threshold for treatment decisions. Several different criteria have been proposed. Because age-related fractures are uncommon until bone mass falls substantially below the peak levels seen in young adults, it has been suggested that the diagnosis of osteopenia be established by a "fracture threshold," based on either the distribution of bone mineral density in young normal persons (2 SDs below the mean [21]) or the distribution among patients with fractures (90th percentile [22] or 65th percentile [23]). This approach does not permit patients with fractures to be discriminated from age- and sex-matched controls (Figure 2); however, discrimination is not necessary, because bone mass measurements are not intended as a diagnostic test for fractures (24). Indeed, serum cholesterol tests do not discriminate between

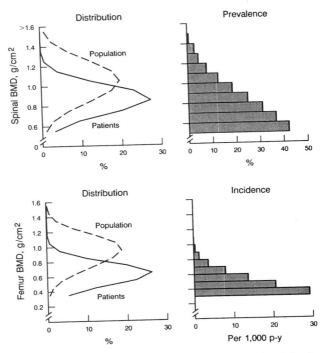

Figure 2. Comparison of the distribution of spinal bone mineral density (*BMD*) of patients with vertebral fracture and controls with vertebral fracture prevalence and the distribution of hip BMD of patients with intertrochanteric hip fracture and controls compared with hip fracture incidence by BMD among women from Rochester, Minnesota.

men with and without coronary heart disease; the distribution of cholesterol values in these two groups is almost identical (25). Nor is the distribution of blood pressure very different between stroke patients and controls (Melton LJ III. Unpublished data). However, all three measurements (bone mass, cholesterol, and blood pressure) predict adverse health outcomes.

Bone mass measurement is the only way to stratify patients by fracture risk. Roentgenograms are needed for diagnosing fractures, but the roentgenographic appearance of the skeleton is an unreliable guide to bone mass (26, 27). Osteoporosis does not consistently cause metabolic abnormalities that can be detected with standard laboratory tests, and there is no evidence that new measurements, such as measurements of bone Gla protein, can predict fracture risk. Although it is generally believed that osteoporosis-prone persons can be identified through common clinical observations (28, 29), several studies have shown that no item from an individual patient's history or physical examination is an accurate predictor of bone mass (30-36) or fractures (37). The risk factors that have been identified account for only about a third of the variability in bone mass and are not precise enough for stratifying patients (38). Further, no unique set of risk factors is consistently found in all studies. Thus, if the prevailing level of bone mass is pertinent to treatment decisions, it must be measured directly rather than estimated indirectly.

Nonetheless, the use of bone mineral density measurements to establish a diagnosis of osteopenia in the absence of fracture is complicated by several factors. First, gradual loss of bone mass occurs in almost everyone, and some find it philosophically distasteful to label such a condition a disease. If intervention can improve health outcomes, however, this objection seems irrelevant. Second, because bone loss at various skeletal sites occurs at different rates (39), one of a patient's bones might be considered osteoporotic and another not. Furthermore, measurement of bone mass at one site (for example, the midradius) does not accurately predict bone mass at another (for example, the proximal femur or spine), though there is clearly a correlation between sites (40). Finally, the availability of many techniques for measuring bone mass makes standardization difficult. Despite these theoretical concerns, recent prospective studies have shown that bone mass measurements made with various techniques and at various skeletal sites can identify persons at the greatest risk for fracture and who should benefit most from therapy.

Screening Tests for Osteopenia

Many different techniques have been used to assess bone mass. The most widely available, accurate, and precise methods are single-photon absorptiometry, dual-photon absorptiometry, and quantitative computed tomography. These methods have been the subject of numerous recent reviews (38, 41-45); we summarize only those aspects especially pertinent to screening and discuss the newest modality, dual-energy x-ray absorptiometry (45-47). Other technologies are available, including neutron activation analysis, Compton scattering, radiogrammetry, radiographic densitometry, and several ultrasound techniques, but these methods are less well developed in clinical practice, and we do not consider them further.

Single-Photon Absorptiometry

This widely used technique involves passing a highly collimated monoenergetic beam of photons (using ^{125}I as the source) across a limb and monitoring the transmitted radiation with a sodium iodide scintillation detector. Differential photon absorption between bone and soft tissue allows calculation of total bone mineral content in the path of the beam, measured as grams per centimeter. Limited to peripheral sites like the radius or os calcis, this technique cannot measure bone density in the hip or spine, nor can it discriminate between cortical and trabecular bone.

The accuracy error (ability of the measurement to reflect the true bone mass value) of single-photon absorptiometry is approximately 4% to 5%, and the precision error (reproducibility of the value upon repeat measurement) of the latest technology, rectilinear single-photon absorptiometry, is approximately 1% to 2% in clinical settings. Patient acceptance is very good and scan times are relatively short; for a typical examination, the patient sits for approximately 10 to 20 minutes. The radiation dose is low (20 to 100 μSv), with a negligible whole-body dose. Charges per scan range from $35 to $120.

Dual-Photon Absorptiometry

This technique emits photons at two different energies (using [153]Gd as the source), permitting direct measurement of bone mineral density (area density in grams per square centimeter) in the proximal femur and lumbar spine. However, dual-photon absorptiometry cannot distinguish between cortical and trabecular bone at those sites. The accuracy error of dual-photon absorptiometry is approximately 3% to 6% for the spine and 3% to 4% for the femoral neck, and the estimated precision error is approximately 2% to 4% for measurements of the lumbar spine and approximately 4% for the femoral neck. Patient acceptance is good, but rectilinear scanning times are long, varying from 20 or more minutes for regional measurements to approximately 60 minutes for total body measurement. A regional scan entails only 50 μSv exposure, although use of spine films to rule out fractured vertebrae increases the radiation dose substantially. Charges for dual-photon absorptiometry vary widely but usually exceed $100.

Dual-Energy X-ray Absorptiometry

In this new absorptiometry technique, an x-ray source

highest quartile, whereas women in the lowest quartile for spinal bone mass were at 3 times greater risk. For vertebral fractures alone, women in the lowest quartile of spinal bone mass had almost a 14 times greater risk.

Preliminary data have also been reported from a new, multicenter, prospective study of 9704 nonblack women 65 or more years of age. Single-photon absorptiometry of the proximal radius, ultradistal radius, and os calcis predicted wrist, humerus, and hip fractures in this population over a mean follow-up of 1.6 years. Each standard deviation decrement of bone mineral density in the ultradistal radius was associated with a 1.9-fold increase in wrist fractures, a 2.7-fold increase in humerus fractures (53), and a 1.6-fold increase in hip fractures (54), even after adjusting for age. One-third of the hip fractures occurred in women whose bone mass was in the lowest decile for their age.

While bone mass measurements of the radius and os calcis predict fracture risk, hip fractures are more strongly associated with bone mass in the proximal femur than in the radius (22, 55), and vertebral fractures are more closely associated with bone mass in the spine (22, 56, 57). Consequently, the bone mass measurements that are now possible in the spine and hip may have even greater predictive accuracy for fractures at these sites. Although the relatively recent introduction of hip measurements has precluded long-term follow-up studies until now, theoretical models indicate that such measurements will predict lifetime hip fracture risk (15, 58). In short, there is very good evidence that bone mass measurements can stratify patients according to their risk for fractures of all types.

Do Risk Categories Determine Treatment Strategies?

Specific treatment regimens are available for using estrogen, calcium, and calcitonin (20) as well as various investigational drugs to treat osteopenia and prevent fractures. The first issue is at what point should treatment be started; however, no universally accepted protocol specifies the degree of osteopenia or the level of fracture risk at which treatment should be initiated. At present, this decision is made on an individual basis by physicians and patients. The lack of generally accepted guidelines is the weakest link in the chain of inference that osteoporosis screening would effectively reduce fracture incidence (59). Before a population-wide program of mass screening of asymptomatic women can be recommended, specific screening protocols must be defined. These protocols must include acceptable approaches to the screening itself as well as treatment guidelines for persons in different fracture-risk categories as determined by screening. A formal assessment of the costs and potential benefits of various screening strategies would also be appropriate.

The use of these treatments for reasons unrelated to bone mass is another issue. Long-term estrogen replacement therapy, for example, is the most effective means to reduce bone loss and minimize subsequent fracture incidence (*see* below) but has other potential benefits as well (60). Because estrogen replacement therapy entails risks and costs, it should be used only for women who are most likely to benefit; thus, bone mass measurements may play an important role in deciding on this therapy. For some women, however, prevention of bone loss and fractures might not be the major determinant of estrogen use. Indeed, estrogens are most commonly prescribed for menopausal symptoms, primarily hot flashes. About one-third of postmenopausal women are given estrogen replacement therapy for this purpose (61, 62). However, most of this use is short-term and relatively ineffective in preventing bone loss and fractures.

This situation could change dramatically if estrogen is shown to have a beneficial effect on cardiovascular disease (63, 64). Most studies, including two population-based cohort studies (65, 66), but not a third (62), have found a decreased risk for cardiovascular disease in unopposed estrogen users. However, the addition of progestins to reduce the risk for endometrial cancer and other adverse gynecologic sequelae (60, 67) could conceivably negate the cardioprotective effects of estrogen alone (63, 64). Moreover, there is the possibility of an increased risk for breast cancer with hormone replacement therapy (64, 68), though the increase appears relatively small and has not been found in all studies (69). Although the potential benefits of heart disease prevention would be greater than the benefits of fracture reduction, prevention of heart disease is not yet an approved indication for estrogen replacement therapy, and many unanswered questions remain.

Bone mass measurements will not affect treatment decisions if a woman is going to receive long-term estrogen replacement therapy for reasons other than bone loss prevention, such as for menopausal symptoms or to prevent cardiovascular disease. At present, however, only about 15% of estrogen-treated women (70, 71) or about 5% of all postmenopausal women get long-term estrogen replacement therapy (10 or more years) for reasons unrelated to osteoporosis, therapy that is, consequently, unaffected by bone mass measurements.

Does Treatment Reduce Bone Loss and Fracture Incidence?

Several treatments have been proposed to reduce bone loss and prevent fractures from osteoporosis. Of these treatments, the evidence best supports estrogen replacement therapy. Many trials (72-89) have compared estrogens with placebos and other treatments, and nearly all indicate that estrogens are effective in maintaining bone mass. For example, in one randomized, controlled trial (73) of three groups of patients followed from 6 weeks, 3 years, or 6 years after oophorectomy, estrogen therapy retarded bone loss for up to 10 years. Such results (90) are independent of the duration of ovarian insufficiency preceding the onset of treatment, and recent data (91) suggest that estrogen replacement therapy may be effective in slowing bone loss until age 70, although questions remain about the persistence of this effect. Because treatment slows the rate of bone loss, however, greater benefits are achieved with earlier treatment because bone mass is maintained at a higher level.

Of even greater importance in the context of screening is the effectiveness of estrogens in preventing fractures. The only randomized, controlled trial (79) showed that only 4% of oophorectomized women receiving estrogen lost height compared with 38% of women not on treatment. Almost 90% of the group not on treatment and with height loss had evidence of vertebral fractures. Moreover, five women in the placebo group had vertebral crush fractures compared with only one in the treatment group. A larger non-randomized study (92) of postmenopausal estrogen use suggested a 50% reduction in osteoporotic fracture incidence, with the greatest effect in the spine. Estrogen-treated women had fewer vertebral crush fractures than untreated women (2.5% compared with 6.6%) and fewer multiple compression fractures (1.2% compared with 2.9%). Similarly, a retrospective cohort study (93) showed a 35% reduction in hip fracture risk among women who had ever taken postmenopausal estrogens.

Randomized trials of estrogen replacement therapy for hip fracture prevention are unfeasible, but case-control studies consistently show a reduction in the incidence of hip and Colles fractures that is associated with long-term estrogen use. Hutchinson and colleagues (94) found a 30% reduction in the risk for hip or Colles fracture among hospitalized women who had documented, conjugated estrogen use for at least 6 months after menopause; the reduction was 60% in women given estrogen within 5 years of menopause. A comparable reduction in risk was seen in King County, Washington, in women from 50 to 74 years of age with hip or Colles fractures who took postmenopausal estrogen for 6 or more years compared with women who did not use estrogen (95). The risk for hip fracture was reduced about 30% for Kaiser Permanente patients who used estrogens perimenopausally (96) and 50% for women who had estrogen replacement therapy for 6 or more months in Connecticut (97). A 60% reduction in hip fracture risk was also seen in a group of women who used estrogens for 5 or more years in Los Angeles; however, the protective effect was most marked in women who had had oophorectomy (98).

Another therapy for osteoporosis, calcitonin, has not been widely used for preventing bone loss because of its high cost and the need for parenteral administration of most formulations (20); treatment with calcitonin is, however, being re-evaluated (99, 100). Calcium supplements are generally recommended for postmenopausal women, but evidence for their efficacy in prophylaxis is controversial (101, 102). These treatments and investigational drugs like bisphosphonates reduce bone loss. Fluoride, the only preparation known to increase bone mass in the axial skeleton, has little effect on bone mass in the appendicular skeleton. Because fluoride does not reduce hip fracture risk and may increase it somewhat, fluoride has no role in osteoporosis prophylaxis (103).

Evidence indicates that long-term treatment with estrogen replacement therapy will reduce the incidence of fracture at virtually all sites. However, only a small proportion of postmenopausal women currently receive long-term estrogen therapy. The reluctance of physicians to prescribe and of women to comply with such therapy may be related to uncertainty about the therapy's benefits and risks (104-108). Although no studies have specifically examined the effect of treatment on women with low bone mass (identified through screening), long-term estrogen use may be effective in these patients. Analyses indicate that widespread use of estrogen replacement therapy could extend quality-adjusted years of life (109-112).

Estimated Effect of Screening

There is no prospective evidence on which to base estimates of the potential impact of screening on fracture incidence. Using indirect evidence and various assumptions (38), very rough estimates can be made of the effectiveness of a one-time screening conducted at the menopause to identify women with osteopenia who would be candidates for estrogen therapy, as shown in Figure 4 for fracture of the hip. As previously noted, about 5% of 50-year-old women would receive long-term estrogen therapy for reasons unrelated to osteoporosis. In the absence of bone mass measurements, it is estimated that only about 10% of the remaining women would comply with estrogen replacement therapy for 5 to 10 years, based on the low proportion of women receiving estrogen therapy at present. However, the lifetime risk for hip fracture (15) would be reduced by 50% in women receiving long-term estrogen replacement. Under this scenario, about 15% of 50-year-old white women would be treated, and the overall lifetime risk for hip fracture would be 10%. If, on the other hand, treatment were guided by bone mineral density measurements in the proximal femur, the proportion of 50-year-old women receiving long-term estrogen might increase from 15% to 19%, and lifetime hip fracture risk could conceivably fall from 10% to 8%, an absolute reduction of 2% and a relative reduction of 20%. This is based on the assumptions that the 70% of 50-year-old women with hip bone density over 1.0 g/cm^2 (10) would not be prescribed estrogen for fracture prevention and that 40% of the intermediate risk group (0.85 to 1.0 g/cm^2) would comply with therapy. In the small subset of women whose bone mineral density of the hip is less than 0.85 g/cm^2, it is assumed that knowledge of a 42% lifetime risk for hip fracture would induce more physicians to prescribe and twice as many women (80%) to comply with estrogen therapy long enough to reduce that risk by 50%. Analogous calculations suggest a 12% relative reduction in the lifetime risk for vertebral fractures in this group of women and a similar reduction in risk for all other limb fractures combined (38). These calculated benefits are, however, sensitive to the assumptions that are made about the level of compliance with therapy.

Ross and colleagues (113) also modeled the savings that might result from treating 50-year-old women with a regimen that slowed bone loss by 50%. They estimated that the incidence of all osteoporotic frac-

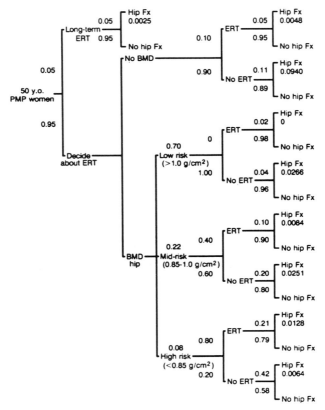

Figure 4. Risk for hip fracture using two alternative patient management systems: with bone mineral density measurements of the proximal femur (*BMD hip*) and without such measurements (*no BMD*). (Reprinted with permission from the *Journal of Bone and Mineral Research.* **Johnston CC, Melton LJ, Lindsay R.** Clinical indications for bone mass measurements. Report of the Scientific Advisory Committee of the National Osteoporosis Foundation. 1989;4(Suppl 2):25.

tures could be reduced by 33% if the women with the lowest 47% of bone mass were selectively treated. Without using specific bone mass levels, Cummings and colleagues (5) calculated a 25% reduction in hip fracture incidence in white women by the year 2020, if 50% of these women accepted long-term estrogen use beginning at age 50.

Although these estimates indicate the general magnitude of the effect of a one-time screening at the menopause, a formal analysis of the benefits and costs of screening should be done using recently available data on bone loss and fracture risk in the population. Earlier cost-effectiveness analyses showed little change in life expectancy but some improvement in quality-adjusted life with estrogen replacement therapy in 55- to 70-year-old women with osteoporosis (109). The cost for each quality-adjusted year of life gained was $5460 to $15 100 for women with a uterus, depending on whether or not endometrial biopsies were done periodically, and $3250 for women without a uterus. These figures were said to be comparable to the benefits of treating moderate to severe hypertension. However, osteoporosis was defined in that study on the basis of vertebral fractures rather than low bone mass or other fractures, so the benefits were probably understated. By considering the risks for hip, wrist, pelvis, humerus, and spine fractures, possible adverse effects on cancer risk, and potential beneficial effects on cardiovascular disease, Hillner and colleagues (111) found that 15 years of estrogen therapy in a 50-year-old woman was associated with an additional 0.67 quality-adjusted years of life. This benefit increased by 0.17 quality-years for each 10% decrease achieved in fracture rates.

Other Recommendations

Single- and dual-photon absorptiometry, quantitative computed tomography, and dual-energy x-ray absorptiometry have all been approved by the Food and Drug Administration for measurement of bone mineral density and monitoring of individual patients over time. However, a position paper by the Health and Public Policy Committee of the American College of Physicians concluded that "neither dual-photon absorptiometry nor computed tomographic techniques can accurately predict the tendency to fracture" (41); however, this conclusion predated the recent prospective studies summarized earlier. These non-invasive techniques were said to be of value in patients with metabolic bone diseases, but no technique was recommended as a general screening test for osteoporosis.

A National Institutes of Health Consensus Conference on Osteoporosis stated that the use of bone mass measurements "will depend on their availability, cost, and further studies of their discriminatory capabilities and sensitivity" (114). No recommendation was made that any of these techniques be used to screen asymptomatic women for osteoporosis. However, estrogen replacement therapy was encouraged, at least for women at high risk for osteoporosis, and a more recent European Consensus Conference echoed that recommendation (115). As previously noted, however, new studies indicate that risk factors cannot replace bone mass measurements in assessing the likelihood of fractures. Indeed, the Food and Drug Administration has approved the use of conjugated estrogen for "post-menopausal women with evidence of loss or deficiency of bone mass, to retard further loss and estrogen deficiency-induced osteoporosis" (116). Because this indication is for "abnormally low bone mass," estrogens cannot be used in the approved manner without bone mass measurements. (Estrogen replacement therapy is also approved to reduce perimenopausal symptoms, but this use is generally for a limited time and is not sufficient to protect against osteoporosis.)

Although it recognizes that osteoporosis is an important problem, the Canadian Task Force on Periodical Health Examinations (117) did not include osteoporosis among the conditions warranting routine periodic screening. The more recent United States Preventive Services Task Force report also recommended against routine screening of asymptomatic women but did indicate that "In perimenopausal women who are at increased risk for osteoporosis and for whom estrogen therapy would otherwise not be recommended, a measurement of bone mineral content may help the patient and clinician determine whether such therapy is appropriate" (118). The Royal College of Physicians, on the other hand, recommends that "Women aged about 50 years should have their bone density measured either radiographically or by photon absorptiometry. Estrogens should be offered to those whose bone mineral density is below a specified cutoff level. Women with low density in the intermediate range might attend for further screening 5 or 10 years after the initial examination" (119). No cutoff level of bone mass was specified in the report, which called for further research on the subject.

Several earlier technology assessments were somewhat more cautious. In evaluations of dual-photon absorptiometry (42) and single-photon absorptiometry (43), the Office of Health Technology Assessment concluded that the ability of bone mass measurements "to predict who is at risk of subsequently developing fractures (screening) has not yet been shown." It also recommended that "These methods for predicting fractures should be tested in prospective studies before they are allocated for widespread use or before they are employed as a basis for recommending specific types of therapy." Such prospective studies have now been published. The Clinical Efficacy Assessment Project (44) reiterated the importance of these prospective data: "If prospective studies establish that densitometry is valuable in predicting hip and vertebral fractures, then screening may be valuable for the postmenopausal woman whose decision about taking estrogen therapy depends on an assessment of her risk of fracture.''

Recommendations

Although our analysis suggests that bone mass measurements might be of value in screening unselected, asymptomatic women for osteoporosis, we cannot recommend mass screening until a specific program has been formulated and justified. However, there are other indications for bone mass measurements besides screening, and a number of these indications have been documented (38). In treating perimenopausal women who are concerned about osteoporosis and considering long-term estrogen replacement therapy, physicians need bone mass measurements to select those women most likely to benefit from treatment. Bone mass measurements are also indicated in patients with equivocal vertebral abnormalities on roentgenogram to document spinal osteoporosis. Measurements should be taken before initiating an extensive evaluation to exclude treatable causes of accelerated bone loss or beginning aggressive therapy to augment spinal bone mass. Similarly, some but not all patients have dramatic bone loss and fractures while receiving corticosteroid therapy, and bone mass measurements may permit adjustments in the corticosteroid regimen to achieve therapeutic benefits while minimizing skeletal side effects. Likewise, parathyroidectomy may stop bone loss induced by hyperparathyroidism, but asymptomatic hyperparathyroidism, uncomplicated by osteopenia, is relatively benign and may not require surgery. Thus, bone mass measurements may provide a basis for decisions on surgery for primary hyperparathyroidism.

Indeed, bone mass measurements are needed whenever the decision to treat is based on bone mass or fracture risk. Additional indications await only better documentation (120). One of the most controversial uses of bone mass measurements is for assessing response to therapeutic measures. Because of the inherent error rate of the measurements themselves, several authors (121, 122) have concluded that estimated rates of bone loss would be too imprecise for use in managing the care of individual patients. However, the improved precision offered by dual-energy x-ray absorptiometry promises to allow such assessments, at least during periods of more rapid bone loss such as at menopause or after initiation of steroid therapy (38,

45, 123). Repeated measures will also increase radiation exposure and costs, but the role of bone mass measurements in detecting nonresponse to therapy is likely to be resolved in the near future.

On the other hand, bone mass measurements are not indicated unless they will influence patient or physician behavior. If, for example, all postmenopausal women were to be given estrogen replacement therapy for prevention of coronary heart disease, bone mass measurements would not be needed to decide about estrogen therapy. Likewise, women in whom estrogen is contraindicated or who refuse to consider estrogen or some other therapy to slow bone loss do not need bone mass measurements. Isolated bone mass screening programs without an organized plan for patient management and referral cannot be supported either. Finally, bone mass measurements are contraindicated when standardization and quality control procedures are insufficient to ensure accurate results.

Discussion

Osteoporosis is a complex, multifactorial chronic disease that may progress silently for decades until characteristic fractures result late in life. Because there are no symptoms until fractures occur, relatively few people are diagnosed in time for effective therapy to be administered. Consequently, many persons experience the pain, expense, disability, and decreased quality of life caused by these age-related fractures. This important public health problem will worsen as the population ages, unless proper intervention can be applied.

Detection of osteoporosis appears to have the potential to reduce fracture incidence in postmenopausal women. Bone mass measurement meets some of the criteria for a mass screening test. Specifically, the disease (osteoporosis) is common and is an important cause of morbidity and mortality; tests are available that are safe, acceptable to patients, and sufficiently accurate in detecting low bone mass; at least one effective therapy (estrogen) is available for patients with abnormal tests; and treatment can be expected to reduce the clinically important manifestation of the disease, the incidence of fracture. Although preventing excessive bone loss is the only action that can be taken now to reduce risk for fractures in the future, no consensus has been reached on a specific screening program for use in the general population.

References

1. **Cummings SR, Kelsey JL, Nevitt MC, O'Dowd KJ.** Epidemiology of osteoporosis and osteoporotic fractures. *Epidemiol Rev.* 1985;7:178-208.

2. **Melton LJ III.** Epidemiology of fractures. In: Riggs BL, Melton LJ III, eds. *Osteoporosis: Etiology, Diagnosis, and Management.* New York: Raven Press; 1988:133-54.

3. Osteoporosis. In: Cassels JS, ed. *Health Promotion and Disability Prevention for the Second Fifty. Institute of Medicine.* Washington, DC: National Academy Press; 1990 [In press].

4. **Holbrook TL, Grazier K, Kelsey JL, Stauffer RN.** *The Frequency of Occurrence, Impact, and Cost of Selected Musculoskeletal Conditions in the United States.* Chicago: American Academy of Orthopedic Surgeons; 1984.

5. **Cummings SR, Rubin SM, Black D.** The coming epidemic of hip fractures in the United States. *Clin Orthop.* [In press].

6. **U.S. Preventive Services Task Force.** Counseling to prevent household and environmental injuries. *Guide to Clinical Preventive Services: Report of the U.S. Preventive Services Task Force.* Baltimore: Williams & Wilkins; 1989:321-9.

7. **Parfitt AM.** Bone remodeling: relationship to the amount and structure of bone, and the pathogenesis and prevention of fractures. In: Riggs BL, Melton LJ III, eds. *Osteoporosis: Etiology, Diagnosis, and Management.* New York: Raven Press; 1988:45-93.

8. **Hayes WC, Gerhart TN.** Biomechanics of bone: applications for assessment of bone strength. In: Peck WA, ed. *Bone and Mineral Research/3.* Amsterdam: Elsevier Science Publishers; 1985:259-94.

9. **Melton LJ III, Chao EY, Lane J.** Biomechanical aspects of fractures. In: Riggs BL, Melton LJ III, eds. *Osteoporosis: Etiology, Diagnosis, and Management.* New York: Raven Press; 1988:111-31.

10. **Melton LJ III, Wahner HW, Richelson LS, O'Fallon WM, Riggs BL.** Osteoporosis and the risk of hip fracture. *Am J Epidemiol.* 1986;124:254-61.

11. **Hui SL, Slemenda CW, Johnston CC Jr.** Age and bone mass as predictors of fracture in a prospective study. *J Clin Invest.* 1988;81:1804-9.

12. **Eastell R, Riggs BL, Wahner HW, O'Fallon WM, Amadio PC, Melton LJ III.** Colles' fracture and bone density of the ultradistal radius. *J Bone Miner Res.* 1989;4:607-13.

13. **Ross PD, Wasnich RD, Vogel JM.** Detection of prefracture spinal osteoporosis using bone mineral absorptiometry. *J Bone Miner Res.* 1988;3:1-11.

14. **Melton LJ III, Kan SH, Frye MA, Wahner HW, O'Fallon WM, Riggs BL.** Epidemiology of vertebral fractures in women. *Am J Epidemiol.* 1989;129:1000-11.

15. **Melton LJ III, Kan SH, Wahner HW, Riggs BL.** Lifetime fracture risk: an approach to hip fracture risk assessment based on bone mineral density and age. *J Clin Epidemiol.* 1988;41:985-94.

16. **Melton LJ III, Riggs BL.** Risk factors for injury after a fall. *Clin Geriatr Med.* 1985;1:525-39.

17. **Cummings SR.** Epidemiology of hip fractures. In: Christiansen C, Johansen JS, Riis BJ, eds. *Osteoporosis 1987.* v 1. Kobenhavn, Denmark: Osteopress; 1987:40-4.

18. **Tinetti ME, Speechley M.** Prevention of falls among the elderly. *N Engl J Med.* 1989;320:1055-9.

19. **Gibson MJ.** The prevention of falls in later life. A report of the Kellogg International Work Group on the Prevention of Falls by the Elderly. *Dan Med Bull.* 1987;34(Suppl 4):1-24.

20. **Riggs BL.** Practical management of the patient with osteoporosis. In: Riggs BL, Melton LJ III, eds. *Osteoporosis: Etiology, Diagnosis, and Management.* New York: Raven Press; 1988:481-90.

21. **Nordin BE.** The definition and diagnosis of osteoporosis [Editorial]. *Calcif Tissue Int.* 1987;40:57-8.

22. **Riggs BL, Wahner HW, Seeman E, et al.** Changes in bone mineral density of the proximal femur and spine with aging. Differences

between the postmenopausal and senile osteoporosis syndromes. *J Clin Invest.* 1982;**70**:716-23.

23. **Mazess RB.** Bone density in diagnosis of osteoporosis: thresholds and breakpoints [Editorial]. *Calcif Tissue Int.* 1987;**41**:117-8.

24. **Davis JW, Vogel JM, Ross PD, Wasnich RD.** Disease versus etiology: the distinction should not be lost in the analysis [Editorial]. *J Nucl Med.* 1989;**30**:1273-6.

25. **Rose G.** Sick individuals and sick populations. *Int J Epidemiol.* 1985;**14**:32-8.

26. **Hurxthal LM, Vose GP, Dotter WE.** Densitometric and visual observations of spinal radiographs. *Geriatrics.* 1969;**24**:93-106.

27. **Stulberg BN, Bauer TW, Watson JT, Richmond B.** Bone quality. Roentgenographic versus histologic assessment of hip bone structure. *Clin Orthop.* 1989;**240**:200-5.

28. **Davis MR.** Screening for postmenopausal osteoporosis. *Am J Obstet Gynecol.* 1987;**156**:1-5.

29. **Heidrich F, Thompson RS.** Osteoporosis prevention: strategies applicable for general population groups. *J Fam Pract.* 1987;**25**:33-9.

30. **Yano K, Wasnich RD, Vogel JM, Heilbrun LK.** Bone mineral measurements among middle-aged and elderly Japanese residents in Hawaii. *Am J Epidemiol.* 1984;**119**:751-64.

31. **Evers SE, Orchard JW, Haddad RG.** Bone density in postmenopausal North American Indian and Caucasian females. *Hum Biol.* 1985;**57**:719-26.

32. **Sowers MR, Wallace RD, Lemke JH.** Correlates of mid-radius bone density among postmenopausal women: a community study. *Am J Clin Nutr.* 1985;**41**:1045-53.

33. **Ismail F, Epstein S, Pacifici R, Droke D, Thomas SB, Avioli LV.** Serum bone gla protein (BGP) and other markers of bone mineral metabolism in postmenopausal osteoporosis. *Calcif Tissue Int.* 1986;**39**:230-3.

34. **Jones KP, Ravnikar VA, Tulchinsky D, Schiff I.** Comparison of bone density in amenorrheic women due to athletics, weight loss, and premature menopause. *Obstet Gynecol.* 1987;**66**:5-8.

35. **Citron JT, Ettinger B, Genant HK.** Prediction of peak premenopausal bone mass using a scale of weighted clinical variables. In: Christiansen C, Johansen JS, Riis BJ, eds. *Osteoporosis 1987.* v 1. Kobenhavn, Denmark: Osteopress; 1987:146-9.

36. **Stevenson JC, Lees B, Devenport M, Cust MP, Ganger KF.** Determinants of bone density in normal women: risk factors for future osteoporosis. *Br Med J [Clin Res].* 1989;**298**:924-8.

37. **Wasnich RD, Ross PD, Vogel JM, MacLean CJ.** The relative strengths of osteoporotic risk factors in a prospective study of postmenopausal osteoporosis. *J Bone Miner Res.* 1987;**2**(Suppl 1):343.

38. **Johnston CC, Melton LJ III, Lindsay R, Eddy DM.** Clinical indications for bone mass measurements. A report from the Scientific Advisory Board of the National Osteoporosis Foundation. *J Bone Miner Res.* 1989;**4**(Suppl 2):1-28.

39. **Riggs BL, Wahner HW, Melton LJ III, Richelson LS, Judd HL, Offord KP.** Rates of bone loss in the appendicular and axial skeletons of women. Evidence of substantial vertebral bone loss before menopause. *J Clin Invest.* 1986;**77**:1487-91.

40. **Ott SM, Kilcoyne RF, Chesnut CH III.** Ability of four different techniques of measuring bone mass to diagnose vertebral fractures in postmenopausal women. *J Bone Miner Res.* 1987;**2**:201-10.

41. **Health and Public Policy Committee, American College of Physicians.** Radiologic methods to evaluate bone mineral content. *Ann Intern Med.* 1984;**100**:908-11.

42. **Erlichman M.** *Dual Photon Absorptiometry for Measuring Bone Mineral Density (Number 6). Health Technology Assessment Reports, 1986.* Rockville, MD: U.S. Department of Health and Human Services, Public Health Service, National Center for Health Services Research and Health Care Technology Assessment; 1986.

43. **Erlichman M.** *Single Photon Absorptiometry for Measuring Bone Mineral Density (Number 7). Health Technology Assessment Reports, 1986.* Rockville, MD: U.S. Department of Health and Human Services, Public Health Service, National Center for Health Services Research and Health Care Technology Assessment; 1986.

44. **Health and Public Policy Committee, American College of Physicians.** Bone mineral densitometry. *Ann Intern Med.* 1987;**107:**932-6.
45. **Genant HK, Block JE, Steiger P, Glueer CC, Ettinger B, Harris ST.** Appropriate use of bone densitometry. *Radiology.* 1989;**170:**817-22.
46. **Wahner HW, Dunn WL, Brown ML, Morin RL, Riggs BL.** Comparison of dual-energy x-ray absorptiometry and dual photon absorptiometry for bone mineral measurements of the lumbar spine. *Mayo Clin Proc.* 1988;**63:**1075-84.
47. **Mazess R, Collick B, Trempe J, Barden H, Hanson J.** Performance evaluation of a dual-energy x-ray bone densitometer. *Calcif Tissue Int.* 1989;**44:**228-32.
48. **Hui SL, Berger JO.** Empirical Bayes estimation of rates in longitudinal studies. *J Am Stats Assoc.* 1983;**78:**753-60.
49. **Smith DM, Khairi MR, Johnston CC Jr.** The loss of bone mineral with aging and its relationship to risk of fracture. *J Clin Invest.* 1975;**56:**311-8.
50. **Hui SL, Slemenda CW, Johnston CC Jr.** Baseline measurement of bone mass predicts fracture in white women. *Ann Intern Med.* 1989;**111:**355-61.
51. **Gärdsell P, Johnell O, Nilsson BE.** Predicting fractures in women by using forearm bone densitometry. *Calcif Tissue Int.* 1989;**44:**235-42.
52. **Wasnich RD.** Fracture prediction with bone mass measurements. In: Genant HK, ed. *Osteoporosis Update 1987.* San Francisco: Radiology Research and Education Foundation; 1987:95-101.
53. **Browner WS, Cummings SR, Genant HK, et al.** Bone mineral density and fractures of the wrist and humerus in elderly women: a prospective study. *J Bone Miner Res.* 1989;**4**(Suppl 1):S171.
54. **Cummings SR, Black DM, Nevitt MC, et al.** Appendicular bone density and age predict hip fractures in women. *JAMA.* 1990 [In press].
55. **Mazess RB, Barden H, Ettinger M, Schultz E.** Bone density of the radius, spine, and proximal femur in osteoporosis. *J Bone Miner Res.* 1988;**3:**13-8.
56. **Nordin BE, Wishart JM, Horowitz M, Need AG, Bridges A, Bellon M.** The relation between forearm and vertebral mineral density and fractures in postmenopausal women. *Bone Miner.* 1988;**5:**21-33.
57. **Eastell R, Wahner HW, O'Fallon WM, Amadio PC, Melton LJ III, Riggs BL.** Unequal decrease in bone density of lumbar spine and ultradistal radius in Colles' and vertebral fracture syndromes. *J Clin Invest.* 1989;**83:**168-74.
58. **Horsman A, Birchall MN.** Assessment and modification of hip fracture risk: predictions of a stochastic model. In: Deluca HF, Mazess RB, eds. *Osteoporosis: Physiological Basis, Assessment, and Treatment: Proceedings of the Nineteenth Steenbock Symposium. Held June 5 through June 8, 1989 at the University of Wisconsin-Madison, U.S.A.* New York: Elsevier Science Publishers; 1990.
59. **Kanouse DE, Jacoby I.** When does information change practitioners' behavior? *Int J Technol Assess Health Care.* 1988;**4:**27-33.
60. **Judd HL, Meldrum DR, Defton LJ, Henderson BE.** Estrogen replacement therapy: indications and complications. *Ann Intern Med.* 1983;**98:**195-205.
61. **Bush TL, Cowan LD, Barrett-Connor E, et al.** Estrogen use and all-cause mortality. Preliminary results from the Lipid Research Clinics Program Follow-up Study. *JAMA.* 1983;**249:**903-6.
62. **Wilson PW, Garrison RJ, Castelli WP.** Postmenopausal estrogen use, cigarette smoking, and cardiovascular morbidity in women over 50. The Framingham Study. *N Engl J Med.* 1985;**313:**1038-43.
63. **Bush TL, Barrett-Connor E.** Noncontraceptive estrogen use and cardiovascular disease. *Epidemiol Rev.* 1985;**7:**89-104.
64. **Henderson BE, Ross RK, Lobo RA, Pike MC, Mack TM.** Re-evaluating the role of progestogen therapy after the menopause. *Fertil Steril.* 1988;**49** (5 Suppl 2):9S-15S.
65. **Stampfer MJ, Willett WC, Colditz GA, Rosner B, Speizer FE, Hennekens CH.** A prospective study of postmenopausal estrogen

therapy and coronary heart disease. *N Engl J Med.* 1985;**313**:1044-9.

66. **Bush TL, Barrett-Connor E, Cowan LD, et al.** Cardiovascular mortality and noncontraceptive use of estrogen in women: results from the Lipid Research Clinics Program Follow-up Study. *Circulation.* 1987;**75**:1102-9.

67. **Ettinger B, Golditch IM, Friedman G.** Gynecologic consequences of long-term, unopposed estrogen replacement therapy. *Maturitas.* 1988;**10**:271-82.

68. **Bergkvist L, Adami HO, Persson I, Hoover R, Schairer C.** The risk of breast cancer after estrogen and estrogen-progestin replacement. *N Engl J Med.* 1989;**321**:293-7.

69. **Barrett-Connor E.** Postmenopausal estrogen replacement and breast cancer [Editorial]. *N Engl J Med.* 1989;**321**:319-20.

70. **Rosenberg L, Shapiro S, Kaufman DW, Slone D, Miettinen OS, Stolley PD.** Patterns and determinants of conjugated estrogen use. *Am J Epidemiol.* 1979;**109**:676-86.

71. **Wingo PA, Layde PM, Lee NC, Rubin G, Ory HW.** The risk of breast cancer in postmenopausal women who have used estrogen replacement therapy. *JAMA.* 1987;**257**:209-15.

72. **Meema S, Bunker ML, Meema HE.** Preventive effect of estrogen on postmenopausal bone loss. *Arch Intern Med.* 1975;**135**:1436-40.

73. **Lindsay R, Hart DM, Aitken JM, MacDonald EB, Anderson JB, Clarke AC.** Long-term prevention of postmenopausal osteoporosis by oestrogen. Evidence for an increased bone mass after delayed onset of oestrogen treatment. *Lancet.* 1976;**1**:1038-40.

74. **Horsman A, Gallagher JC, Simpson M, Nordin BE.** Prospective trial of oestrogen and calcium in postmenopausal women. *Br Med J [Clin Res].* 1977;**2**:789-92.

75. **Recker RR, Saville PD, Heaney RP.** Effect of estrogens and calcium carbonate on bone loss in postmenopausal women. *Ann Intern Med.* 1977;**87**:649-55.

76. **Lindsay R, Hart DM, Purdie D, Ferguson MM, Clark AS, Kraszewski A.** Comparative effects of oestrogen and a progestogen on bone loss in postmenopausal women. *Clin Sci Mol Med.* 1978;**54**:193-5.

77. **Nachtigall LE, Nachtigall RH, Nachtigall RD, Beckman EM.** Estrogen replacement therapy I: a 10-year prospective study in the relationship to osteoporosis. *Obstet Gynecol.* 1979;**53**:277-81.

78. **Christiansen C, Christensen MS, McNair P, Hagen C, Stocklund KE, Transbøl I.** Prevention of early postmenopausal bone loss: controlled 2-year study in 315 normal females. *Eur J Clin Invest.* 1980;**10**:273-9.

79. **Lindsay R, Hart DM, Forrest C, Baird C.** Prevention of spinal osteoporosis in oophorectomised women. *Lancet.* 1980;**2**:1151-4.

80. **Nordin BE, Horsman A, Crilly RG, Marshall DH, Simpson M.** Treatment of spinal osteoporosis in postmenopausal women. *Br Med J [Clin Res].* 1980;**280**:451-5.

81. **Christiansen C, Christensen MS, Transbøl I.** Bone mass in postmenopausal women after withdrawal of oestrogen/gestagen replacement therapy. *Lancet.* 1981;**1**:459-61.

82. **Genant HK, Cann CE, Ettinger B, Gordan GS.** Quantitative computed tomography of vertebral spongiosa: a sensitive method for detecting early bone loss after oophorectomy. *Ann Intern Med.* 1982;**97**:699-705.

83. **Jensen GF, Christiansen C, Transbøl I.** Treatment of postmenopausal osteoporosis. A controlled therapeutic trial comparing oestrogen/gestagen, 1,25-dihydroxy-vitamin D_3 and calcium. *Clin Endocrinol (Oxf).* 1982;**16**:515-24.

84. **Christiansen C, Rødbro P.** Does oestriol add to the beneficial effect of combined hormonal prophylaxis against early postmenopausal osteoporosis? *Br J Obstet Gynaecol.* 1984;**91**:489-93.

85. **Lindsay R, Hart DM, Clark DM.** The minimum effective dose of estrogen for prevention of postmenopausal bone loss. *Obstet Gynecol.* 1984;**63**:759-63.

86. **Gotfredsen A, Nilas L, Riis BJ, Thomsen K, Christiansen C.** Bone changes occurring spontaneously and caused by estrogen in early postmenopausal women: a local or generalised phenomenon? *Br*

Med J [Clin Res]. 1986;**292**:1098-100.

87. **Riis B, Thomsen K, Christiansen C.** Does calcium supplementation prevent postmenopausal bone loss? A double-blind, controlled clinical study. *N Engl J Med*. 1987;**316**:173-7.

88. **Riis BJ, Thomsen K, Strøm V, Christiansen C.** The effect of percutaneous estradiol and natural progesterone on postmenopausal bone loss. *Am J Obstet Gynecol*. 1987;**156**:61-5.

89. **Munk-Jensen N, Pors Nielsen S, Obel EB, Bonne Eriksen P.** Reversal of postmenopausal vertebral bone loss by oestrogen and progestogen: a double blind placebo controlled study. *Br Med J [Clin Res]*. 1988;**296**:1150-2.

90. **Abdalla H, Hart DM, Lindsay R.** Differential bone loss and effects of long-term estrogen therapy according to time of introduction of therapy after oophorectomy. In: Christiansen C, Arnaud CD, Nordin BE, Parfitt AM, Peck WA, Riggs BL, eds. *Osteoporosis 2.* Copenhagen, Denmark: Aalborg Stifsbogtrykkeri; 1984:621-3.

91. **Quigley ME, Martin PL, Burnier AM, Brooks P.** Estrogen therapy arrests bone loss in elderly women. *Am J Obstet Gynecol*. 1987;**156**:1516-23.

92. **Ettinger B, Genant HK, Cann CE.** Long-term estrogen replacement therapy prevents bone loss and fractures. *Ann Intern Med*. 1985;**102**:319-24.

93. **Kiel DP, Felson DT, Anderson JJ, Wilson PW, Moskowitz MA.** Hip fracture and the use of estrogens in postmenopausal women. The Framingham Study. *N Engl J Med*. 1987;**317**:1169-74.

94. **Hutchinson TA, Polansky SM, Feinstein AR.** Post-menopausal oestrogens protect against fractures of hip and distal radius. A case-control study. *Lancet*. 1979;**2**:705-9.

95. **Weiss NS, Ure CL, Ballard JH, Williams AR, Daling JR.** Decreased risk of fractures of the hip and lower forearm with postmenopausal use of estrogens. *N Engl J Med*. 1980;**303**:1195-8.

96. **Johnson RE, Specht EE.** The risk of hip fracture in postmenopausal females with or without estrogen drug exposure. *Am J Public Health*. 1981;**71**:138-44.

97. **Kreiger N, Kelsey JL, Holford TR, O'Connor T.** An epidemiologic study of hip fracture in postmenopausal women. *Am J Epidemiol*. 1982;**116**:141-8.

98. **Paganini-Hill A, Ross RK, Gerkins VR, Henderson BE, Arthur M, Mack TM.** Menopausal estrogen therapy and hip fractures. *Ann Intern Med*. 1981;**95**:28-31.

99. **Reginster JY, Denis D, Albert A, et al.** 1-Year controlled randomised trial of prevention of early postmenopausal bone loss by intranasal calcitonin. *Lancet*. 1987;**2**:1481-3.

100. **MacIntyre I, Stevenson JC, Whitehead MI, Wimalawansa SJ, Banks LM, Healy MJ.** Calcitonin for prevention of postmenopausal bone loss. *Lancet*. 1988;**1**:900-2.

101. **Kanis JA, Passmore R.** Calcium supplementation of the diet–I. *Br Med J [Clin Res]*. 1989;**298**:137-40.

102. **Kanis JA, Passmore R.** Calcium supplementation of the diet–II. *Br Med J [Clin Res]*. 1989;**298**:205-8.

103. **Melton LJ III.** Fluoride in the prevention of osteoporosis and fractures. *J Bone Miner Res*. 1990 [In press].

104. **Holzman GB, Ravitch MM, Metheny W, Rothert ML, Holmes M, Hoppe RB.** Physicians' judgments about estrogen replacement therapy for menopausal women. *Obstet Gynecol*. 1984;**63**:303-11.

105. **Leiblum SR, Swartzman LC.** Women's attitudes toward the menopause: an update. *Maturitas*. 1986;**8**:47-56.

106. **Elstein AS, Holzman GB, Ravitch MM, et al.** Comparison of physicians' decisions regarding estrogen replacement therapy for menopausal women and decisions derived from a decision analytic model. *Am J Med*. 1986;**80**:246-58.

107. **Ravnikar VA.** Compliance with hormone therapy. *Am J Obstet Gynecol*. 1987;**156**:1332-4.

108. **Grisso JA, Baum CR, Turner BJ.** What do physicians in practice do to prevent osteoporosis? *J Bone Miner Res*. 1990 [In press].

109. **Weinstein MC.** Estrogen use in postmenopausal women–costs, risks, and benefits. *N Engl J Med*. 1980;**303**:308-16.

110. **Weinstein MC, Schiff I.** Cost-effectiveness of hormone replacement

therapy in the menopause. *Obstet Gynecol Surv.* 1983;**38**:445-55.

111. **Hillner BE, Hollenberg JP, Pauker SG.** Postmenopausal estrogens in prevention of osteoporosis. Benefit virtually without risk if cardiovascular effects are considered. *Am J Med.* 1986;**80**:1115-27.

112. **Tosteson AA, Rosenthal DI, Weinstein MC.** Cost-effectiveness of screening women for osteoporosis [Abstract]. *Legal Issues in Medical Decision Making.* 1987;**7**:281.

113. **Ross PD, Wasnich RD, MacLean CJ, Hagino R, Vogel JM.** A model for estimating the potential costs and savings of osteoporosis prevention strategies. *Bone.* 1988;**9**:337-47.

114. Consensus conference: osteoporosis. *JAMA.* 1984;**252**:799-802.

115. Consensus development conference: prophylaxis and treatment of osteoporosis. *Br Med J [Clin Res].* 1987;**295**:914-5.

116. *Physicians' Desk Reference.* Oradell, New Jersey: Medical Economics; 1988:665.

117. **Canadian Task Force on the Periodic Health Examination.** The periodic health examination: 2. 1987 update. *Can Med Assoc J.* 1988;**138**:618-26.

118. **U.S. Preventive Services Task Force.** Screening for postmenopausal osteoporosis. *Guide to Clinical Preventive Services: report of the U.S. Preventive Services Task Force.* Baltimore: Williams & Wilkins; 1989:239-43.

119. Fractured neck of femur. Prevention and management. Summary and recommendations of the Royal College of Physicians. *J R Coll Physicians Lond.* 1989;**23**:8-12.

120. **Riggs BL, Wahner HW.** Bone densitometry and clinical decision making in osteoporosis [Editorial]. *Ann Intern Med.* 1988;**108**:293-5.

121. **Heaney RP.** En recherche de la différence (*P* less than 0.05). *Bone Miner.* 1986;**1**:99-114.

122. **Cummings SR, Black D.** Should perimenopausal women be screened for osteoporosis? *Ann Intern Med.* 1986;**104**:817-23.

123. **Mazess RB, Gallagher C, Notelovitz M, Schiff I.** Monitoring skeletal response to estrogen. *Am J Obstet Gynecol.* [In press].

Screening for Breast Cancer

DAVID M. EDDY, MD, PhD

In 1989 approximately 114 000 women in the United States will be diagnosed with new primary breast cancer, and about 48% of these women will eventually die of the disease. Breast cancer is the commonest cancer in women (except skin cancer), the second commonest cause of death from cancer in women (lung cancer recently passed breast cancer), and the commonest cause of death from cancer in women 40 to 50 years old.

Several methods are available to screen for breast cancer, and breast cancer screening is the most intensively evaluated of all screening procedures. This paper reviews aspects of the disease pertinent to decisions about screening, the available screening methods, and the evidence that screening is effective in reducing breast cancer mortality. This paper also estimates the magnitudes of the benefits, harms, and costs of different screening strategies.

Probability of Developing Breast Cancer

The probability that a woman will develop breast cancer in the coming year depends on age and risk factors. Table 1 shows the probabilities for women at average risk in various age groups (age-specific incidence rates). Based on current incidence rates, the lifetime probability that a woman at average risk will develop breast cancer is approximately 9.3%.

Several factors are associated with a higher-than-average risk for developing breast cancer. Perhaps the most important factor for practitioners to consider in making a screening decision is that the risk for breast cancer is approximately twice the average in women whose mothers or sisters have had breast cancer and approximately three times the average for women whose mothers and sisters have had breast cancer (1). Conversely, women without any first-degree relative with breast cancer have a risk for breast cancer slightly below average.

▶ This chapter was originally published in *Annals of Internal Medicine.* 1989;111:389-99.

Table 1. *Annual Age-Specific Incidence Rates of Breast Cancer from 1983 to 1985**

Age, y	Incidence Rates†
0 to 4	0.0
5 to 9	0.0
10 to 14	0.0
15 to 19	0.08
20 to 24	1.06
25 to 29	7.81
30 to 34	24.59
35 to 39	62.97
40 to 44	111.67
45 to 49	159.18
50 to 54	185.36
55 to 59	227.26
60 to 64	261.60
65 to 69	297.12
70 to 74	316.45
75 to 79	327.00
80 to 84	336.86
85 or older	312.48

* Data are from reference 30.
† Per 100 000 persons.

The importance of analyzing risk factors lies in identifying a collection of factors that concentrate a high proportion of cases into a small group. The actual degree of concentration depends on the particular definitions of the risk categories. One risk-classification scheme concentrated 80% of breast cancer cases in 60% to 65% of women (2), implying a relative risk (compared with average) of 1.33 in the "high-risk" group and 0.5 in the "low-risk" group. Schechter and colleagues (3) were able to define a high-risk subgroup that concentrated more than 85% of breast cancer cases in 40% of women, implying a relative risk (compared with average) of approximately 2 in the "high-risk" group and a relative risk of approximately 0.25 in the "low-risk" group. Additional analyses of risk factors are discussed by Schechter and colleagues (3).

Screening Procedures

Two main procedures have been proposed to screen for breast cancer: breast physical examination by a trained practitioner and mammography. Thermography, ultrasonography, computed tomography, and photoluminescence have also been proposed for breast cancer screening, but the initial experience with such procedures was discouraging; these procedures are not used widely, and there is little experience on which to base estimates of effectiveness. Breast self-examination has also been proposed to detect breast cancers early; it has been discussed by O'Malley and Fletcher (4) and Hill and colleagues (5), and will not be analyzed in this paper.

Breast Physical Examination

The sensitivity of breast physical examination, or any cancer screening test, depends on the size of the lesions searched for, which in turn depends on the other tests used and the frequency of screening. In this paper, sensitivity is defined as the number of cancers detected by the screening test at an annual examination (for example, breast physical examination) divided by the number of cancers detected at the screening sessions by all the examinations offered (for example, breast physical examination and mammography) plus the number of cancers that become clinically apparent in the interval between scheduled examinations. By this definition, the sensitivity of breast physical examination in the Health Insurance Plan of Greater New York (HIP) study and the Breast Cancer Detection Demonstration Project (BCDDP) was about 50%. The specificity of breast physical examination depends on a woman's age and ranges from 98% (for younger women) to 99% (for older women) (6).

Charges for breast physical examination vary widely. The marginal cost of a breast physical examination is minimal when a woman is receiving health care for other purposes; one group estimated the marginal cost to be less than $3.50 (2). However, if a woman sees her physician solely to have a breast physical examination, the fee could be $10 to $60. The cost analysis that follows will use a $25 fee as a baseline estimate.

Mammography

Two types of mammography are currently used for screening. Screen-film mammography uses a conventional roentgen-ray film plus an intensifying screen to record the image. Xeromammography is done with a tungsten-target tube or a molybdenum target that has been heavily filtered with aluminum. The image is recorded on an electrostatic plate rather than on conventional film. Although the two methods have different sensitivities for different types of lesions, their overall sensitivities are very similar, and reports of results of large programs (for example, the BCDDP) usually do not separate data for the two methods (6). The sensitivity of mammography was approximately 50% and approximately 70% in the HIP study and the BCDDP, respectively. The specificity of mammography in the BCDDP was approximately 99% for women of all ages.

The cost of mammography also varies widely; charges range from $25 to more than $200. The average charge in 1985 for the screening centers that grew out of BCDDP was estimated to be $100 (Baker LH. Personal communication.). However, many centers have shown that screening mammography can be profitably offered at a charge of about $40 to $50. Assuming that about half of women will seek the low-cost screening mammogram, this analysis uses a $75 fee as a baseline estimate for calculating the effect of screening on costs.

Evidence of Effectiveness

Seven controlled studies and one uncontrolled study provide information about the reduction in mortality achieved by breast cancer screening with breast physical examination or mammography, or both, at various time intervals. The data on women 40 to 50 years of age is summarized elsewhere (7). This paper summarizes the results for that age group and adds results for women 50 to 65 years of age and 65 to 75 years of age.

The Health Insurance Plan Study

The randomized, controlled trial by The Health Insurance Plan of Greater New York (HIP) offered approximately 31 000 women (age, 40 to 64 years) four successive annual screenings with mammography (two views) and breast physical examination (the "study group"). Approximately 67% of the women accepted, and approximately 50% received at least three screenings (8-10). The trial showed a statistically significant reduction in mortality in women who were over 50 years of age at entry into the study. Five years after entry, the reduction in mortality was about 50%, gradually decreasing to about 20% at 18 years after entry. For women 40 to 50 years old at entry, the reduction in mortality was small (about 5%) at 5 years, gradually increasing to about 25% after 18 years of follow-up. Depending on the methods used in the calculations, the reduction can be claimed to be statistically significant (11).

Calculation Methods

The range of values shown in Table 2 can be used to estimate the effect of breast cancer screening on morbidity, mortality, and financial costs for an individual woman or a population of women in a specific age group. The calculations were done using a computer model called CAN*TROL (26, 27).

CAN*TROL consists of five submodels. A population submodel starts with a population specified by sex, 5-year age group, and cancer status and uses estimates of future birth and death rates to estimate the population for each future year. The effects on an individual woman or group are estimated by defining the "population" to be a person or a cohort of persons of the same age and relative risk. The effects on women in the United States are estimated by defining the population to be the U.S. population. A cancer-incidence submodel uses information on age- and sex-specific cancer incidence rates and relative risk to estimate the number of new primary cases of cancer that will occur in each future year. A disease submodel uses data on the proportion of cancers detected in each stage and on stage-specific relative survival rates to estimate the probability that a cancer patient will die from cancer for each year after the diagnosis. The core model for doing the calculations is a set of 100 nine-state Markov processes (one for each age group). The effect of screening on cancer mortality is calculated by changing the proportion of cancers detected in each stage, and (optionally) by altering stage-specific relative survival rates. A fourth submodel keeps track of the probabilities that both cancer patients and persons without cancer will die of other causes. Finally, a cost submodel keeps track of the costs of screening, workups, initial treatment, continuing care, terminal care for patients dying of cancer, and terminal care for patients dying from other causes. The CAN*TROL model is described in detail elsewhere (26).

For this analysis, to simulate the implications of the HIP data, stage proportions were set to achieve the actual mortality reductions observed in that trial in various years (at 2, 5, 10, 14, and 18 years). For the estimates based on the BCDDP, stage proportions and stage-specific relative survival rates were set to the values observed in the BCDDP (incorporating a 1-year lead time) and the SEER program as analyzed by Seidman and colleagues (19). Additional U.S. data on the age distribution of the population, projected birth rates, age-specific breast cancer incidence rates, age-specific mortality from breast cancer, age-specific mor-

Table 3. The Benefits and Risks of Breast Cancer Screening for Asymptomatic Average-Risk Women of Various Ages*

Variable	Age Group, y					
	40 to 50		55 to 65		65 to 75	
	HIP	BCDDP	HIP	BCDDP	HIP	BCDDP
Probability of developing breast cancer during the coming 10 years	133 (in 10 000)		233 (in 10 000)		279 (in 10 000)	
Probability of dying from breast cancer diagnosed in the next 10 years	86 (in 10 000)		123 (in 10 000)		120 (in 10 000)	
Decrease in probability of death from breast cancer achieved by screening 10 years with BPE	15	29 (in 10 000)	20	41 (in 10 000)	21	42 (in 10 000)
Additional decrease in probability of death from breast cancer achieved by adding 10 years of MGY to BPE	8	29 (in 10 000)	10	41 (in 10 000)	10	42 (in 10 000)
Increase in life expectancy achieved by 10 years of BPE, d	13	27	13	26	10	18
Discounted 5%	4	8	6	10	5	9

Additional increase in life expectancy achieved by adding 10 years of						
MGY to BPE, *d*	7	27	7	26	5	18
Discounted 5%	2	8	3	10	2	9
Increase in net charges due to BPE (discounted 5%), $	331	319	243	232	233	226
Additional increase in net charges due to adding MGY to BPE (discounted 5%), $	666	647	644	621	616	598
Probability that 10 MGY examinations will cause breast cancer in remaining years of a woman's life	< 1 in 25 000		< 1 in 50 000		< 1 in 50 000	
Probability of a false-positive BPE or MGY examination during the next 10 years	30 in 100		20 in 100		20 in 100	

* BPE = breast physical examination; MGY = mammography; HIP = Health Insurance Plan of Greater New York; BCDDP = Breast Cancer Detection Demonstration Project. All answers assume perfect compliance.

tality from other causes of death, proportion of breast cancers found in various stages in the absence of screening, and survival rates by stage were drawn from standard sources described elsewhere (28). Additional information about the model, assumptions, and results are available on request.

Outcomes for an Individual Woman

Application of the model to the results of the HIP study and BCDDP indicates the following benefits, harms, and costs of various screening strategies. Table 3 estimates answers to questions that apply to average-risk, asymptomatic women of different ages (ages 40, 55, and 65) who are contemplating annual breast cancer screening with breast physical examinations or with the combination of breast physical examination and mammography for the coming 10 years (ages 40 to 50, 55 to 65, and 65 to 75). The 10-year period from age 55 to 65 was chosen rather than the 15-year period from age 50 to 65 to simplify comparisons among age groups. Results for a woman 50 to 60 years of age are slightly lower. The answers assume that the woman is screened in each of the 10 years.

In general, the probability that an asymptomatic woman at average risk will develop breast cancer in the coming 10 years varies from about 130 per 10 000 or 1.3% (for a 40-year-old woman) to about 280 per 10 000 or 2.8% (for a 65-year-old woman). The probability that such a woman will ever die of a cancer that occurs in the coming 10 years is correspondingly low—varying from about 90 to 125 per 10 000 depending on age (Table 3).

Annual breast physical examinations for 10 years can be expected to decrease the chance that a woman will die of breast cancer by about 15 to 40 per 10 000. Stated another way, for every 10 000 women screened annually for 10 years with breast physical examinations, screening will make the difference between life and death from breast cancer for about 25 women. The increase in life expectancy achieved by 10 years of screening with breast physical examinations ranges from 10 to 30 days (4 to 10 days if discounted 5%). Adding mammography to breast physical examinations for 10 years will decrease the chance of death from breast cancer by an additional 8 to 40 per 10 000 and increase life expectancy an additional 5 to 30 days (2 to 10 days if discounted 5%).

These projections of the reduction in probability of

parameter, the effectiveness of breast physical examination and mammography, is indicated in the tables
by showing the implications of two programs, the HIP
study and the BCDDP. The effect of different assumptions can be explored. Table 6 indicates the sensitivity
of results to different assumptions about various parameters. It gives the approximate percent change in
number of deaths from breast cancer, net costs, and
cost per year of life caused by a 10% change in various
factors. The effects are different for different screening
strategies (for example, breast physical examination
alone or combined breast physical examination and
mammography) and vary slightly for different age
groups. Additional instructions for a sensitivity analysis are presented elsewhere (7).

Additional Options

The estimates in Tables 3, 4, and 5 pertain to a woman
at average risk who will receive annual breast physical
examinations alone or in combination with annual
mammograms. Additional options include focusing on
high-risk women or changing the frequency of examinations.

High-Risk Women

Women who have a family history of breast cancer
have about twice the risk for developing breast cancer
compared with the average risk; women with a personal history of breast cancer have about three times the
average risk. In high-risk women, the probability of
developing breast cancer, the probability of dying
from breast cancer, and the difference in probability of
dying caused by screening are all increased in proportion to the woman's relative risk (compared with all
women). For example, considering women between
ages 40 and 50 (see Table 3), if a woman's risk is
twice the average, her chance of developing a breast
cancer in the fifth decade of age is 256 in 10 000. Her
chance of eventually dying from a breast cancer developed in that age decade in the absence of screening is
194 in 10 000. The chance that the woman will die
from breast cancer if she is screened with breast physical examination is 140 to 162 in 10 000 (or 84 to 148
in 10 000 if she is screened with both breast physical
examination and mammography). The effect of a
woman's risk on the chance of having a false-positive
screening test, the possibility of radiation hazard, and
costs are negligible. Thus, the figures in Table 3 can be

Table 6. *Effect on Base-Case Estimate of Number of Breast Cancer Deaths and Net Costs in the Year 2000 Caused by Changing Reference Assumptions by 10 Percent**

Factor	Reference Assumption	Approximate Effect of Changing Reference Assumption by 10%		
		In Breast Cancer Deaths	In Net Costs	In Marginal Cost per Year of Life
		%———		
Proportion of women who accept screening	25%	10	10	0
Relative risk of women who accept screening	1	10	0.43	10
False-positive rate of BPE				
< 50 years old	2%	0	1.4 to 4	1.4 to 4
> 50 years old	1%	0	0.7 to 2	0.7 to 2
False-positive rate of MGY	1%	0	0.7	0.7
Cost				
Screening BPE	$25	0	5.6 to 1.9	5.6 to 1.9
Screening MGY	$75	0	7.7	7.7
Workup	$900	0	2.0 to 4	2.0 to 4
Initial treatment (average)	$9000	0	0.015	0.015
Terminal care (breast cancer)	$24 500	0	0.5	0.5
Terminal care (other causes)	$25 000	0	0.02	0.02

* BPE = breast physical examination; MGY = mammography. The base-case estimates apply to screening 25% of average-risk women who are 40 to 75 years old with the combination of mammography and breast physical examination annually from 1989 to 2000. The base-case estimates are given in Table 5.

tailored to a given woman's risk by multiplying the appropriate entries in the table by the relative risk. Precise adjustment of Tables 4 and 5 for different risk groups is more complicated and requires additional calculations.

An additional factor to consider for high-risk women is the effect of being high risk on the degree of reassurance gained from a negative examination and the willingness to tolerate a false-positive examination and workup. Whether it is justified by the actual probabilities, women with visible risk factors, such as breast cancer in a mother or sister, might perceive themselves to be at very high risk and therefore might derive inordinate relief from a negative examination or be unusually willing to accept a false-positive result. These perceptions could have a greater effect on the perceived balance of benefits and harms than the actual effect of the risk factors on breast cancer mortality. The effect of these risk factors will depend strongly on their visibility—on how much they cause the woman to worry. From this point of view, the most important risk factors by far are a personal history of breast cancer and a history of breast cancer in a sister or mother.

Low-Risk Women

Similarly, screening will have less effect on women who do not have any risk factors. For example, if a low-risk group has a relative risk of 0.25, the benefits are one fourth those shown in Table 3 and the cost per year of life is four times that shown in Table 4.

Frequency

The relative value of screening at different time intervals is determined by the natural history of breast cancer: that is, the interval between a cancer's initial detectability and the development of obvious signs and symptoms of breast cancer in the patient. The longer this "preclinical interval," the greater the proportion of effectiveness retained as the screening interval is lengthened. Calculating the actual effect of screening at various time intervals is very complicated, but some general rules apply. A lower bound is that whatever the natural history, doubling the screening interval will do no worse than cut the effectiveness in half (for example, screening will be approximately 50% as effective as if done annually), tripling the interval will do no worse than cut the effectiveness to a third, and so forth.

The actual effect of screening frequency appears to depend considerably on the woman's age. For women 40 to 50 years of age, the preclinical interval appears to be short (less than 2 years), so the degree of effectiveness retained will be only slightly better than the lower bound. It is pertinent that 2-year screening in Sweden has shown no beneficial effect on mortality in women 40 to 50 years of age after 6 years. Thus, it appears that if mammographic screening is to be done in women under 50 years of age, it should be done annually. In the case of breast cancer in women over 50 years of age, the preclinical interval appears to be longer, so the degree of effectiveness retained will be considerably better than the worst case. A 2-year interval between screenings will retain a high proportion of the effectiveness of an annual screening for this age group.

Recommendations of Organizations

Women Over 50 Years of Age

The American Cancer Society recommends annual breast physical examinations and annual mammograms for this age group. The National Cancer Institute recommends breast physical examinations at every periodic examination and mammography annually. The American College of Obstetricians and Gynecologists recommends mammograms and breast physical examinations at a frequency determined by a woman's physician. The American College of Radiology recommends annual mammograms and breast physical examinations. The American College of Physicians recommends mammograms for women between the ages of 50 and 59 "on a routine basis." Mammograms are recommended for women 60 years of age and over, with the screening interval chosen by the physician and patient. The U.S. Preventive Services Task Force recommends annual mammograms and clinical breast examinations for women over 50 years of age.

Women 40 to 50 Years of Age

The American Cancer Society recommends a baseline mammogram for women between the ages of 35 and 40, annual breast physical examinations from age 40 to age 50, and a mammogram every 1 to 2 years from age 40 to age 50. Women who are 20 to 40 years of age are recommended to see their physicians every 3 years for breast physical examination. The National Cancer Institute recommends breast physical examinations at every periodic examination, encourages mammography every 1 to 2 years starting at age 40, and encourages annual mammograms for women with a personal history of breast cancer. The American College of Obstetricians and Gynecologists recommends a baseline mammogram for women between the ages of 35 and 50, and a breast physical examination in the same age group. At any age, mammograms are recommended if there are strong indications such as a family or personal history of breast cancer, breast augmentation implants, or first pregnancy after age 30. The American College of Radiology recommends a baseline mammogram before the age of 40 years and subsequent mammograms every 1 to 2 years or more frequently based on the physician's assessment. The American College of Physicians does not recommend mammography for women below 50 years of age. The U.S. Preventive Services Task Force recommends annual clinical breast examinations for women 40 to 49 years of age but does not recommend mammograms for this age group.

Discussion

There is excellent evidence that breast cancer screening with a combination of mammography and breast physical examinations reduces mortality from breast cancer for women over 50 years of age. Although 5- to 10-year results of three controlled studies raise doubts about the effectiveness of screening in women under 50 years of age, long-term results of one trial and results of an uncontrolled project suggest it might be effective for women in that age group as well.

The relative reduction in breast cancer mortality is impressive. For women destined to develop breast cancer, a reduction in mortality from 10% to 60% can be expected, depending on the specific program (for example, breast physical examinations alone or breast physical examinations and mammography), the woman's age, and the source of the estimate (for example, HIP study or BCDDP). However, the actual magnitude of the effect is less impressive; annual screening with breast physical examinations for 10 years can be expected to decrease the probability that a woman will die of breast cancer by approximately 25 in 10 000 or increase her life expectancy approximately 25 days.

Adding mammography will further decrease the probability of death from breast cancer by about 25 in 10 000 and increase life expectancy an additional 20 days. Balanced against these benefits are the chance of a false-positive result (20% to 30% for 10 examinations) and the cost of screening (which can vary from about $400 to more than $2000 for 10 examinations). The carcinogenic effect is small.

The decision to screen for breast cancer and the choice of specific screening strategies requires making value judgments about the quality of the evidence of effectiveness and the estimated health and economic outcomes (Tables 3, 4, and 5). It is not known how women would respond if actually presented information on the magnitudes of the expected benefits, harms, and costs. One clue, albeit a very imperfect one, is that despite the nearly unanimous recommendations by several national organizations that all women over age 50 be screened annually, only about 10% of women actually choose to do so.

Eliciting the preferences of a large and representative group of women is clearly a high-priority research project. In the meantime, an appropriate approach for practitioners is to discuss the estimated outcomes for breast cancer screening (for example, those given in Table 3) with women and help them decide for themselves based on their own preferences.

Recommendation

It is recommended that practitioners present the estimates of benefits, harms, and costs to their patients and let them choose a screening strategy that suits their personal history and preferences. To the extent that a general recommendation is needed, it is reasonable to suggest that women at average risk have breast physical examinations annually after age 40 and mammography every 1 to 2 years starting at age 50. For hish-risk women, mammography can be recommended annually starting at age 40. If mammography is to be used in women under age 50, it should be done annually.

References

1. **Lynch HT, Guirgis H, Lynch J, et al.** Genetic factors in breast cancer. In: Lynch, HT, ed. *Cancer Genetics.* Springfield, Illinois: C.C. Thomas; 1976:389-423.
2. **Carter AP, Thompson RS, Bourdeau RV, et al.** A clinically effective breast cancer screening program can be cost-effective, too. *Prev Med.* 1987;**16**:19-34.
3. **Schechter MT, Miller AB, Baines CJ, Howe GR.** Selection of wom-

en at high risk of breast cancer for initial screening. *J Chronic Dis.* 1986;**39**:253-60.

4. **O'Malley MS, Fletcher SW.** US Preventive Services Task Force. Screening for breast cancer with breast self-examination. A critical review. *JAMA.* 1987;**257**:2196-203.

5. **Hill D, White V, Jolley D, Mapperson K.** Self examination of the breast: is it beneficial? Meta-analysis of studies investigating breast self examination and extent of disease in patients with breast cancer. *BMJ.* 1988;**297**:271-5.

6. **Baker LH.** Breast Cancer Detection Demonstration Project: five-year summary report. CA. 1982;**32**:194-225.

7. **Eddy DM, Hasselblad V, McGivney W, Hendee W.** The value of mammography screening in women under age 50 years. *JAMA.* 1988;**259**:1512-9.

8. **Shapiro S, Venet W, Strax P, Venet L, Roeser R.** Ten- to fourteen-year effect of screening on breast cancer mortality. *J Natl Cancer Inst.* 1982;**69**:349-55.

9. **Shapiro S, Venet W, Strax P, Venet L, Roeser R.** Selection, follow-up, and analysis in the Health Insurance Plan Study: a randomized trial with breast cancer screening. *Natl Cancer Inst Monogr.* 1985;**67**:65-74.

10. **Shapiro S, Venet W, Strax P, Venet L.** *Periodic Screening for Breast Cancer: The Health Insurance Plan Project and Its Sequelae.* Baltimore: Johns Hopkins University Press; 1988.

11. **Chu KC, Smart CR, Tarone RE.** Analysis of breast cancer mortality and stage distribution by age for the Health Insurance Plan clinical trial. *J Natl Cancer Inst.* 1988;**80**:1125-32.

12. **Tabar L, Faberberg G, Day NE, Holmberg L.** What is the optimum interval between mammographic screening examinations? An analysis based on the latest results of the Swedish two-county breast cancer screening trial. *Br J Cancer.* 1987;**55**:547-51.

13. **UK Trial of Early Detection of Breast Cancer Group.** First results on mortality reduction in the UK trial of early detection of breast cancer. *Lancet.* 1988;**2**:411-6.

14. **Andersson I, Aspergren K, Janzon L, et al.** Mammographic screening and mortality from breast cancer: the Malmö mammographic screening trial. *BMJ.* 1988;**297**:944-8.

15. **Verbeek AL, Hendriks JH, Holland R, et. al.** Reduction of breast cancer mortality through mass screening with modern mammography. First results of the Nijmegen project, 1975-1981. *Lancet.* 1984;**1**:1222-4.

16. **Verbeek AL, Hendriks JH, Holland R, Mravunac M, Sturmans F.** Mammographic screening and breast cancer mortality: age-specific effects in Nijmegen Project, 1975-82 [Letter]. *Lancet.* 1985;**1**:865-6.

17. **Palli D, Del Turco MR, Buiatti E, et al.** A case-control study of the efficacy of a non-randomized breast cancer screening program in Florence (Italy). *Int J Cancer.* 1986;**38**:501-4.

18. **Collette HJ, Day NE, Rombach JJ, deWaard F.** Evaluation of screening for breast cancer in a non-randomised study (the DOM project) by means of a case-control study. *Lancet.* 1984;**1**:1224-6.

19. **Seidman H, Gelb SK, Silverberg E, LaVerda N, Lubera JA.** Survival experience in the Breast Cancer Detection Demonstration Project. *CA.* 1987;**367**:258-90.

20. **Miller AB, Howe GR, Wall C.** The National Study of Breast Cancer Screening Protocol for a Canadian Randomized Controlled trial of screening for breast cancer in women. *Clin Invest Med.* 1981;**4**:227-58.

21. **Bailar JC 3d.** Mammography: a contrary view. *Ann Intern Med.* 1976;**84**:77-84.

22. **Eddy DM.** *Screening for Cancer: Theory, Analysis and Design.* Englewood Cliffs, New Jersey: Prentice-Hall Inc.; 1980.

23. **Shapiro S.** Evidence on screening for breast cancer from a randomized trial. *Cancer.* 1977;**39**(6 Suppl):2772-82.

24. **Shwartz M.** An analysis of the benefits of serial screening for breast cancer based upon a mathematical model of the disease. *Cancer.* 1978;**51**:1550-64.

25. **Gohagan JK, Darby WP, Spitznagel EL, Monsees BS, Tome AE.** Radiogenic breast cancer effects of mammographic screening. *J Natl Cancer Inst.* 1986;**77**:71-6.

26. **Eddy DM.** A computer-based model for designing cancer control strategies. *Natl Cancer Inst Monogr.* 1986;**2**:75-82.

27. **Eddy DM.** Breast cancer screening for women over age 65. Report prepared for U.S. Congress, Office of Technology Assessment for their report, *Breast Cancer Screening for Medicare Beneficiaries: Effectiveness, Costs to Medicare and Medical Resources Required.* Washington, DC: U.S. Government Printing Office, 1987.

28. **Greenwald P, Sondik EJ, eds.** Cancer control objectives for the nation: 1985-2000. *Natl Cancer Inst. Monogr.* 1986;**2**:59-67.

29. **Keeler EB, Cretin S.** Discounting of life-saving and other nonmonetary effects. *Manage Sci.* 1983;**29**:300-6.

30. **Sondik E, ed.** Annual Cancer Statistics Review, 1988. Washington, DC: Division of Cancer Prevention and Control, National Cancer Institute; [In press].

Screening for Cervical Cancer

DAVID M. EDDY, MD, PhD

Approximately 13 000 cases of and 7000 deaths from cervical cancer were expected to occur in the United States in 1988 (1). Although these figures are low compared with the other cancers for which screening is commonly recommended, the natural history of cervical cancer, with a long preinvasive stage, and the availability of a simple test make cervical cancer ideal for screening. We review current information on incidence and risk factors; evidence of effectiveness; and magnitudes of benefits, harms, and costs.

Probability of Developing Cervical Cancer

Compared with other cancers for which screening is frequently recommended, the probability an individual woman will develop invasive cervical cancer in the coming year (incidence) is low. Annual incidence rates rise slowly beginning at about age 35 to 39 and quickly plateau at about 20 per 100 000 (2). Incidence rates of carcinoma in situ are higher, peaking at about 130 per 100 000 in the age decade 25 to 35, then declining to about 20 per 100 000 by age 50 (3). (For comparison, the incidence of breast cancer in a 65-year-old woman is approximately 292 per 100 000.) On the basis of these age-specific incidence rates, the lifetime probability that an average-risk woman in the United States will develop invasive cervical cancer was estimated in 1985 to be about 0.7%. The lifetime probability of developing carcinoma in situ was estimated at that time to be about 2% (4).

These incidence rates are strongly affected by screening, and do not represent the rates that would occur in an unscreened population. In unscreened women, the incidence of carcinoma in situ would be far lower, and the incidence of invasive cancer would be higher. Although it is impossible to know for certain what the incidence rates would be in the United States without screening, a reasonable estimate, based on observations of how rates have changed historically after the intro-

▶ This chapter was originally published in *Annals of Internal Medicine*. 1990;**113:**214-26.

duction of screening, and based on observed incidence rates of preinvasive lesions, is that in the absence of screening, rates of invasive cervical cancer in the United States would be approximately two to three times those actually observed.

Risk factors for cervical cancer have been well reviewed by Brinton and Fraumeni (5). Incidence rates are approximately two times higher for blacks, Hispanics, and Native Americans than for whites, whereas Orientals have rates similar to those of whites. The two most important factors affecting risk are early age at first intercourse and number of sexual partners. Several studies indicate that women with more than one partner have approximately two to three times the risk compared with women who have had only one partner (6, 7).

Several studies that controlled for the number of sexual partners or age at first intercourse, or both, found an association between smoking and the incidence of cervical cancer (8-12). Recent data from a five-center study in the United States (13) support an independent effect; after adjusting for confounding factors, smokers were found to have about a 50% higher risk for developing squamous cell cancer of the cervix than nonsmokers. The risk increases for long-term smokers, high-intensity smokers, and users of unfiltered cigarettes.

Although early studies failed to associate use of oral contraceptives with cervical cancer, more recent studies indicate both an increased risk for noninvasive cervical abnormalities as well as invasive neoplasms for long-term pill users (10, 14-17). The World Health Organization (WHO) Collaborative Study of Neoplasia and Steroid Contraceptives (18) controlled for a number of confounding variables and found an adjusted relative risk of 1.2 associated with any use of oral contraceptives, and an adjusted relative risk of 1.5 associated with 5 or more years of use of oral contraceptives (18). Another study in five geographic areas in the United States found a 50% excess risk in all users of oral contraceptives, and a twofold increased risk in long-term users (19).

Screening Tests

The main test used to screen for cervical cancer is the Papanicolaou smear, developed by Dr. George Papanicolaou in the 1930s and introduced for widespread screening in the 1940s by Drs. Papanicolaou and Traut. Other procedures, such as colposcopy and cervigrams (20), have been used for screening but at this time are not widely available or proposed, have not been fully researched, and will not be analyzed here.

The probability that a particular Papanicolaou smear will fail to detect an existing lesion (dysplasia, carcinoma in situ, or invasive cancer) depends on technical factors related to sampling, slide preparation, laboratory accuracy, and reporting. "False-negative rates" due to these causes are reported to range from less than 5% to more than 50% (21-32). The wide discrepancy is explained in part by the different definitions of false-negative rate and different methods used by various investigators. For example, Berkowitz and colleagues (22) calculated not the false-negative rate as it is technically defined (the probability of a negative result in a woman who actually has a cancer or preinvasive lesion), but rather reported the proportion of women with invasive cancer who had recently had a negative examination. Rylander (28) reported the rate of misclassified smears in women who developed invasive cancer within 4 to 5 years of a "negative" smear. Morell and colleagues (27) calculated the false-negative rate in women who developed invasive cancer, which is biased by not including women who had true-positive examinations that detected lesions before invasion. All of these approaches tend to overestimate the true false-negative rate. Most other studies are not population-based. Two of the most useful papers, because they are population-based and current, are by Yobs and colleagues (32) and van der Graaf and Vooijs (31).

Yobs and colleagues (32) calculated a "relative" laboratory false-negative rate by having two laboratories trade 20 000 slides and comparing their diagnoses. Depending on which laboratory is considered the "truth," the rate of undercalling a carcinoma in situ or invasive cancer ranged from 34% to 57%. These figures overestimate the true false-negative rate because some of the reference laboratories' "positives" could have been "false-positives." Van der Graaf and Vooijs (31), defining a Papanicolaou smear as falsely negative if a woman developed a confirmed lesion within 2 years of a negative smear, calculated a false-negative rate of 17%. This definition also overestimates the false-negative rate because it includes cases not actually present at the time of screening but that developed rapidly to signs or symptoms within 2 years.

Fortunately, if there is empiric evidence about how screening affects incidence and mortality from invasive cervical cancer, it is not necessary to establish exactly what the false-negative rate is. Nature integrates all the pertinent information on natural history, progression times, regression rates, false-negative rates, stage progression, and other factors to produce the true effect of screening. To the greatest extent possible, choices among strategies should be based on these empiric observations, as will be done in this paper, rather than on theories developed from individual factors such as false-negative rates, however defined. The main reasons to study false-negative rates are to compare the quality of providers and laboratories in different settings and to seek ways to reduce the errors.

False-positive Papanicolaou smears can occur in two ways. A laboratory report can incorrectly state that a specimen contains abnormal cells when it does not. Although there are few good data on false-positive rates, the study by Yobs and colleagues (32) calculated "relative" false-positive rates. Depending on which laboratory is considered the "truth," the false-positive rate for diagnosing a lesion as carcinoma in situ or invasive cancer was 0.24% to 0.6%. The relative false-positive rate for diagnosing a lesion as moderate dysplasia or worse was between 0.5% and 1.3%.

A second type of "false positive" can occur if the examination detects a case of dysplasia or carcinoma in situ that would have regressed spontaneously had the woman not been examined. These results can be considered false-positive in the sense that the woman will receive an unnecessary workup and possibly treatment. Several studies have reported spontaneous regression rates for dysplasia diagnosed cytologically in the range of 6% to 60% (33-39).

Evidence of Effectiveness

Evidence about the effectiveness of cervical cancer screening is provided by historical studies, case-control studies, analysis of data from large screening programs, and analysis of the natural history of cervical cancer with mathematic models.

Historic Studies

More than a dozen regions ranging in size from cities to countries have reported declines in both incidence and mortality of invasive cervical cancer after the introduction of large-scale screening programs. Data from Iceland are illustrative (40). Before screening was introduced in 1964, the mortality from cervical cancer had been rising, and continued to rise during the first few years of screening. Beginning in 1970, however, the annual mortality rate began to decline and by 1974 was about half the rate in the late 1960s (a decrease from 23.1 per 100 000 from 1965 to 1969 to 14.6 per 100 000 from 1970 to 1974). Similar observations have been made in the Nordic countries (41, 42), Germany (43), Scotland (44), as well as in the United States (45) and Canada. Supporting epidemiologic evidence is the observation that in Canada the reduction in mortality from cervical cancer correlated with the intensity of screening (as measured by the proportion of the population screened) across communities (46). The correlation coefficient was 0.72.

Case-Control Studies

A large number of case-control studies have been done, all of which showed that screening reduces the incidence of invasive cervical cancer. Clarke and Anderson (47) evaluated the effectiveness of cervical cancer screening in women diagnosed with invasive cervical cancer in the Toronto area in the mid-1970s. Two hundred twelve cases were matched by age with five controls drawn from neighbors. They found a relative risk for invasive cancer of 0.37 ($P < 0.0001$) in women who had been screened with Papanicolaou smears compared with those who had not. The results persisted after stratification by age, income, education, marital history, smoking habit, employment status, and access to medical care.

A case-control study from Milan (48) involved 191 women with invasive cancer detected between 1981 and 1983, matched by age and hospital admission. Compared with women with no previous screening, screened women had a relative risk for invasive cervical cancer of 0.44 (95% confidence interval [CI], 0.25 to 0.8) for those who had one smear, and 0.2 (CI, 0.13 to 0.32) for those who had had two or more smears. The relative risk varied with the time since the last smear: 0.36 for intervals of more than 5 years, 0.18 for intervals of 3 to 5 years, and 0.1 for intervals of less than 3 years. The investigators estimated that invasive cervical cancer could be reduced 64% by screening every 5 years, an additional 18% by screening every 3 to 5 years, and an additional 8% by screening at intervals of less than 3 years.

A case-control study of screening in Cali, Columbia (49) involved 204 patients with cervical cancer and two sets of matched controls. The most pessimistic estimate, based on neighborhood controls, was a relative risk of 0.1 in women screened compared with those never screened.

A study by MacGregor and colleagues (50) of women with invasive cancer in northeastern Scotland estimated the relative risk for invasive cervical cancer in each year after a negative screening result. One hundred fifteen women with invasive cancers diagnosed between 1968 and 1982 were matched by age with 5 controls each. They found a relative risk for invasive cancer of 0.11 for 12 to 23 months after a Papanicolaou smear, 0.28 for 24 to 35 months, 0.43 for 36 to 47 months, 0.63 for 47 to 71 months, and 1 for more than 72 months. They concluded that the degree of "protection" was high for the first 3 years after a negative smear.

A more recent case-control study analyzed a screening program in the Netherlands (51). Thirty-six women with invasive cervical cancer were matched by age with 120 controls. The relative risk for invasive cervical cancer for women screened at least once compared with women never screened was 0.32. After correcting for age at first intercourse (the major risk factor found in this study), the relative risk decreased to 0.22. The investigators also analyzed the effect of the length of time since the last smear; the relative risk was 0.18 when the last smear was done between 2 and 5 years earlier, and 0.3 when the smear was more than 5 years earlier. They concluded that "even an interval of more than five years seems to provide considerable protection" (51).

A very recent nationwide case-control evaluation from Denmark (52) reported data on 428 women with invasive cancer and matched controls. When only asymptomatic patients were considered, the relative risk was reduced to 0.15 for women screened every 3 years compared with those never screened. Even screening every 5 or more years reduced the relative risk to 0.33, compared with no screening. The authors concluded that the greatest need is to screen unscreened women and that increasing the number of screens had only marginal benefit.

Finally, Shy and colleagues (53) reported that the risk of invasive cervical cancer (all cell types) was increased 3.9 times (CI, 1.2 to 12.3) with screening every 3 years compared with every 1 year, but there was no increase in risk associated with screening every 2 years compared with every 1 year, even after adjustment for age, education, marital status, age at first intercourse, and number of sexual partners.

The case-control studies, from various settings, all indicate that screening for cervical cancer with Papanicolaou smears is highly effective, decreasing the occurrence of invasive cancer by 60% to more than 90%.

Table 1. *Percent Reduction in Cumulative Rate of Invasive Cervical Cancer in Women Screened from Age 35 to 64 at Different Frequencies**

Interval between Screenings	Reduction in Cumulative Incidence	Tests
y	%	*n*
1	93.5	30
2	92.5	15
3	90.8	10
5	83.6	6
10	64.1	3

* Assumes a woman has had at least one previous screen. Source: reference 54.

They also all indicate that the degree of protection is related to the interval between examinations, and considerable protection is present even with long intervals (for example, 3 to 5 years).

Analysis of Data from Large Screening Programs

Recently, a working group of the International Agency for Research on Cancer (IARC) conducted a comprehensive analysis of data from several of the largest screening programs in the world (54). The group analyzed data from screening programs conducted in the 1960s and 1970s in eight countries in North America and Europe to determine the reduction in probability of invasive cancer caused by screening and the relative reduction caused by screening at different frequencies. Most of the data come from centrally organized screening programs, and incorporated results from programs previously analyzed by case-control studies in Scotland (50) and Toronto (47).

The estimated reduction in probability of developing invasive cancer as a function of the interval between examinations, for women between ages 35 and 64, is shown in Table 1. In general, screening reduced the probability a woman would develop invasive cervical cancer by approximately 90% for frequencies up to every 3 years. Screening every 2 to 3 years was found to be almost as effective by this measure as screening every year (within 3%). The effectiveness dropped more sharply when screening intervals are extended beyond 3 to 5 years, although a 10-year frequency still reduced the incidence of invasive cervical cancer by 64%.

The expected effect on incidence of other combinations of ages and frequencies based on the results of the IARC study have been calculated by Miller (55) (Table 2). Again, virtually all strategies provide a similar high degree of protection against invasive cervical cancer, although they have very different requirements for patient visits and resources (reflected in the number of tests). Shun-Zhang and colleagues (56) conducted a similar analysis based on Canadian data and derived similar results.

Mathematic Models

Mathematic models have been developed to simulate the natural history of cervical cancer: the incidence, natural history, detectability, and survival with treatment (56-62). These models all indicate that Papanicolaou smear screening, even at frequencies of more than 5 years, should be quite effective in reducing mortality, yielding reductions in the range of 60% to 90% over the period of screening.

Risks

A Papanicolaou smear by itself carries virtually no direct risk. The main risks are those of a false-positive result due to overreading by the laboratory or the detection of a lesion that would have regressed spontaneously. The seriousness of these events depends on the subsequent workup and treatment. If patients diagnosed with early dysplasia are merely followed with repeated Papanicolaou smears, the outcome is anxiety and inconvenience. Treatment with conization or hysterectomy involves more serious risks. Another possible risk is a false sense of security. Women who have recently been screened and had a negative test might tend to ignore signs and symptoms, allowing an invasive cancer to develop to an advanced stage. There are no data on the frequency with which this occurs or the consequences.

Costs

Laboratory charges for a Papanicolaou smear are approximately $3. When institution charges and physician fees are included, however, the cost is considerably higher. The actual fees charged have never been systematically surveyed. A sense of the range and approximate magnitude of charges is revealed by an informal telephone survey of 20 institutions and physicians; the total charge for a Papanicolaou smear (including any

Table 2. *The Effect of Different Screening Strategies on the Cumulative Incidence of Invasive Cancer of the Uterine Cervix**

Screening Schedule	Reduction in Rate	Tests
	%	n
Every 5 years, age 20 to 64	83.6	9
Every 5 years, age 25 to 64	81.8	8
Every 5 years, age 35 to 64	69.6	6
Every year, age 20 to 34, then every 5 years, age 35 to 64	85.5	21
Age 25, 26, 30, then every 5 years	82.6	9
Every 3 years, age 20 to 64	91.2	15
Every 3 years, age 26 to 64	89.8	13
Every 3 years, age 35 to 64	77.6	10
Every year, age 20 to 34, then every 3 years, age 35 to 64	91.7	25
Ages 25, 26, 29, then every 3 years	90.1	14
Screening every year, age 20 to 64	93.3	35

* Source: reference 55.

physician or clinic fees required before a woman can obtain a Papanicolaou smear) averaged $76, with a range from $34 to more than $100. An article from the Kaiser Permanente Medical Center in Los Angeles (a health maintenance organization) reported a cost for a Papanicolaou smear of $62 (20).

For decisions by individual practitioners, the pertinent costs are their own charges and depend on the circumstances in which screening is being offered. If the practitioner is already seeing the woman for other reasons and the Papanicolaou smear is an incidental test, the appropriate charge does not include the office visit fee. On the other hand, if the practitioner recommends that a woman be seen specifically for a Papanicolaou smear or if a woman comes to see her physician primarily for a Papanicolaou smear, the charge includes the office visit fee.

Choosing a Screening Strategy

The American Cancer Society, the National Cancer Institute, and the American College of Obstetricians and Gynecologists recently issued recommendations that women who are 18 years of age or sexually active have Papanicolaou smears annually for 3 years. After three satisfactory negative annual examinations, the frequency can be reduced at the discretion of their physicians.

If these recommendations are used as a starting point, they raise several important questions for the practicing physician. First, what is the expected effect of screening? For example, how important is it to ensure that all women receive some screening? How important is it to start at age 18? What are the consequences if a woman waits until age 20—or later? How important are the three initial annual negative examinations? For example, what if a woman has received negative examinations at ages 20, 23, and 26; does she still require three annual examinations, or can she wait until, say, age 29 and continue with 3-year examinations? After several negative examinations, what are the consequences of reducing the frequency, and, if it is to be reduced, what should the new frequency be? At what age is it appropriate to stop receiving Papanicolaou smears? If a woman has been screened to age 62, can she stop? If not, can she stop at age 74, 86, or some other age? What if it is suspected that a laboratory has a higher than average false-negative rate? How will this change the expected outcomes of different strategies? Finally, should different screening strategies be recommended for low-risk or for high-risk women?

It is not possible to answer these questions with empiric experiments such as controlled trials. The outcomes can be estimated, however, from existing empiric data with mathematic models calibrated to fit those data. For this analysis, the consequences of different options were estimated with a mathematic model that was calibrated to reproduce the empirically observed IARC results (60). The model and main assumptions are described in the Appendix. The IARC data were chosen as the basis for the model because they encompass by far the largest population, being based on five case-control studies conducted within cohort studies as well as five additional cohort studies. Altogether, the screened populations that contributed data to this study comprise more than 1 million women. Potential limitations of these data are that the IARC analysis was conducted for women from 35 to 64 years of age, and that the screening programs used centralized laboratories.

Because charges for Papanicolaou smears vary so much from practitioner to practitioner and setting to setting (for example, a visit primarily for a Papanicolaou smear compared with an "incidental" Papanicolaou smear done while a patient is seeing a physician for other reasons), it is impossible to calculate costs or costs per year of life expectancy that are broadly applicable to all settings. As a reference, this analysis will give the cost per year of life expectancy assuming a $75 charge, as might occur if it is recommended that a woman see her physician primarily for a Papanicolaou smear. If the charges are lower (or higher) in particular settings, the cost per year of life expectancy will be correspondingly, but not strictly proportionately, lower or higher.

Reference

Without screening, a 20-year-old average-risk asymptomatic woman has about a 250 in 10 000 (2.5%) chance of ever developing invasive cervical cancer during the rest of her life, and about a 118 in 10 000 (1.18%) chance of dying from cervical cancer. Cervical cancer reduces the average-risk woman's life expectancy by about 109 days.

Magnitude of Effect

Table 3 shows the effect of six screening options, presented from the perspective of a 20-year-old average-risk asymptomatic woman. The six columns of the table estimate the effects of a woman being screened from age 20 to about age 75 every 4 years, every 3 years to age 74, every 3 years after four initial annual negative examinations, every 2 years to age 74, every 2 years after three initial annual negative examinations, and every year to age 75. Figure 1 compares the effectiveness (measured as the decrease in probability of dying from cervical cancer) and cost (measured as net financial costs, discounted 5%) (63), for the six strategies. Screening with any of these strategies can be expected to decrease the probability a woman will ever develop invasive cervical cancer by about 215 in 10 000, and to decrease the probability a woman will die from cervical cancer by about 107 in 10 000. Stated differently, for a group of 10 000 women screened for 55 years from age 20 to 74, screening will make a difference between life and death from cervical cancer in about 107 women. Screening from age 20 to 74 will increase a woman's life expectancy by about 96 days. After discounting 5%, the increase in life expectancy caused by screening is approximately 10 days. The discounted costs and the marginal costs per year of life expectancy (without quality adjustment) are given in the fifth and sixth rows. For calculating marginal costs per year of life expectancy, both health effects and costs are discounted 5% (63).

The difference in effectiveness between the strategies

Table 3. *Estimated Outcomes of Cervical Cancer Screening for an Average-Risk Asymptomatic 20-year-old Woman Screened from Age 20 to 75**

Estimated Outcome	Papanicolaou Smear					
	Every 4 Years	Every 3 Years	Every 3 Years after Four Annual Negative Smears	Every 2 Years	Every 2 Years after Three Annual Negative Smears	Every Year
Decrease in probability of developing invasive cervical cancer†, /10 000	207	210	211	216	216	222
Decrease in lifetime probability of death from cervical cancer‡, /10 000	104.3	105.2	105.4	106.7	106.8	108.5
Increase in life expectancy, d	93.8	95.4	95.7	96.9	97.0	98.6
Increase in life expectancy, discounted 5%, d	9.54	9.72	9.78	9.88	9.9	10.07
Net costs, discounted 5%, $	264	355	467	439	597	1093
Marginal cost per year of life expectancy§, $	10 000‖	184 528¶	681 336**	262 800**	>1 000 000††	>1 000 000††

* All estimates are approximate. Decimal points are retained to avoid roundoff errors.
† Reference probability without screening: 250 in 10 000.
‡ Reference probability without screening: 118 in 10 000.
§ Health effects and costs are discounted 5%.
‖ Compared with no screening.
¶ Compared with screening every 4 years.
** Compared with screening every 3 years.
†† Compared with screening every 2 years.

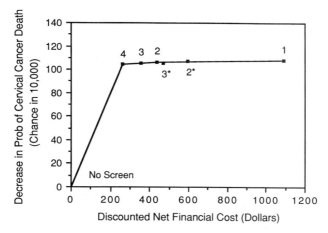

Figure 1. Graph of decrease in the probability of dying from cervical cancer (per 10 000) compared with net financial cost (discounted 5%) for an average-risk woman screened from 20 to 75 years of age at various frequencies. 1 = Papanicolaou smear every year (to age 75); 2 = Papanicolaou smear every 2 years (to age 74); 2* = Papanicolaou smear every 2 years after three initial negative Papanicolaou smears (to age 74); 3 = Papanicolaou smear every 3 years (to age 74); 3* = Papanicolaou smear every 3 years after four initial negative Papanicolaou smears (to age 74); 4 = Papanicolaou smear every 4 years (to age 76).

is very small. For example, compared with a 3-year frequency, screening annually from ages 20 to 74 (36 additional screens) decreases the probability that an average-risk woman will die from cervical cancer by about 4 in 10 000, and increases her life expectancy by about 3 days. After discounting, the difference in life expectancy between annual compared with triennial screening is on the order of 9 hours.

Age to Start Screening

Table 4 shows the differences in probabilities of ever developing or dying from invasive cervical cancer if screening is begun at different ages and continued every 3 years until age 74. If screening is begun at age 17 instead of 20, for example, the probability of developing invasive cervical cancer will be decreased an additional 3 in 10 000 (213 − 210 = 3), the probability of dying from cervical cancer will be decreased an additional 2 in 10 000 (107 − 105 = 2), and the woman's life expectancy will be increased about 3 days (about 10 hours, with discounting). The effects of starting at ages other than those shown in Table 4 can be estimated by inter-

Table 4. *Estimated Outcomes of Cervical Cancer Screening for an Average-Risk Asymptomatic Woman Screened Every 3 Years to Age 74**

Estimated Outcome
Decrease in probability of developing invasive cervical cancer†, /10 000
Decrease in probability of dying from cervical cancer‡, /10 000
Increase in life expectancy, *d*
Increase in life expectancy, discounted 5%, *d*
Net costs, discounted 5%, $
Marginal cost of adding an additional year of life expectancy§, $

* All estimates are approximate. Decimal points are retained to avoid roundoff errors.

† Reference probability without screening: 250 in 10 000.

polation. Thus the difference made by initiating screening at 17 years of age compared with 20 or 23 is very small.

Effect of Initial Annual Examinations

The possible need for several annual negative examinations before decreasing the frequency of screening is examined in Table 3. Comparing the second and third columns indicates that for a woman who starts screening at age 20 and is screened every 3 years until age 74, receiving four initial annual examinations will decrease her probability of ever developing invasive cervical cancer by about 1 in 10 000, will decrease her chance of dying from cervical cancer by about 0.2 in 10 000 (2 in 100 000), and will increase her life expectancy by about 0.3 days (about 7 hours). The effect of requiring two or three initial annual negative examinations (instead of four as shown in the third column) is proportionately less. After discounting, the marginal cost per year of life expectancy of requiring four initial annual negative examinations before switching to a 3-year frequency (compared with a straight 3-year frequency) is about $681 000. Similarly, if screening is done every 2 years, requiring three initial annual examinations before moving to a 2-year frequency has very little effect.

To answer a question previously raised, if a woman is screened at 20, 23, and 26 years of age, the effect of requiring three annual examinations (ages 27, 28 and 29) before returning to a 3-year frequency is to decrease her chances of developing or dying from invasive cervical cancer by 0.7 in 10 000 (7 in 100 000), and 0.2 in 10 000

Table 4. (*Continued*)

Age at which Screening Is Begun, y				
17	20	23	26	29
213	210	206	199	190
107	105	103	100	96
98	95	92	87	80
10.1	9.7	9.1	8.2	7.2
423	355	297	249	209
50 095	33 078	20 612	14 747	10 537

‡ Reference probability without screening: 118 in 10 000.
§ Comparisons are 29 versus no screening, 26 versus 29, and so forth. Health effects and costs are discounted 5%.

(2 in 100 000), respectively. The effect on life expectancy is 0.3 days (approximately 7 hours without discounting, 1 hour with discounting), and the marginal cost per year of life expectancy achieved by requiring three annual examinations is about $721 310. The requirement that the three initial screens be done annually has great cost but little effect on health outcomes.

Choice of a Reduced Frequency

If a woman has had four initial negative examinations starting at 20 years of age, the effect of reducing the frequency to every 3 years after that is shown by comparing the third and sixth columns of Table 3. The IARC results imply that whether the outcome is incidence of invasive cervical cancer, mortality from cervical cancer, or life expectancy, a 3-year frequency retains about 96% of the effect of an annual frequency. The improvements in probabilities of developing or dying from invasive cervical cancer with annual screening compared with a 3-year frequency are 11 in 10 000 and 3.1 in 10 000, respectively. The improvement in life expectancy is less than 2.9 days without discounting (7 hours with discounting). The marginal cost per year of life expectancy achieved by retaining an annual frequency is about $794 000. The effect of a 2-year frequency is shown in the fourth column.

Age to End Screening

The effect of screening older women depends heavily on their previous screening histories. Consider first a 65-year-old woman who has had negative examinations

Table 5. *Estimated Outcomes of Cervical Cancer Screening for a Previously Screened Average-Risk Asymptomatic Woman Screened Every 3 Years for Four Additional Examinations**†

Estimated Outcome	Starting at	
	Age 65	Age 74
Decrease in probability of developing invasive cervical cancer‡, *per 10 000*	45.7	17.7
Decrease in probability of dying from invasive cervical cancer§, *per 10 000*	17.9	6.2
Increase in life expectancy, *d*	3.1	1.1
Increase in life expectancy, discounted 5%, *d*	1.6	0.5
Net costs, discounted 5%, *$*	229	220
Marginal cost per year of life expectancy (compared with no further screening)‖, *$*	52 241	160 000

* All estimates are approximate. Decimal points are retained to avoid roundoff errors.

† Assumes the woman was screened previously every 3 years for at least 12 years (at least five previous examinations).

‡ Reference probability without screening: 94.5 in 10 000 for women age 65; 61.2 in 10 000 for women age 74.

§ Reference probability without screening: 39.8 in 10 000 for women age 65; 24 in 10 000 for women age 74.

‖ Health effects and costs are discounted 5%.

every 3 years for the previous several screenings (for example, at ages 53, 56, 59, and 62), and is considering continuing triennial examinations for another 9 years (four more examinations). The first column of Table 5 pertains to such a woman at age 65, showing the effects of continuing screening with four additional triennial examinations to age 74. Continuing screening will decrease the chance of death from cervical cancer by about 18 in 10 000, and increase life expectancy by about 3 days. The second column of the table shows the same information from the viewpoint of a 74-year-old woman who has been screened over the past 10 years (at ages 62, 65, 68, and 71), and who is considering having four more examinations over the next 9 years (to age 83). The effect on life expectancy is about a third of that for a 65-year-old woman.

If a woman has never been screened previously, the effect is roughly twice as great, depending on the outcome of the examination. Table 6 shows the outcomes of four triennial examinations starting at ages 65 and 74 for women who have never before been screened.

False-Negative Rates

Tables 3 to 6 are based on data obtained from large

screening programs with centralized laboratories in North America and Europe. A frequently expressed concern is that the quality of cytology laboratories in the United States might not be as high as the quality of the laboratories analyzed in the IARC study, although there is virtually no experimental evidence for this. Indeed, studies of some U.S. laboratories have shown that false-negative rates due to laboratory errors are low (26). If any practitioner suspects his or her laboratory has a higher than average false-negative rate, the obvious course is to switch to a laboratory with better quality control. A list of laboratories that participate in the voluntary accreditation program of the American Society of Cytology can be obtained from that organization (1015 Chestnut Street, Suite 1518, Philadelphia PA 19107).

If for some reason a practitioner cannot avoid using a laboratory that he or she suspects has worse than average quality, the consequences can be estimated. Table 7 shows the effects of some of the screening strategies shown in Table 3, but assumes Papanicolaou smears are processed by a laboratory that has a false-negative rate 15% higher (that is, worse) than the laboratories involved in the IARC study. (This assumption can be considered pessimistic; for example, Gay and col-

Table 6. *Estimated Outcomes of Cervical Cancer Screening for an Average-Risk Asymptomatic Woman (Never Previously Screened) Screened Every 3 Years for 12 Years**

Estimated Outcome	Starting at	
	Age 65	Age 74
Decrease in probability of developing invasive cervical cancer†, *per 10 000*	59	32
Decrease in probability of dying from invasive cervical cancer‡, *per 10 000*	29	16
Increase in life expectancy, *d*	9.2	3.3
Increase in life expectancy, discounted 5%, *d*	4	1.7
Net costs, discounted 5%, *$*	246	233
Marginal cost per year of life expectancy (compared with no further screening)§, *$*	22 448	50 026

* All estimates are approximate. Decimal points are retained to avoid roundoff error.

† Reference probability without screening: 94.5 in 10 000 for women age 65; 61.2 in 10 000 for women age 74.

‡ Reference probability without screening: 39.8 in 10 000 for women age 65; 24 in 10 000 for women age 74.

§ Health effects and costs are discounted 5%.

Table 7. *Estimated Outcomes of Cervical Cancer Screening Every 3 Years from Age 20 to 74 for an Average-Risk Asymptomatic 20-year-old Woman, Assuming the False-Negative Rate is 15% Higher than in Centralized Laboratories in Europe and Canada**

Estimated Outcome

Decrease in probability of developing invasive cervical
    cancer†, */10 000*
Decrease in lifetime probability of death from cervical cancer‡,
    /10 000
Increase in life expectancy, *d*
Increase in life expectancy, discounted 5%, *d*
Net costs, discounted 5%, *$*
Marginal cost per year of life expectancy§, *$*

* All estimates are approximate. Decimal points are retained to avoid
roundoff errors.
    † Reference probability without screening: 250 in 10 000.
    ‡ Reference probability without screening: 118 in 10 000.

leagues [26] found that the laboratory false-negative rate was approximately 10%.)

Even assuming this higher false-negative rate, the overall value of screening still shows about an 88% reduction in mortality. Further, the difference between annual and triennial examinations remains small. For example, the difference in life expectancy achieved by screening every year compared with every 3 years is about 2.5 days greater for the centralized laboratories (Table 3) compared with laboratories that have a 15% higher false-negative rate (Table 7). (After discounting, the difference between annual and triennial screening caused by the higher false-negative rate is about 6.5 hours.)

Screening Low-Risk and High-Risk Women

Because Tables 1 and 2 give the decrease in probability of invasive cancer in women who are otherwise destined to develop invasive cancer (that is, without screening), they apply to women in any risk group. However, the absolute reduction in probability caused by screening of developing or dying from invasive cancer is affected by a woman's risk. Tables 3 to 7 apply to average-risk women. The effect of screening strategies for women at lower than average risk or higher than

Table 7. *(Continued)*

Papanicolaou Smear			
Every 3 Years	Every 3 Years after Four Annual Negative Smears	Every 2 Years	Every Year
200	202	210	219
102	102	105	108
92.0	92.9	95.0	97.6
9.3	9.5	9.6	9.9
357	468	540	1094
13 996‖	253 219¶	208 734¶	674 033**

§ Health effects and costs are discounted 5%.
‖ Compared with no screening.
¶ Compared with screening every 3 years.
** Compared with screening every 2 years.

average risk can be estimated by multiplying the appropriate entries in Tables 3 to 7 by the relative risk (relative to the risk of the total population). For example (*see* Table 3), a woman with twice the average risk would have about a 400 in 10 000 chance of developing cervical cancer, and 3-year screening from age 20 to 74 can be expected to reduce the probability by about 420 in 10 000 (210 × 2 = 420). The difference between a 3-year frequency and an annual frequency is to increase the chance she will develop invasive cervical cancer by approximately 24 in 10 000. If a low-risk woman has a risk about half the average risk, the entries in Tables 3 to 7 should be divided by two.

When tailoring these tables to apply to individual women, it is important not to mis-estimate a woman's relative risk. For example, the simple fact that a woman has had more than one sexual partner does not automatically place her at higher than average risk because the average number of sexual partners is more than one. (Two or more sexual partners carries a higher risk than zero or one partner, but not necessarily a higher risk than the average woman, because the average woman has had multiple partners.) There are few good data on the relative risk for different categories of numbers of sexual partners (for example, 0, 1 to 3, 4 to 6, 7 to 10, and so on.) One approach to estimating an upper limit for a woman's relative risk is to estimate what percentile she is in with respect to the number of sexual partners. For example, consider a particular woman in the top 30%. If all the cases of cervical cancers occurred in women in that percentile (with no cancers at all occurring in women with fewer sexual partners), the relative risk would be given by the reciprocal of the percentile (1 divided by the percentile). For a woman in the top 30%, for example, the maximum value for her relative risk is less than 3.3 (1/0.3 = 3.3). This is an overestimate, however, because cervical cancers do occur in women with fewer sexual partners.

Cost-Effectiveness

The marginal cost-effectiveness of different strategies depends greatly on Papanicolaou smear charges, which vary widely, and depends somewhat on the false-positive rate and the cost of working up a false-positive test result. To provide a reference, the sixth rows of Tables 3 to 7 show the implications of a $75 charge (the average value obtained in the informal survey), and a 0.5% rate of false-positive examinations that require a repeat Papanicolaou smear. Both health effects and estimated costs are discounted 5% (63).

These estimates include expected savings from finding lesions in earlier, usually preinvasive stages, in which treatment costs are low, and include expected savings from reduced costs for terminal care. Not included are continuing care costs, any costs of treating noninvasive lesions that would regress spontaneously, and the cost of lost time from work, travel expenses, or other indirect costs. Further, any anxiety, discomfort, or inconvenience of examinations or workups are not included. Taken together, these factors indicate that the cost estimates understate the cost per year of quality-adjusted life expectancy.

Tables 3 to 7 show that the cost-effectiveness of different strategies varies tremendously. For example, whereas a 4-year Papanicolaou smear delivers a year of life expectancy (not adjusted for quality) for about $10 000 (discounting both health effects and costs 5%), the marginal cost of adding an additional year of life expectancy by increasing the frequency or requiring initial annual negative examinations is exceedingly high—in the hundreds of thousands of dollars.

Given the importance of Papanicolaou smear charges and given the high variability in current fees, it is important to explore the consequences of different fees. In general, changing the assumed charge for Papanicolaou smears by 10% changes the discounted net costs about 10%, which in turn changes the cost per year of life expectancy by about 10%. If an examination is $37.50 instead of $75, for example, the marginal cost per year of life expectancy will be approximately 50% of the values shown in the tables. The effect of different assumptions about the false-positive rate is negligible.

Change in Incidence or Natural History of Cervical Cancer

Some authors have raised the possibility that there is an increased frequency of preinvasive cancers in younger women or that there is an etiologically distinct subgroup of lesions that have rapid progression times (so-called "fast movers") or both. These were apparently important considerations in the revised screening recommendations of the Canadian Task Force on Cervical Cancer Screening (64).

There is little empiric evidence for either hypothesis. First, a comparison of 1975 and 1986 data from the Surveillance, Epidemiology, and End Results Program (SEER) of the National Cancer Institute shows a decrease in incidence of invasive cervical cancer in all age groups but one—80 to 84 years—and there the increase was trivial (25.66 per 100 000 in 1975 compared with 25.81 per 100 000 in 1986). For carcinoma in situ, the incidence increased for only three age groups—15 to 19 years, 20 to 24 years, and 80 to 84 years. However, these findings must be interpreted with great caution. The increase was observed for only 2 years (1985, 1986); it is not adjusted for any changes in screening or diagnostic techniques (for example, colposcopy); not all cases of carcinoma in situ progress to invasive cancer; and it is not matched by any increase in incidence of invasive cervical cancers. Further, the actual magnitude of the increase in carcinoma in situ is very small, on the order of 8 cases in 100 000 women. Even if the observations are considered real and assumed to imply an eventual increase in occurrence of invasive cervical cancers, the effect on the merits of screening at different frequencies is very small (a few minutes of life expectancy). In any event, even the most pessimistic interpretation would have no implications for the frequency of screening after age 25.

Regarding the question of an increasing frequency of "fast movers" that progress rapidly from carcinoma in situ to invasion, a critical evaluation of the evidence does not support the clinical impression. For example, a Task Force of the International Union Against Cancer

Table 8. *Estimated Outcomes of Cervical Cancer Screening for an Average-Risk Asymptomatic 20-year-old Woman Screened from Age 20 to 74, Assuming a High Laboratory False-Negative Rate, an Increase in Incidence in Younger Women, and Rapid Progression to Invasion of 20% of Lesions**

Estimated Outcome

Decrease in probability of developing invasive cervical
   cancer†, /10 000
Decrease in lifetime probability of death from cervical cancer‡,
   /10 000
Increase in life expectancy, *d*
Increase in life expectancy, discounted 5%, *d*
Net costs, discounted 5%, *$*
Marginal cost per year of life expectancy§, *$*

  * All estimates are approximate. Decimal points are retained to avoid
roundoff errors.
  † Reference probability without screening: 250 in 10 000.
  ‡ Reference probability without screening: 118 in 10 000.

(UICC) did not agree with the conclusions of the Canadian Task Force, pointing out that there was little evidence to support more rapid progression in women at younger ages and that, indeed, potentially the reverse was true (54). A recent case-control study found no evidence of a distinctive subgroup of rapidly progressing lesions, related either to demographic characteristics or specific risk factors (65). Another quantitative analysis found no support for the hypothesis of a new fast-growing cervical cancer in younger women (66).

"Worst Case" Scenario

Nonetheless, it is possible to estimate the consequences of pessimistic assumptions about an increasing incidence of rapidly progressing cancers. Table 8 shows the implications of assuming that the incidence of invasive cervical cancers is three times the rates currently observed in the United States; the observed increase in carcinoma in situ in 1985 and 1986 in women from 15 to 24 years of age implies a real increase in invasive cancer in the future; 20% of lesions are an etiologically distinct subgroup that progresses rapidly to invasion (in less than 2 years); and the false-negative rate of the average laboratory in the United States is 15% worse

Table 8. *(Continued)*

	Papanicolaou Smear		
Every 3 Years	Every 3 Years after Four Annual Negative Smears	Every 2 Years	Every Year
171	173	182	196
92.7	93.3	97	101
84	85	88	92
8.5	8.7	8.9	9.3
361	473	545	1097
15 501‖	204 400¶	167 900¶	503 700**

§ Health effects and costs are discounted 5%.
‖ Compared with no screening.
¶ Compared with screening every 3 years.
** Compared with screening every 2 years.

than in Canada and Europe. These results should be interpreted with great caution as there is no evidence for these assumptions; they are presented as a "worst case" scenario. Even with these assumptions, screening is highly effective, the marginal gains with increasing frequencies remain small, and the marginal cost per year of life expectancy achieved by more frequent screening remains high (Table 8).

Compliance

Another frequently expressed concern is that women cannot remember the 3-year frequency, or "if you tell them every 3 years, they will do it every 6." Questions of paternalism aside, there is a considerable amount of leeway in advising a frequency in the sense that the effectiveness of screening is not very sensitive to the actual frequency of screening. For example, Table 3 shows the outcomes of a 4-year frequency, which is 99% as effective as a 3-year frequency. Thus, it is not critical that a woman be screened at precisely 3-year intervals; any interval from 1 to 4 years will deliver virtually the same benefits. Even with some slippage in compliance, a 3-year frequency will be highly effective.

Detection of Other Conditions

A possible indirect benefit of periodic Papanicolaou smears is the incidental discovery of other conditions. There is virtually no published information on the value of finding and treating other conditions in asymptomatic women being seen primarily for cervical cancer screening, and thus no basis for estimating the potential magnitude of this benefit. Nor is there any basis for determining if the potential detection of other conditions should affect the frequency of visits for Papanicolaou smears. There might be value to seeing women more frequently for conditions other than for Papanicolaou smears. However, the specific conditions; their frequencies of occurrence; the detection procedures; the benefits, harms, and costs of early detection and treatment; and the appropriate frequency of examinations remain to be specified.

Summary

The available empiric evidence, and inferences drawn from that evidence, support the following conclusions.

It is important that women be screened for cervical cancer. The evidence, although indirect, that cervical cancer screening is effective is extremely strong. Whereas incidence rates of the disease are low (compared with other cancers for which screening is recommended), the potential reduction in mortality with screening is high (approximately 90%), having the potential to almost eliminate the disease. If a screening strategy is chosen with care, screening for cervical cancer can be very cost-effective—costing in the range of $10 000 per year of life expectancy (both health effects and costs discounted 5%).

The incidence of either invasive cervical cancer or carcinoma in situ is extremely low in young women. Even if the observed rates are thought to be artificially low by a factor of two to three due to previous screening in the population and cohort effects (for example, changes in sexual habits), very good protection is achieved by starting screening at any age from 17 to 26. The additional benefit from starting at age 17 instead of, for example, 20 or 23, is very small (Table 4).

The effect of having four initial annual examinations before reducing the frequency is very small (Table 3), even if the laboratory processing the slides is thought to have a higher than average false-negative rate (Table 7). The number of initial negative examinations obtained before decreasing the frequency and the actual timing of repeat examinations also have very little effect on outcomes.

The differences in effectiveness between 1-year, 2-year, 3-year, or 4-year frequencies are also small (Table 3). The largest collection of data indicates that a 3-year frequency will achieve the overwhelming percentage (about 96%) of the benefit of annual examinations, with a great reduction (by about two thirds) in inconvenience, risk, and cost. The actual frequency of screening within 1 to 4 years is not critical.

If a woman has been screened regularly (for example, every 3 years), and if she does not have numerous partners, the value of continuing screening beyond her mid-60s is fairly small (Table 5). The benefits of screening such a woman in her 70s are very small.

For women in their 60s who have not been screened in the previous dozen years, and who have had multiple sexual partners during those years, the value of screening might be considered sufficiently high to justify three or four examinations over the next 10 years (Table 6).

The greatest impact by far on the incidence and mortality of cervical cancer can be achieved by ensuring that all women are screened. Screening a previously unscreened woman has about 20 times the effect of screening annually compared with every 3 years.

Recommendation

The current recommendations of major organizations properly give practicing physicians considerable flexibility. Choosing an appropriate strategy involves two steps. First, the outcomes of different options must be estimated; then the desirability of the outcomes must be assessed. The first step is a question of evidence. The second is a question of personal values and preferences. Because different people have different preferences, it is appropriate to keep the two steps separate.

Tables 3 to 8 provide estimates of the consequences of different options under different assumptions. In general, as screening becomes more intensive (more frequent), the gains become smaller while the costs and inconvenience grow. The question is where to draw the line. Ideally, this should be decided by women themselves.

To the extent that a general recommendation is required, a reasonable recommendation is that women should be screened at least every 3 years starting in their early 20s, and continuing into their 60s. For most women, a 3-year frequency is appropriate. Some women, however, might prefer more intensive screening (for example, every 2 years or even annually). If there are questions, women should be given information on the expected benefits, risks, and costs (Table 3), and allowed to choose.

Appendix: Mathematic Model of Cervical Cancer Screening

The model is a nine-state time-varying Markov chain. The states represent persons who are alive and "well" (no diagnosis of cervical cancer), persons who have cancer diagnosed in various stages, persons who have died from cervical cancer, and persons who have died from other causes. Movement between states each year is controlled by transition probabilities. For each year in a woman's life, the model calculates five main probabilities: the probability a woman who is alive and "well" has an asymptomatic but potentially detectable cervical cancer or precancerous lesion (for example, carcinoma in situ); the probability that a Papanicolaou smear, if done, would detect an existing cancer or precancerous lesions in such a woman; for women who have cancers or precancerous lesions detected, the stage of the cancer at the time of detection; for women with cancers diagnosed in various stages, the probability of dying from cancer in the coming year; and, finally, the probability a woman will die from other causes in the coming year. The first probability is calculated from age-specific and sex-specific incidence rates, risk factors, the "preclinical interval," and the history of previous screening tests. The preclinical interval is the time required for a lesion to develop from first being potentially detectable by screening (for example, an early dysplasia) to the appearance of signs and symptoms. The second probability is determined by the state of development of the lesion at the time the screening test is done (for example, its size), and the random false-negative rate of the Papanicolaou smear. The third probability is determined by the rate of development of the lesion, the patient's history of previous screening examinations, and the random false-negative rate of the Papanicolaou smear. The fourth probability is determined by stage-specific relative survival rates, and the fifth probability is determined by age-specific and sex-specific rates of mortality from other causes. Formulas for calculating these and other probabilities are described elsewhere (59). The model incorporates the following features:

Natural History
1. Cervical cancers can develop from two sources: one with a relatively long preinvasive stage, the other with a relatively short preinvasive stage.
2. Not all cases of dysplasia or carcinoma in situ develop into invasive cancers.

Screening Procedures
1. The Papanicolaou smear can have two types of false-negative results, nonrandom and random. Nonrandom false-negative results are due to biologic features of a lesion such as its location and size. These false-negatives

are beyond the control of the practitioner or laboratory. If an examination is negative due to a nonrandom cause, immediate repetition of the test will remain negative. Random false-negative results are due to random or technical factors such as the examiner's technique, sampling, fixing of slides, laboratory errors, reporting, and follow-up. If an examination is negative due to random causes, repeat examinations could be positive, subject to the random false-negative rate.

2. The Papanicolaou smears can give false-positive test results, warranting follow-up diagnostic procedures.

Clinical History and Treatment

1. The effect of therapy for a cervical cancer, as expressed by relative case-survival rates, depends on the stage of the cancer.
2. Signs or symptoms might lead a woman to seek care in the interval between screening examinations.
3. People are subject to death from causes other than cervical cancer.

The model includes financial charges for the following events: the Papanicolaou smear, work-ups of false-positive test results, initial care and terminal care for cervical cancer, and terminal care for other causes of death. The present value of a lifetime of expected costs can be calculated, taking into account the probabilities each of these costs will occur at any time in the future. Any discount rate can be specified. The model can also discount future health outcomes.

The model can calculate the outcomes of screening with any combination of tests, in any order and frequency, starting and stopping at any age, for women in any risk category. The outcomes include the probability a woman will develop an invasive cervical cancer, the probability of dying from cervical cancer, life expectancy, the chance of a false-positive test result, the chance of a specified risk (for example, detection of a lesion that would have regressed spontaneously), the expected cost of screening, the expected cost of a false-positive test result, the expected savings in treatment costs, and net or total costs.

The values assigned to various parameters for a base case as well as the principal sources are given in the next section. The model reproduces these numbers exactly (for example, incidence rates, case-survival rates by stage). The most critical factors for comparing different screening strategies are the preclinical interval of lesions that develop slowly, the preclinical interval of lesions that develop rapidly, the proportion of lesions that develop rapidly, and the random false-negative rate. These parameters were estimated to fit the results of the large screening programs analyzed by a workgroup of the IARC. The model has been calibrated to fit these results within 1% (60).

Assumptions of the Mathematic Model

Natural History

1. Age-specific incidence rates for invasive cervical cancer were estimated by multiplying the incidence rates observed in the United States by a factor of three, to adjust for the prevalence of screening and cohort effects (67).

2. Ninety-five percent of cervical cancers have a long pre-clinical interval, 5% a short preclinical interval.* The consequences of 20% of invasive cancers having a short preinvasive stage were also calculated. These parameters were estimated to fit IARC data (54).
3. For lesions with a long preclinical interval, the average time to grow from first time of detectability into an invasive cancer is 8 years, with a range of 0 to 16 years.* These parameters were estimated to fit IARC data (54).
4. For lesions with a short preclinical interval, the average time to grow from first time of detectability into an invasive cancer is 1 year, with a range of 0 to 2 years.* These parameters were estimated to fit IARC data (54).

Screening Procedures

1. The random false-negative rate is 3%* (*see* page 224 for footnote). Parameters were estimated to fit IARC data (54).
2. The false-positive rate of the Papanicolaou smear is 0.5% (32).
3. The charge for the Papanicolaou smear is $75, from an informal survey of 20 physicians, clinics, and hospitals.
4. The charge for working up a person with a false-positive Papanicolaou smear is $150, assuming a repeat Papanicolaou smear and colposcopy.
5. The charge for treating a lesion that would have regressed spontaneously is $5641, assuming the cost of treating a preinvasive lesion (68).

Clinical History and Treatment

1. Relative case-survival rates for cervical cancers detected and treated in various stages were estimated for all years following diagnosis. The 5-year survival rates are 86%, 59%, 40%, and 18%, for stages 1 through 4, respectively (68).
2. The cost of initial therapy is as follows: in situ: $5641; stage 1: $11 600; stage 2: $16 891; stage 3: $16 891; stage 4: $18 587 (68).
3. The cost of terminal care for a patient dying of cervical cancer is $22 150 (68).
4. Without screening, about 46% of patients seek care for stage 1 invasive cancer, about 26% for stage 2 invasive cancer, about 16% for stage 3 invasive cancer, and about 12% for stage 4 invasive cancer (69).
5. Age-specific and sex-specific mortality rates for cervical cancer were estimated from reference 67.

---

* Given the inherent range of uncertainty in any experiment, the IARC results are compatible with a range of assumptions about the three critical factors. Most important, the IARC data are compatible with a longer preclinical interval of lesions that develop slowly, coupled with a lower proportion of rapidly developing lesions and a higher random false-negative rate. For this analysis, the values for these parameters were chosen to be conservative in the sense of underestimating the value of longer intervals between examinations compared with annual examinations.

References

1. **Silverberg E, Lubera JA.** Cancer statistics, 1988. *Ca.* 1988;**38**:5-22.
2. **Horm JW, Asire AJ, Young JL Jr, Pollack ES.** SEER Program: cancer incidence and mortality in the United States 1973-81. Bethesda, Maryland: U.S. Department of Health and Human Services, Public Health Service, National Institutes of Health, National Cancer Institute; 1984. NIH publication no. 85-1837.
3. **Young JL Jr, Percy CL, Asire AJ.** Surveillance, epidemiology, and end results (SEER): incidence and mortality data, 1973-77. Bethesda, Maryland: U.S. Department of Health and Human Services, Public Health Service, National Institutes of Health, National Cancer Institute; 1981. NIH publication no. 81-2330.
4. **Seidman H, Mushinski MH, Gelb SK, Silverberg E.** Probabilities of eventually developing or dying of cancer—United States, 1985. *Ca.* 1985;**35**:36-56.
5. **Brinton LA, Fraumeni FJ Jr.** Epidemiology of uterine cervical cancer. *J Chronic Dis.* 1986;**39**:1051-65.
6. **Rotkin ID.** Adolescent coitus and cervical cancer: associations of related events with increased risk. *Cancer Res.* 1967;**27**:603-17.
7. **Kessler II, Kilcar Z, Zimola A, et al.** Cervical cancer in Yugoslavia. II. Epidemiologic factors of possible etiologic significance. *J Natl Cancer Inst.* 1974;**53**:51-60.
8. **Clarke EA, Morgan RW, Newman AM.** Smoking as a risk factor in cancer of the cervix: additional evidence from a case-control study. *Am J Epidemiol.* 1982;**115**:59-66.
9. **Greenberg ER, Vessey M, McPherson K, Yeates D.** Cigarette smoking and cancer of the uterine cervix. *Br J Cancer.* 1985;**51**:139-41.
10. **Harris RW, Brinton LA, Cowdell RH, et al.** Characteristics of women with dysplasia or carcinoma in situ of the cervix uteri. *Br J Cancer.* 1980;**42**:359-69.
11. **Lyon JL, Gardner JW, West DW, Stanish WM, Hebertson RM.** Smoking and carcinoma in situ of the uterine cervix. *Am J Public Health.* 1983;**73**:558-62.
12. **Trevathan E, Layde P, Webster LA, Adams JB, Benigno BB, Ory H.** Cigarette smoking and dysplasia and carcinoma in situ of the uterine cervix. *JAMA.* 1983;**250**:499-502.
13. **Brinton LA, Schairer C, Hasenszel W, et al.** Smoking and invasive cervical cancer. *JAMA.* 1986;**255**:3265-9.
14. **Ebeling K, Nischan P.** Assessing the effectiveness of a cervical cancer screening program in the German Democratic Republic. *Intl J Tech Assess Health Care.* 1987;**3**:137-47.
15. **Meisels A, Begin R, Schneider V.** Dysplasias of uterine cervix: epidemiological aspects: role of age at first coitus and use of oral contraceptives. *Cancer.* 1977;**40**:3076-81.
16. **Peritz E, Ramcharan S, Frank J, Brown WL, Huang S, Ray R.** The incidence of cervical cancer and duration of oral contraceptive use. *Am J Epidemiol.* 1977;**106**:462-9.
17. **Stern E, Forsythe AB, Youkeles L, Coffelt CF.** Steroid contraceptive use and cervical dysplasia: increased risk of progression. *Science.* 1977;**196**:1460-2.
18. Invasive cervical cancer and combined oral contraceptives. WHO collaborative study of neoplasia and steroid contraceptives. *Br Med J [Clin Res].* 1985;**290**:961-5.
19. **Brinton LA, Huggins GR, Lehman HF, et al.** Long-term use of oral contraceptives and risk of invasive cervical cancer. *Int J Cancer.* 1986;**38**:339-44.
20. **Tawa K, Forsythe A, Cove JK, Saltz A, Peters HW, Watring WG.** A comparison of the Papanicolaou smear and the cervigram: sensitivity, specificity, and cost analysis. *Obstet Gynecol.* 1988;**71**:229-35.
21. **Anderson GH, Flynn KJ, Hickey LA, et al.** A comprehensive internal quality control system for a large cytology laboratory. *Acta Cytol.* 1987;**31**:895-9.
22. **Berkowitz RS, Ehrmann RL, LaVizzo-Mourey R, Knapp RC.** Invasive cervical carcinoma in young women. *Gynecol Oncol.* 1979;**8**:311-6.
23. **Cecchini S, Palli D, Casini A.** Cervical intraepithelial neoplasia. III. An estimate of screening error rates and optimal screening interval. *Acta Cytol.* 1985;**29**:329-33.

24. **Davis JR, Hindman WM, Paplanus SH, Trego DC, Wiens JL, Suciu TN.** Value of duplicate smears in cervical cytology. *Acta Cytol.* 1981;**25**:533-8.
25. **Figge DC, Bennington JL, Schweid AI.** Cervical cancer after initial negative and atypical vaginal cytology. *Am J Obstet Gynecol.* 1970; **108**:422-8.
26. **Gay JD, Donaldson LD, Goellner JR.** False-negative results in cervical cytologic studies. *Acta Cytol.* 1985;**29**:1043-6.
27. **Morell ND, Taylor JR, Snyder RN, Ziel HK, Saltz A, Willie S.** False-negative cytology rates in patients in whom invasive cervical cancer subsequently developed. *Obstet Gynecol.* 1982;**60**:41-5.
28. **Rylander E.** Negative smears in women developing invasive cervical cancer. *Acta Obstet Gynecol Scand.* 1977;**56**:115-8.
29. **Husain OA.** Quality control in cytologic screening for cervical cancer. *Tumori.* 1976;**62**:303-14.
30. **Shulman JJ, Leyton M, Hamilton R.** The Papanicolaou smear: an insensitive case-finding procedure. *Am J Obstet Gynecol.* 1974; **120**:446-51.
31. **van der Graaf Y, Vooijs GP.** False negative rate in cervical cytology. *J Clin Pathol.* 1987;**40**:438-42.
32. **Yobs AR, Plott AE, Hicklin MD, et al.** Retrospective evaluation of gynecologic cytodiagnosis. II. Interlaboratory reproducibility as shown in rescreening large consecutive samples of reported cases. *Acta Cytol.* 1987;**31**:900-10.
33. **Campion MJ, McCance DJ, Cuzick J, Singer A.** Progressive potential of mild cervical atypia: prospective cytological, colposcopic, and virological study. *Lancet.* 1986;**2**:237-40.
34. **Fox CH.** Biologic behavior of dysplasia and carcinoma in situ. *Am J Obstet Gynecol.* 1967;**99**:960-74.
35. **Hulka BS.** Cytologic and histologic outcome following an atypical cervical smear. *Am J Obstet Gynecol.* 1968;**101**:190-9.
36. **MacGregor JE, Teper S.** Uterine cervical cytology and young women. *Lancet.* 1978;**1**:1029-31.
37. **Richart RM, Barron BA.** A follow-up study of patients with cervical dysplasia. *Am J Obstet Gynecol.* 1969;**105**:386-93.
38. **Rummel HH, Fick R, Heberling D, Schubert D.** Cytologic follow-up examination of patients with a suspicious Papanicolaou type 3D smear. *Geburtshilfe Frauenheilkd.* 1977;**37**:521-6.
39. **Svirannaboon S, Bhamanapravati N.** Prevalence and outcome of dysplasia of the cervix in self-selected population of Thailand. *J Med Assoc Thai.* 1974;**57**:351-6.
40. **Johannesson G, Geirsson G, Day N.** The effect of mass screening in Iceland, 1965-1974, on the incidence and mortality of cervical carcinoma. *Int J Cancer.* 1978;**21**:418-25.
41. **Day NE.** Effect of cervical cancer screening in Scandinavia. *Obstet Gynecol.* 1984;**63**:714-8.
42. **Hakama M, Chamberlain J, Day NE, Miller AB, Prorok PC.** Evaluation of screening programmes for gynaecological cancer. *Br J Cancer.* 1985;**52**:669-73.
43. **Ebeling K, Nischan P, Schindler C.** Use of oral contraceptives and risk of invasive cervical cancer in previously screened women. *Int J Cancer.* 1987;**39**:427-30.
44. **Duguid HL, Duncan ID, Currie J.** Screening for cervical intraepithelial neoplasia in Dundee and Angus 1962-81 and its relation with invasive cervical cancer. *Lancet.* 1985;**2**:1053-6.
45. **Dunn JE Jr, Schweitzer V.** The relationship of cervical cytology to the incidence of invasive cervical cancer and mortality in Alameda County, California, 1960 to 1974. *Am J Obstet Gynecol.* 1981; **139**:868-76.
46. **Miller AB, Lindsay J, Hill GB.** Mortality from cancer of the uterus in Canada and its relationship to screening for cancer of the cervix. *Int J Cancer.* 1976;**17**:602-12.
47. **Clarke EA, Anderson TW.** Does screening by "Pap" smears help prevent cervical cancer? A case-control study. *Lancet.* 1979;**2**:1-4.
48. **LaVecchia C, Franceschi S, Decarli A, et al.** "Pap" smear and the risk of cervical neoplasia: quantitative estimates from a case-control study. *Lancet.* 1984;**2**:779-82.

49. **Aristizabal N, Cuello C, Correa P, Collazos T, Haenszel W.** The impact of vaginal cytology on cervical cancer risks in Cali, Colombia. *Int J Cancer.* 1984;**34**:5-9.

50. **MacGregor JE, Moss SM, Parkin DM, Day NE.** A case-control study of cervical cancer screening in north east Scotland. *Br Med J [Clin Res].* 1985;**290**:1543-6.

51. **van der Graaf Y, Zielhuis GA, Peer PG, Vooijs PG.** The effectiveness of cervical screening: a population-based case-control study. *J Clin Epidemiol.* 1988;**41**:21-6.

52. **Olesen F.** A case-control study of cervical cytology before diagnosis of cervical cancer in Denmark. *Int J Epidemiol.* 1988;**17**:501-8.

53. **Shy K, Chu J, Mandelson M, et al.** Papanicolaou smear screening interval and risk of cervical cancer. *Obstet Gynecol.* 1989;**74**:838-43.

54. Screening for squamous cervical cancer: duration of low risk after negative results of cervical cytology and its implication for screening policies. IARC Working Group on evaluation of cervical cancer screening programmes. *Br Med J [Clin Res].* 1986;**293**:659-64.

55. **Miller AB.** Screening for cancer: issues and future directions. *J Chronic Dis.* 1986;**39**:1067-77.

56. **Shun-Zhang Y, Miller AB, Sherman GJ.** Optimising the age, number of tests, and test interval for cervical screening in Canada. *J Epidemiol Community Health.* 1982;**36**:1-10.

57. **Albert A, Gertman P, Louis T.** Screening for the early detection of cancer. I. The temporal natural history of a progressive disease state. *Math Biosci.* 1978;**40**:1-59.

58. **Albert A, Gertman P, Louis T, et al.** Screening for the early detection of cancer. II. The impact of screening on the natural history of the disease. *Math Biosci.* 1978;**40**:61-109.

59. **Eddy DM.** *Screening for Cancer: Theory, Analysis, and Design.* Englewood Cliffs, New Jersey: Prentice-Hall; 1980.

60. **Eddy DM.** The frequency of cervical cancer screening: comparison of a mathematical model with empirical data. *Cancer.* 1987;**60**: 1117-22.

61. **Galliher HP.** Optimizing ages for cervical smear examinations in followed healthy individuals. *Gynecol Oncol.* 1981;**12**:S188-S205.

62. **Parkin DM, Moss SM.** An evaluation of screening policies for cervical cancer in England and Wales using a computer simulation model. *J Epidemiol Community Health.* 1986;**40**:143-53.

63. **Keeler EB, Cretin S.** Discounting of life-saving and other nonmonetary effects. *Manage Sci.* 1983;**29**:300-6.

64. Cervical cancer screening programs. Summary of the 1982 Canadian Task Force report. *Can Med Assoc J.* 1982;**127**:581-9.

65. **Peters RK, Thomas D, Skultin G, Henderson BE.** Invasive squamous cell carcinoma of the cervix after recent negative cytologic tests results—a distinct subgroup? *Am J Obstet Gynecol.* 1988;**158**:926-35.

66. **Silcocks PB, Moss SM.** Rapidly progressive cervical cancer: is it a real problem? *Br J Obstet Gynaecol.* 1988;**95**:1111-6.

67. **Sondik E, ed.** *Annual Cancer Statistics Review, 1988.* Washington, DC: Division of Cancer Prevention and Control, National Cancer Institute; 1989.

68. **Baker MS, Kessler LG, Smucker RC.** Analysis of the continuous Medicare history sample file: the cost of treating cancer. In: *Proceedings of Cancer Care and Costs, a meeting of the American Cancer Society, San Diego California, May 1987.* 1989.

69. **Bearman DM, MacMillan JP, Creasman WT.** Papanicolaou smear history of patients developing cervical cancer: an assessment of screening protocols. *Obstet Gynecol.* 1987;**69**:151-5.

Screening for Colorectal Cancer

DAVID M. EDDY, MD, PhD

Colorectal cancer is the most common of the lethal cancers, striking both men and women at approximately equal rates. In 1990, approximately 150 000 new cases of and 60 900 deaths from colorectal cancer are expected to occur in the United States (1). Colorectal cancer's prevalence and natural history make it a prime candidate for screening. Evidence on screening's effectiveness, however, is incomplete, and the magnitude of screening's benefits and harms is uncertain. This article reviews aspects of the disease that are important to making decisions about screening; describes the available screening tests; presents evidence on the effectiveness of screening; and interprets the available indirect evidence to estimate the benefits, harms, and costs of various screening strategies.

The Probability of Developing Colorectal Cancer

The probability that a person at average risk will be diagnosed as having cancer of the colon or rectum in the coming year is shown for various age groups in Table 1. The lifetime probability that a person will develop colorectal cancer is approximately 6% (2). Several factors modify a person's probability of developing colorectal cancer. These factors include inflammatory bowel disease (chronic ulcerative colitis and Crohn colitis), familial polyposis syndromes (for example, inherited adenomatosis of the colon and rectum, the Gardner syndrome, the Turcot syndrome, the Oldfield syndrome), family cancer syndromes, a history of colorectal cancer in a first-degree relative, and a previous personal history of neoplasms.

The highest risk is found in patients with familial adenomatosis; persons with this condition have approximately a 50% probability of developing colorectal cancer by 40 years of age if they have not been treated (3). Altogether, inherited forms of polyposis account for

▶ This chapter was originally published in *Annals of Internal Medicine*. 1990;**113**:373-84.

Table 1. *Age-Specific Incidence Rates (per 100 000 Persons) for Cancers of the Colon and Rectum**

Age, y	Men	Women
0-4	0.0	0.0
5-9	0.0	0.0
10-14	0.0	0.0
15-19	0.2	0.1
20-24	0.4	0.4
25-29	1.2	1.1
30-34	2.5	2.4
35-39	5.9	5.9
40-44	12.3	11.9
45-49	27.7	24.6
50-54	57.2	46.3
55-59	102.6	76.7
60-64	164.9	105.7
65-69	243.9	155.5
70-74	320.5	226.9
75-79	411.3	293.6
80-84	463.5	365.5
85 +	497.6	391.5

* From reference 37.

approximately 1% of all large-bowel cancers. Persons with a long history (greater than 10 years) of ulcerative colitis involving more than the rectum are estimated to have approximately 20 times the average annual risk for developing an invasive cancer of the colon (4). The risk for persons with ulcerative colitis involving only the rectum is elevated, but not as much. The increased risk for colorectal cancer in patients with Crohn disease is less than in patients with ulcerative colitis, and it increases with the duration of disease. Inherited conditions that are not associated with polyposis (such as having a first-degree relative with colorectal cancer) account for 12% to 26% of colorectal cancers (5). Patients with a first-degree relative with colorectal cancer are thought to have a two- to threefold increased risk for developing colorectal cancer, compared with the general population (6-8). These and other risk factors are well described by Winawer and colleagues (3).

This article focuses on screening for persons at average risk and persons at high risk because of having a first-degree relative with colorectal cancer. Persons with inflammatory bowel disease and hereditary syndromes (for example, familial polyposis), those with a personal history of colorectal cancer, and those with signs or symptoms of colorectal cancer require individualized management and are not the subject of this article.

Screening Tests

Several tests and procedures have been proposed to screen for colorectal cancer. The most commonly recommended are the digital examination, the fecal occult blood test, and various types of sigmoidoscopy. Air-contrast barium enemas and colonoscopy have been recommended for screening high-risk persons. The reach, sensitivity, specificity, perforation rates, and costs of these tests were estimated by the Patient Care Subcommittee of the National Digestive Diseases Advisory Board, based on the literature and a questionnaire sent to experts in various aspects of colorectal cancer. This process was described by Eddy and colleagues (reference 9 contains sources for the estimates used in this article).

Sigmoidoscopy

An estimated 30% of adenomas and cancers develop within the region of the bowel typically reached by the rigid sigmoidoscope. Within that portion of the bowel, sensitivity is approximately 85%. The main drawback of using this instrument is patient discomfort. Approximately 55% of adenomas and de-novo cancers develop within the 60-cm flexible sigmoidoscope's typical reach. The sensitivity of this instrument within its reach is approximately 85%. The flexibility as well as the smaller diameter of the instrument tends to cause the patient slightly less discomfort than does the rigid sigmoidoscope. To reduce the cost and increase patient acceptance of flexible sigmoidoscopy, a 35-cm flexible sigmoidoscope was developed (10). This sigmoidoscope reaches an estimated 40% of neoplastic lesions and has a sensitivity within its reach of approximately 85%. False-positive rates for all types of sigmoidoscopy are negligible, due to the opportunity these procedures provide to do a biopsy of any lesion that is visualized.

Fecal Occult Blood Test

Many fecal occult blood tests are available. One of the most common is the Hemoccult II (SmithKline Diagnostics, Sharon Hill, Pennsylvania). Almost 20 other brands are also used in the United States and around the world. Most of these tests are based on guaiac undergoing phenolic oxidation and turning blue in the presence of hemoglobin (a pseudoperoxidase) and hydrogen peroxide. The Hemoccult II thus involves smearing stool on a slide impregnated with guaiac, adding hydrogen peroxide, and looking for a color change. Because rectal bleeding is often intermittent, the most common protocol for screening with these tests is to take two samples on 3 different days, for a total of six samples. A test result is considered "positive" if one or more slides is positive.

Important considerations in administering these tests are that, at least in theory, true-positive and false-positive rates are affected by diet and rehydration of the stool specimen. Peroxidase activity is not limited to human hemoglobin; it is also found in fresh fruits and vegetables and bacteria as well as in animal hemoglobin and myoglobin. For example, turnips, horseradishes, broccoli, cauliflower, and radishes have high peroxidase activity, and cabbage, potatoes, cucumbers, mushrooms, and artichokes have moderate peroxidase activity. In addition, reducing agents such as ascorbic acid might interfere with the oxidation of guaiac, resulting in a false-negative reaction. For these reasons, it is frequently recommended that persons having fecal occult blood testing by most guaiac tests observe a diet designed to minimize the chances of false-positive and false-negative results. However, some studies have shown that a meat-free diet has no effect on results (11).

With the Hemoccult II, both true-positive and false-positive rates are increased if the slides are rehydrated, with a resulting decrease in the predictive value of a positive result. In a controlled setting, Kewenter and colleagues (12) found the rate of positivity to be significantly higher with rehydration (5.8%) than without rehydration (1.9%), as was the number of neoplasms detected (50 compared with 24). The sensitivities for neoplasms with and without rehydration were 93% and 28%, and the predictive values positive for neoplasms were 22% and 32%, respectively.

An immunochemical test proposed by Songster and colleagues (13) uses antisera to intact human hemoglobin to increase the test's specificity to human hemoglobin. This test is considerably more sensitive than the usual guaiac-based tests. For example, in a study of 150 patients with colon cancer, the test produced positive results in 65% compared with 40% with Hemoccult slides (13). Its main disadvantage is its lengthy and complex processing. Another fecal occult blood test under investigation, the HemoQuant, is a fluorescent assay based on hemoglobin-derived porphyrin in stool. This quantitative test determines both the fecal hemoglobin and the fraction of hemoglobin converted to porphyrin by intestinal bacteria.

The fecal occult blood test analyzed in this article

parallels the Hemoccult II, with two samples obtained per day on 3 different days. For reliable results, patients must adhere to a diet designed to minimize false-positive and false-negative results, and the slides must be rehydrated before interpretation.

Colonoscopy

Because the colonoscope is designed to reach the cecum, it can potentially detect virtually all adenomatous colon polyps and de-novo cancers. In practice, the proportion of cancers that develop in the region viewed by the instrument is an estimated 95%. Within its reach, the sensitivity of colonoscopy is approximately 95%. The false-positive rate for the colonoscope is negligible, because biopsies can be taken directly through the scope. Its main drawbacks for use in screening are discomfort and cost. In addition to its role in screening, the colonoscope is valuable for evaluating positive or suspicious fecal occult blood test or barium enema results.

Air-Contrast Barium Enema

In practice, the air-contrast barium enema can visualize an estimated 92% of neoplastic lesions of the large bowel and has a sensitivity within its reach of approximately 85%. As with colonoscopy, the main drawbacks are discomfort and expense. Air-contrast barium enemas can play an additional role in the evaluation of patients with positive fecal occult blood test results.

Risks

The main risks associated with using the tests are perforations from the endoscopes and barium enema and false-positive test results with fecal occult blood testing. As already indicated, the false-positive rate of fecal occult blood tests depends on the particular test being used, the protocol (for example, two slides obtained for each of 3 days, rehydration of slides), and, perhaps, diet. The false-positive rate of the guaiac-impregnated slide is approximately 1% to 4%. A series of annual fecal occult blood tests done over 25 years, for persons from 50 to 75 years of age, has a cumulative probability of a false-positive result sometime in that 25-year period of approximately 40%. The work-up of a false-positive test result is extensive, requiring examination of the entire colon with colonoscopy, a barium enema, or both.

The air-contrast barium enema can also yield false-positive results, indicating a lesion when in fact there is no abnormality; such a result could, for example, be caused by residual stool. A positive or suspicious finding on barium enema must be confirmed with sigmoidoscopy or colonoscopy. The false-positive rate of air-contrast barium enema is approximately 3% to 4%. A series of air-contrast barium enemas every 3 years for patients between 50 and 75 years of age has a cumulative probability of a false-positive result of approximately 25%.

Perforation rates have been estimated at 0.0125% for rigid sigmoidoscopy, 0.02% for 35-cm flexible sigmoidoscopy, 0.045% for 60-cm flexible sigmoidoscopy, 0.2% for colonoscopy, and 0.02% for air-contrast barium enema. Perforation usually requires surgery and has a 5% to 10% mortality rate.

Costs

Charges for each procedure vary widely. Approximate charges, based on an informal survey of six institutions, are $5 for a fecal occult blood test, $70 for rigid sigmoidoscopy, $100 for 35-cm flexible sigmoidoscopy, $135 for 60-cm flexible sigmoidoscopy, $500 for colonoscopy, and $200 for an air-contrast barium enema. When making decisions about individual patients, practitioners should refer to the charges in their own practices and institutions.

Evidence of Effectiveness

Digital Rectal Examination

The proposal that the digital rectal examination be used to screen for colorectal cancer is based on its simplicity. Unfortunately, there is virtually no direct evidence that the examination reduces mortality from colorectal cancer. Indirect evidence suggesting such a reduction is based on the estimate that approximately 10% of adenomas and cancers develop within the potential reach of an exploring finger and on the observation that relative case-survival rates are higher for cancers detected in earlier stages.

Fecal Occult Blood Test

Many uncontrolled screening programs have shown that fecal occult blood testing can detect both adenomas and cancers in asymptomatic persons (14-20). These programs also provide information on patient compliance with fecal occult blood testing, the proportion of patients with positive test results, the proportion of patients with positive test results who comply with a work-up, and the approximate yield of neoplasms (adenomas and cancers). In general, on initial (prevalence) examinations, from 1% to 5% of unselected persons tested with fecal occult blood tests have positive test results. Of those with positive test results, approximately 10% have cancer and approximately 20% to 30% have adenomas. The rate of detection of cancers and polyps and the predictive value positive for cancer and polyps can be expected to be lower on re-examination (incidence examinations).

These studies do not indicate the value of fecal occult blood testing in reducing morbidity or mortality from colorectal cancer. Direct evidence of this value requires controlled trials. Five such trials are currently in progress. A controlled trial at the Strang Clinic and Memorial Sloan-Kettering Hospital (with patients allocated to screening or control groups according to month of enrollment) offered screening to more than 22 000 men and women over 40 years of age (3). All patients had a complete history and physical examination as well as rigid sigmoidoscopy. In addition, the screened group received Hemoccult tests. Compliance was 70% to 80% for the fecal occult blood test and approximately 95% for sigmoidoscopy. Overall, approximately 2.5% of Hemoccult slides were positive. However, this figure varied with age; for patients in their 50s, the rate of positive slides was approximately 1.7% whereas, for patients over 70 years of age, the rate of positive slides increased to 4.4%. The predictive value of a positive slide was approximately 12% for carcinoma and 38% for adenoma. The trial's most recent report (3) indicated that 71 cases of colon carcinoma had been diagnosed. A shift toward detecting cancer at earlier stages in the group that was offered fecal occult blood testing has been reported. However, the study has not yet reported complete staging information or mortality results.

Another controlled trial is under way at the University of Minnesota (21). It involves approximately 45 000 persons over 50 years of age randomly assigned to receive annual fecal occult blood testing, biennial fecal occult blood testing, or no special testing (the control group). The rate of positive slides was reported to be 2.4%. Of those persons with positive slides, about 8.2% had colorectal cancer; 78% of these cancers were in either Dukes' A or B stages, or were in situ. This study has not yet reported complete staging information or any reduction in mortality.

A randomized controlled trial of the Hemoccult test was begun in Nottingham, England, in 1981 (22). Of the 52 258 persons between 45 and 75 years of age who were offered screening, 27 651 completed the first screen. Of these persons, 618 (2.3%) had positive test results, and 63 cancers were found. At rescreening every 2 years (9510 persons completed the first rescreen, 3639 completed the second rescreen), the rate of positive results was lower (1.7% and 0.3% for the first and second rescreens, respectively). Cancers detected by screening were at a less advanced stage, but it is too early to show any effect of screening on colorectal cancer mortality.

In a randomized trial in Denmark, the Hemoccult II is being offered to 30 970 persons between 45 and 74 years of age in the county of Funen, and another 30 968 persons are being followed as controls (23). At last report, approximately 20 000 persons had completed the test, and 215 (1%) had positive results; 37 persons had carcinomas and 86 had adenomas. The prevalence of both cancers and adenomas was higher in the group offered screening than in the control group. Mortality results will not be available for approximately 5 years.

Another randomized controlled trial of the Hemoccult II, involving approximately 27 700 persons between 60 and 64 years of age, was recently started in Göteborg, Sweden (12). Of the 13 759 persons invited to receive screening, 9040 completed an initial test, and 7770 completed a second test after 16 to 22 months. At the first screen, the rate of positivity was 1.9% and 5.8%, depending on whether slides were rehydrated. The number of neoplasms detected was significantly higher with rehydration. Significantly more cancers were found in the test group (61 cancers) compared with the control group (20 cancers). Cancer patients in the test group tended to have tumors that were at more favorable stages. Mortality results are not yet available.

Sigmoidoscopy

Two uncontrolled studies and one controlled study have examined sigmoidoscopy. In an uncontrolled study conducted at the Strang Clinic, approximately 26 000 persons were examined, and 58 cancers were detected. After 7 cancers were excluded because they were advanced at diagnosis, approximately 80% of the remaining cancers were observed to be in Dukes' A or B (local) stages. The 15-year survival rate of the patients with nonadvanced cancers was 90%, a rate higher than the investigators expected under ordinary circumstances (24).

Another uncontrolled study, conducted at the University of Minnesota, involved doing several sigmoidoscopies on approximately 18 000 persons. After the initial examination, only 13 additional cancers were found on subsequent examinations. This rate was considerably lower than the investigators expected on the basis of the age and sex distribution of the screened population (approximately 85 cases were expected), leading to the supposition that removal of polyps decreases the incidence of invasive cancers (25). Unfortunately, a lack of controls as well as several biases (length bias, lead time bias, and patient selection bias) render the Strang and Minnesota studies difficult to interpret.

A randomized, controlled trial of multiphasic screening conducted by the Kaiser Foundation Health Plan included the use of rigid sigmoidoscopy (26). One group of approximately 5000 persons was offered multiphasic screening which included sigmoidoscopy (study group) whereas a randomly selected control group was offered "usual care." After 16 years of follow-up, there were 12 deaths from colorectal cancer in the study group compared with 29 in the control group. This result is statistically significant if only colorectal cancer is considered (27). However, some investigators challenge this interpretation because, as part of a multiphasic screening program, many null hypotheses were being tested and, by standard statistical techniques, approximately 5% would be expected to be rejected by chance. The results also have been challenged because the difference in exposure to sigmoidoscopy in the two groups was small: only about a third of the persons in the study group actually accepted and received sigmoidoscopy, whereas approximately 25% of subjects in the control group were examined at least once with sigmoidoscopy. The investigators themselves warn that their results should not be used to draw conclusions, either positive or negative, about the effectiveness of sigmoidoscopy. No completed or ongoing trials involve using flexible sigmoidoscopy, colonoscopy, or barium enemas to screen asymptomatic persons at average risk.

Methods

There is no direct evidence from which to estimate the effectiveness of colorectal cancer screening in reducing mortality. Further, even when the ongoing trials are complete, they will have examined only a small portion of the possible screening strategies. Given the lack of direct evidence, three approaches are possible: Require direct evidence of effectiveness, decline to screen until such evidence is available, and adhere in the future to whatever screening strategy was used in the trials that showed effectiveness; base recommendations on global subjective judgment (a judgment about the overall value of screening, without explicit consideration of individual factors such as incidence, anatomy, natural history, and test effectiveness); or use analytic methods to synthesize the indirect evidence and targeted judgments. (Targeted judgments identify the important factors, focus on each factor separately, and systematically examine evidence for each factor.)

Use of the first approach leads to a recommendation against screening for colorectal cancer. The second approach is subject to obvious biases from incomplete reasoning, errors in reasoning, and personal and professional biases. It also leads to widely varying recommendations, with no basis for reviewing their logic or distinguishing among them. The third approach has the merit of making all assumptions and reasoning explicit, but the results remain projections based on indirect evidence and targeted judgments, not "facts" established through controlled trials.

This article takes the third approach. It reports the results of a mathematic model that takes into account evidence and targeted judgments on such factors as the age- and sex-specific incidence rates of colorectal cancer, the natural history of colorectal cancer (proportions of cancers arising from adenomas or de novo from the mucosa), the anatomy of colorectal cancer (proportion of adenomas and de-novo cancers that arise within reach of various instruments), the sensitivities and specificities of the available screening tests, stage-specific case-survival rates, and deaths from other causes. The model and its main assumptions are summarized in the Appendix.

Estimated Effectiveness of Colorectal Cancer Screening

Without screening, a 50-year-old man at average risk has approximately a 537-in-10 000 (5.37%) chance of developing invasive colorectal cancer sometime in the rest of his life. For a 50-year-old woman at average risk, the chance is approximately 525 in 10 000 (5.25%). Without screening, the probability that a 50-year-old man or woman at average risk will die from colorectal cancer is approximately 277 in 10 000 and 227 in 10 000, respectively. Tables 2 and 3 show some of the important outcomes for 11 possible screening strategies for asymptomatic 50-year-old men and women at average risk. (The strategies are ordered according to their ability to reduce the probability of dying from colorectal cancer.) Two of the strategies are commonly recommended—an annual fecal occult blood test and an annual fecal occult blood test coupled with a 60-cm flexible sigmoidoscopy every 3 years. The other strategies involve air-contrast barium enemas and colonoscopies and are not usually recommended for persons at average risk. They are included because of their high expected effectiveness; their benefits might be worth the inconvenience, discomfort, and costs for high-risk and some average-risk persons.

Table 2. *Estimated Benefits and Risks for Colorectal Cancer Screening at 50 to 75 Years of Age for an Average-Risk Asymptomatic 50-Year-Old Man**

Tests	Decrease in Probability of Invasive Colorectal Cancer†	Decrease in Probability of Death from Colorectal Cancer
	n/10 000	*n/10 000*
Annual FOBT	40	71
Annual FOBT, scope/5 years	138	120
Annual FOBT, scope/3 years	153	126
Annual FOBT, annual scope	196	139
Annual FOBT, barium enema/5 years	314	196
Annual FOBT, barium enema/3 years	339	203
Annual FOBT, scope, barium enema/ 3 years	348	206
Annual FOBT, colonoscopy/5 years	355	212
Annual FOBT, annual barium enema	373	215
Annual FOBT, colonoscopy/3 years	370	215
Annual FOBT, annual colonoscopy	391	224

* FOBT = fecal occult blood test; scope = 60-cm flexible sigmoidoscopy.
† Screening decreases the chance of developing invasive colorectal cancer by finding precancerous adenomas before they become invasive cancers.

The outcomes shown are a decrease in the probability of ever developing an invasive colorectal cancer (due to the removal of adenomas); a decrease in the probability of ever dying from colorectal cancer; an increase in life expectancy, undiscounted; an increase in life expectancy, discounted 5%; net financial costs, discounted 5%; and the probability of a perforation. The logic for discounting health effects is described by Keeler and Cretin (28). The discounted effects on life expectancy and costs can be used to calculate average and marginal cost per year of additional (increased) life expectancy. The decrease in the probabilities of developing and dying from invasive colorectal cancer are given per 10 000 persons screened. For example, an annual fecal occult blood test and an air-contrast barium enema every 5 years decreases the probability that a man at average risk will die from colorectal cancer by approximately 200 in 10 000 or 0.2%. Stated another way, of 10 000 50-year-old men at average risk screened, an annual fecal occult blood test and an air-contrast barium enema every 5 years until the men are 75 years of age will make the difference between life and death from colorectal cancer for approximately 200 men.

Table 2. *(Continued)*

Increase in Life Expectancy	Increase in Life Expectancy (discounted 5%)	Increase in Net Costs (discounted 5%)	Probability of Perforation‡
d	*d*	$	*n/10 000*
30.6	8.8	202	9
44.0	10.8	568	21
45.7	11.1	770	36
50.6	12.2	1828	96
76.2	20.4	682	10
79.6	21.3	1003	23
80.7	21.7	1607	49
82.8	22.3	1492	103
83.9	22.5	2736	50
84.8	22.9	2252	153
87.7	23.7	6236	417

‡ Includes perforations due to colonoscopies done after getting false-positive FOBT results.

Figure 1 plots a measure of effectiveness (the decrease in the probability of dying from colorectal cancer, undiscounted) against a measure of costs (the present value of net financial cost, discounted 5%) for the 11 strategies. If the choice of a strategy is based only on the lifesaving effects of screening compared with costs, the strategies that are connected by the lines in Figure 1 are preferred. For any strategy underneath the boundary, strategies may be found on the boundary that offer greater effectiveness per unit cost. The choice of a strategy not on the boundary must be based on considerations other than lifesaving and cost, such as patient discomfort or access. In general, practitioners should first consider using the strategies on the boundary.

Although these results are based on indirect evidence and have not been verified with direct evidence from controlled studies, some general conclusions can be drawn (Tables 2 and 3). First, the results for men and women, although not identical, are similar. Designing different recommendations for the two groups is not necessary. Second, screening for colorectal cancer can be both effective and, if the strategy is chosen carefully, cost effective. For example, an annual fecal occult blood test in men or women between 50 and 75 years of age (Tables 2 and 3, column 1) decreases the chance of

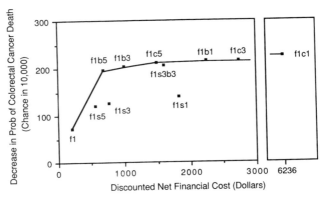

Figure 1. The decrease in the probability of dying from colorectal cancer (chance in 10 000) plotted against net financial cost, discounted 5%, for various screening strategies. f1 = annual fecal occult blood test (FOBT); f1s5 = annual FOBT and 60-cm sigmoidoscopy every 5 years; f1s3 = annual FOBT and 60-cm sigmoidoscopy every 3 years; f1b5 = annual FOBT and barium enema every 5 years; f1b3 = annual FOBT and barium enema every 3 years; f1c5 = annual FOBT and colonoscopy every 5 years; f1s3b3 = annual FOBT, 60-cm sigmoidoscopy, and barium enema every 3 years; f1s1 = annual FOBT and annual 60-cm sigmoidoscopy; f1b1 = annual FOBT and annual barium enema; f1c3 = annual FOBT and colonoscopy every 3 years; and f1c1 = annual FOBT and annual colonoscopy.

dying from colorectal cancer by approximately 65 in 10 000. The annual test (Tables 2 and 3, column 1) delivers a year of life expectancy at a cost of approximately $10 200 (both health effects and costs discounted 5%). Doing a barium enema every 5 years as well increases life expectancy by approximately 180 days (Tables 2 and 3, column 5) and, compared with an annual fecal occult blood test alone, has a marginal cost per additional year of life expectancy of approximately $15 000 (with discounting).

Third, a fecal occult blood test alone (Tables 2 and 3, column 1), although the simplest, most convenient, and least expensive, is the least effective of the available strategies. However, this relatively low effectiveness is similar to that of screening women between 55 and 65 years of age for breast cancer with an annual breast physical examination, both in terms of relative effectiveness (an approximately 25% reduction in mortality) and absolute effectiveness (a decrease in the probability of dying from cancer of approximately 30 in 10 000 and an increase in life expectancy of approximately 20 days) (30).

Fourth, strategies that involve complete visual examinations of the colon, either with barium enemas or colonoscopy, have the greatest effectiveness—more than twice that of the annual fecal occult blood test alone. They are more effective, because they can potentially find lesions throughout the bowel and have a greater ability to detect adenomas and lower random false-negative rates than does the fecal occult blood test. Although they are uncomfortable, require special skill on the part of practitioners, and are not often used for screening, especially for persons at average risk, these strategies are highly effective. They should be considered for patients who are especially concerned about colorectal cancer, and for whom the discomfort and costs are relatively unimportant.

Fifth, if the barium enema or any of the endoscopic procedures is used, a 3- to 5-year frequency preserves approximately 90% of the effectiveness of annual examinations, with much less inconvenience and cost (*compare* Tables 2 and 3, columns 5, 6, and 9). Sixth, if a barium enema is to be used at any interval, doing a sigmoidoscopic examination as well increases effectiveness little (*compare* Tables 2 and 3, column 6 with column 7). Finally, the greatest effectiveness is achieved with colonoscopy. It is approximately 5% more effective than barium enemas offered at comparable frequencies, but costs about twice as much at present (*compare* Tables 2 and 3, columns 6 and 10). Doing a colonoscopy every 3 to 5 years could be considered for persons for whom cost is not an issue.

A reasonable approach to deciding on a screening strategy follows. Starting with the strategy of no screening, consider the strategies shown in Tables 2 or 3 in order of increasing cost (*read* from left to right in Figure 1). Compare each strategy with its predecessor and ask whether the additional benefits are worth the additional inconvenience, discomfort, risks, and costs. If the answer is affirmative, proceed to the next strategy and repeat the questions. For example, suppose an annual fecal occult blood test and a 60-cm flexible sigmoidoscopy every 5 years (Tables 2 and 3, column 2) is considered desirable. Whether the benefits of using an air-contrast barium enema every 5 years instead of a 60-cm flexible sigmoidoscope every five years are worth the harms and costs can then be evaluated. For example, would a further decrease in the probability of developing invasive colorectal cancer of 176 in 10 000, a further decrease in the probability of dying from colorectal cancer of 76 in 10 000, and an additional increase in life expectancy of 32.2 days (*see* Table 2, values

Table 3. *Estimated Benefits and Risks for Colorectal Cancer Screening at 50 to 75 Years of Age for an Average-Risk Asymptomatic 50-Year-Old Woman**

Tests	Decrease in Probability of Invasive Colorectal Cancer†	Decrease in Probability of Death from Colorectal Cancer
	n/10 000	*n/10 000*
Annual FOBT	38	59
Annual FOBT, scope/5 years	140	102
Annual FOBT, scope/3 years	153	106
Annual FOBT, annual scope	191	117
Annual FOBT, barium enema/5 years	301	160
Annual FOBT, barium enema/3 years	320	164
Annual FOBT, scope, barium enema/3 years	329	166
Annual FOBT, colonoscopy/5 years	340	172
Annual FOBT, annual barium enema	354	174
Annual FOBT, colonoscopy/3 years	349	173
Annual FOBT, annual colonoscopy	372	181

* FOBT = fecal occult blood test; scope = 60-cm flexible sigmoidoscopy.

† Screening decreases the chance of developing invasive colorectal cancer by finding precancerous adenomas before they become invasive cancers.

calculated by subtracting column 2 from column 5) be worth the increase in discomfort associated with air-contrast barium enema (compared with 60-cm flexible sigmoidoscopy) and the increase in cost (approximately $65 per examination or $114 for the complete 25-year strategy)? If so, increasing the frequency of the barium enema to every 3 years might be considered. Ideally, these questions should be asked for each patient, as each has different preferences for the potential benefits, harms, and costs.

Age at Which to Begin Screening

The implications of beginning screening at different ages are examined in Table 4. The estimated effects are calculated from the perspective of a 40-year-old man at average risk, assuming his options are to begin screening at 40 years of age, wait 5 years and begin screening at 45 years of age, or wait 10 years and begin screening at 50 years of age. The implications of these three options are shown for the strategy of an annual fecal occult blood test and an air-contrast barium enema ev-

Table 3. *(Continued)*

Increase in Life Expectancy	Increase in Life Expectancy (discounted 5%)	Increase in Net Costs (discounted 5%)	Probability of Perforation‡
d	*d*	*$*	*n/10 000*
30.2	8.3	231	9
42.6	10.3	625	24
43.9	10.6	843	37
48.2	11.5	1995	106
68.3	17.2	785	14
70.9	17.9	1135	26
72.0	18.2	1785	55
73.8	18.6	1663	115
74.6	18.8	3021	56
75.2	19.1	2484	56
77.5	19.6	6812	169

‡ Includes perforations due to colonoscopies done after getting false-positive FOBT results.

ery 5 years. The relative differences between the three age options are similar for other screening strategies (for example, annual fecal occult blood test alone) and for women. Starting screening at 40 as compared with 50 years of age increases the effectiveness (measured as the decrease in the probability of developing invasive colorectal cancer, the decrease in the probability of dying from colorectal cancer, or the increase in life expectancy) very little (Table 4). Delaying screening from 40 to 50 years of age, however, reduces costs by a factor of about two.

Screening High-Risk Persons

The benefits of screening (for example, the decrease in the probability of developing invasive colorectal cancer, the decrease in the probability of dying from colorectal cancer, and the increase in life expectancy) are proportional to a person's risk for developing colorectal cancer. For example, if a person with a first-degree relative with colorectal cancer is thought to have a relative risk that is twice the average risk, the estimates of these outcomes for persons at average risk (Tables 2 and 3) can be multiplied by two. If a person's risk is thought to be three times the average, the estimates of

Table 4. *Estimated Benefits and Risks for Colorectal Cancer Screening Using an Annual FOBT and an Air-Contrast Barium Enema Every 5 Years for an Average-Risk Asymptomatic 40-Year-Old Man**

Benefits and Risks	Age to Begin Screening, y		
	40	45	50
Decrease in probability of developing invasive colorectal cancer, *n/10 000*†	216	214	212
Decrease in probability of death from colorectal cancer, *n/10 000*	124	123	122
Increase in life expectancy, *d*	47	47	47
Increase in life expectancy (discounted 5%), *d*	7	7	7
Increase in net costs (discounted 5%), *$*	997	688	448
Probability of a perforation, *n/10 000*‡	130	100	71

* FOBT = fecal occult blood test.
† Screening decreases the chance of developing invasive colorectal cancer by finding precancerous adenomas before they become invasive cancers.
‡ Includes perforations due to colonoscopies done after getting false-positive FOBT results.

the outcomes are multiplied by three. Because the cost of a strategy is relatively unaffected by a person's individual risk, the cost per year of life expectancy is roughly inversely proportional to a person's individual risk. For example, if the cost per year of life expectancy with an annual fecal occult blood test and a flexible sigmoidoscopy every 3 years is approximately $10 200 for an average-risk man, the cost per year of life expectancy for a high-risk man with a relative risk of two is approximately $5100 (10 200 ÷ 2).

Sensitivity Analysis

The three most critical factors, in terms of their uncertainty and importance, are the proportion of invasive cancers that arise from adenomas, how long a precancerous adenoma takes to progress from being first detectable by an endoscope or barium enema to being an invasive cancer, and how long a precancerous adenoma bleeds sufficiently to be detected by the fecal occult blood test before becoming an invasive cancer.

One of the main potential benefits of screening for this disease is finding and removing precancerous lesions (defined as adenomas destined to become invasive cancers if not removed). The results in Tables 2 and 3 are based on the assumption that 93% of invasive cancers arise from adenomas. Changing this assumption will cause an approximately proportional decrease in the effectiveness of screening. For example, if the true percentage of invasive cancers that arise from adenomas is half of 93% (46.5%), the effectiveness will be about halved.

How long a precancerous adenoma takes to progress from being first detectable by an endoscope or barium enema to being an invasive cancer controls the relative effectiveness of screening with endoscopes and barium enemas at different frequencies. The results in Tables 2 and 3 are based on the assumption that the average time for a 1-cm adenoma to become an invasive cancer is 7 years (range, 0 to 14 years) (distributed approximately normally). If this duration is shorter or longer, more or less frequent screening with these procedures would be required to achieve the degree of effectiveness shown in Tables 2 and 3. This fact has important implications for costs, inconvenience, discomfort, and anxiety. In general, a frequency that preserves approximately 90% of the effectiveness of an annual frequency at a reduced cost can be estimated by dividing the average duration of the preclinical interval by two. In the base case of this analysis (Tables 2 and 3) it was assumed that the average preclinical interval for adenomas was 7 years and that a screening frequency of every 3 to 5 years preserved approximately 90% of the effectiveness of annual screening at about half the cost. If the preclinical interval is thought to be, say, 5 years, screening every 2.5 years would preserve approximately 90% of the effectiveness of screening annually.

How long a precancerous adenoma bleeds sufficiently to be detected by a fecal occult blood test before becoming an invasive cancer controls the effectiveness of the test. Tables 2 and 3 are based on the assumption that only approximately 32% of precancerous adenomas bleed before becoming invasive cancer and, for those that bleed, bleeding begins an average of 2 years before they become invasive (range, 0 to 4 years). The calculations are also based on the assumption that a fecal occult blood test done during this interval has a 60% chance of detecting the bleeding (sensitivity). Although these assumptions appear to be conservative, to the extent that a smaller proportion of precancerous adenomas bleed before invasion and to the extent that these adenomas do not bleed for as long before invasion, the effectiveness of the fecal occult blood test has been overestimated.

The most critical financial factor affecting the choice

of a screening strategy is the cost of a colonoscopy compared with that of a barium enema. The indirect evidence indicates that both procedures should be highly effective in decreasing both the incidence of and mortality from colorectal cancer. The barium enema costs less. If the colonoscopy's cost were reduced to that of the barium enema, it would be competitive.

Recommendations of Major Organizations

The American Cancer Society recommends that men and women over 40 years of age receive annual digital rectal examinations and that persons over 50 years of age receive an annual fecal occult blood test and a sigmoidoscopy every 3 to 5 years after two initial examinations a year apart. For persons at high risk because of a personal family history (not an inherited polyposis syndrome), the Society recommends also examining the total colon by either air-contrast barium enema or colonoscopy every 3 to 5 years. The Canadian Task Force on the Periodic Health Examination includes testing stool for occult blood, not more frequently than annually, in their "health protection packages" for men and women 46 years of age and over. The National Cancer Institute recommends an annual fecal occult blood test and a sigmoidoscopy every 3 to 5 years for "case finding" in asymptomatic persons.

The U.S. Preventive Services Task Force (29) finds that there is insufficient evidence either for or against doing fecal occult blood tests or sigmoidoscopy in asymptomatic patients. It also believes, however, that discontinuing this form of screening where it is currently practiced or withholding it from persons who request it would be inappropriate. The Task Force also suggested that offering screening to persons 50 years of age and older with known risk factors for colorectal cancer may be "clinically prudent" and recommends that physicians give patients current information about the benefits, risks, and uncertainties of the available tests. One of the main purposes of this article is to provide practicing physicians with "best estimates" of the benefits, harms, and costs for use in making decisions.

Discussion

Choosing a screening strategy for colorectal cancer is very difficult. Three main issues must be addressed: the quality of the evidence of benefit; uncertainty about the magnitude of benefit; and the desirability of the estimated benefits compared with the inconvenience, discomfort, risks, and costs. In the case of colorectal cancer screening, these issues are not clearly answered. Little direct evidence of effectiveness exists at present. On the other hand, indirect evidence, based on the natural history and anatomy of the disease and the detection abilities of the screening tests, indicates that screening with various tests would reduce the incidence of and mortality from this disease. A mathematic model that integrates the existing empiric evidence with targeted judgments indicates that the effect of screening would be substantial, within the range of benefit achieved by screening for cancers of the breast or cervix (30, 31). In this sense, screening for colorectal cancer is like many other health activities that are supported by indirect evidence, but that lack "proof" from well-controlled trials.

The nonconclusive evidence of benefit translates into considerable uncertainty about the magnitude of benefit. Tables 2 and 3 present estimates based on the best information available and the judgments of informed persons; however, the degree of uncertainty is high (approximately ± 30%). Different persons react differently to uncertainty—some are eager to pursue any chance of benefit; others want "proof" from randomized controlled trials and certainty before acting.

Even if the estimated benefits and risks presented in Tables 2 and 3 are considered certain, no single screening policy is obviously preferable. For the fecal occult blood test, the main question is whether the benefits shown in the first column of Tables 2 and 3 (that is, a reduction in the chance of ever dying from colorectal cancer of approximately 65 in 10 000 and an increase in life expectancy of approximately 30 days) is worth a 1% to 3% chance of a false-positive result each year for 25 years. The next question is whether either of the procedures that enable visualization of the entire colon (air-contrast barium enema or colonoscopy) should be considered for persons at average risk. Both are specialized procedures, requiring practitioner skill and involving discomfort and higher cost; however, they approximately double the benefit. Their use eliminates the need for rigid or flexible sigmoidoscopy. If they are not used, sigmoidoscopy can be considered. For sigmoidoscopy, the main question is whether the additional benefits are worth the discomforts and costs of an examination.

Different persons react differently to these choices. For some, fear of cancer and stoicism make even barium enemas desirable. For others, denial, inconvenience, and anxiety make even the fecal occult blood test undesirable. In some, but by no means all, cases, a person's relative risk for developing colorectal cancer can shift the balance. For example, a woman might decide that the reduction in the probability of death from colorectal cancer of approximately 160 in 10 000 (approximately 1 in 40) obtained with an annual fecal occult blood test and a barium enema every 5 years is not worth the discomfort. However, if she is at high risk because of colorectal cancer in a close family member, the effect of having a barium enema every 3 years is twice as high—in the range of 320 in 10 000—and might be considered worth the discomfort. Others might find a 320-in-10 000 or even a 500-in-10 000 reduction in the chance of death from colorectal cancer still too small to warrant the discomfort.

Recommendation

Because of the reliance on indirect evidence; uncertainty about the magnitude of the outcomes; and a difficult balance between benefits, risks, and side effects, no obvious recommendation can be applied uniformly to all persons. Ideally, each physician and patient should discuss the issues and select a screening strategy to suit each patient's needs and values. In this sense, screening strategies for colorectal cancer are options (38).

The following explicit guidelines can be offered: Persons who are at average risk and over 50 years of age should have an annual fecal occult blood test and a sigmoidoscopy (preferably with a 70-cm flexible sigmoidoscope) every 3 to 5 years. Persons at high risk for developing colorectal cancer due to a history of colorectal cancer in a first-degree relative should be encouraged to have a complete examination of the colon with an air-contrast barium enema at 3- to 5-year intervals. If cost is not a concern, colonoscopy can be used in place of the barium enema.

It is important to understand, however, that others can (and have) come to different conclusions. Any recommendation, whether for a specific screening strategy or for no screening at all, should be considered a guideline, not a standard. With any recommendation, reviewing new information as it becomes available from ongoing research is important. In particular, the results of controlled trials of the fecal occult blood test currently under way in Minnesota and New York are expected to be available in the next few years.

Appendix Table 1. *Assumptions of the Mathematic Model**

Natural history

1. Age- and sex-specific incidence rates for invasive colorectal cancer for average-risk persons are shown in Table 1. Estimated rates for high-risk persons can be estimated by multiplying the rates for average-risk persons by the relative risk.
2. A high-risk person has twice the risk of an average-risk person.
3. Ninety-three percent of colorectal cancers arise from adenomatous polyps.
4. Of the cancers arising from adenomatous polyps, the average time for a 1-cm adenoma to become an invasive cancer is 7 years (range, 0 to 14 years).
5. Approximately 5% of adenomas that reach 5 mm develop into an invasive cancer.
6. The proportion of adenomatous polyps and de-novo cancers that develop within practical reach of various instruments is as follows: rigid sigmoidoscope, 30%; 35-cm flexible sigmoidoscope, 40%; 60-cm flexible sigmoidoscope, 55%; colonoscope, 95%; and air-contrast barium enema, 92%.
7. On average, an invasive cancer takes 2 years to pass through Dukes' A stage, 1 year to pass through Dukes' B stage, and 1 year to pass through Dukes' C stage.

Screening procedures

1. The nonrandom false-negative rates of the tests are encoded in their effective ranges (*see* item 6, above) and in how long before invasion they can first detect an adenoma or cancer. For adenomas within the effective range of a procedure, sigmoidoscopes and barium enemas were assumed to be able to detect adenomas an average of 7 years before invasion (range, 0 to 14 years). For calculating the probability that a lesion will be detected by a fecal occult blood test, 32% of adenomas larger than 1 cm were assumed to bleed sufficiently to be potentially detectable (subject to the random false-negative rate) for an average of 2 years before becoming invasive cancers (range, 0 to 4 years).
2. Random false-negative rates: fecal occult blood test, 40%; sigmoidoscopy, 15%; colonoscopy, 5%; and air-contrast barium enema, 15%.
3. Perforation rates: rigid sigmoidoscope, 0.0125%; 35-cm flexible sigmoidoscope, 0.02%; 60-cm flexible sigmoidoscope, 0.045%; colonoscope, 0.2%; and air-contrast barium enema, 0.02%.
4. False-positive rates: fecal occult blood test, 2%; and air-contrast barium enema, 3.5%.
5. Charges: fecal occult blood test, $5; rigid sigmoidoscopy, $70; 35-cm flexible sigmoidoscopy, $100; 60-cm flexible sigmoidoscopy, $135; colonoscopy, $500; and air-contrast barium enema, $200.
6. Charge for working up a person with a false-positive fecal occult blood test result: $800.
7. Charge for treating a perforation: $10 000.
8. Charges for initial treatment (39): adenoma, $800; invasive cancer, stage 1, $14 674; invasive cancer, stage 2, $15 928; invasive cancer, stage 3, $16 114; and invasive cancer, stage 4, $20 179.
9. Charge for terminal care: $23 460.

Clinical history and treatment

1. Relative case-survival rates for colorectal cancers detected and treated in various stages were estimated for all years after diagnosis. As an example, 5-year survival rates for men and women, respectively, were as follows: stage 1, 0.86 and 0.88; stage 2, 0.76 and 0.78; stage 3, 0.48 and 0.51; and stage 4, 0.08 and 0.09.
2. Without screening, approximately 50% of patients seek care for local invasive cancer, approximately 30% for regional invasive cancer, and approximately 20% for distant invasive cancer.
3. Age- and sex-specific mortality rates for other causes were estimated by subtracting mortality from colorectal cancer from mortality from all causes.

* From reference 9.

Appendix

The mathematic model used to analyze the effect of different screening strategies on colorectal cancer incidence and mortality is based on a mathematic model of screening described elsewhere (32-34). The model has been applied previously to analyze screening for cancers of the cervix, breast, and colon (32, 35, 36). For this analysis, the model was augmented to permit the analysis of three screening tests delivered separately and to include the possibility of two types of false-negative test results, nonrandom and random. The model adjusts for lead time and length biases.

The model consists of a nine-state time-varying Markov chain. The states represent persons who are alive and "well" (no diagnosis of cancer), who have cancer diagnosed in various stages, who have died from cancer, and who have died from other causes. Movement between states each year is controlled by transition probabilities. For each year in a person's life, the model calculates five main probabilities: the probability that a person who is alive and "well" has an asymptomatic but potentially detectable cancer or precancerous lesion (for example, an adenoma); the probability that a screening test, if applied, would detect an existing cancer or precancerous lesions in such a person; for persons with detected cancers or precancerous lesions, the stage of the cancer when detected; for persons with cancers diagnosed in various stages, the probability of dying from cancer in the coming year; and the probability that a person will die from other causes in the coming year. The first probability is calculated from age- and sex-specific incidence rates, risk factors, the "preclinical interval," and the history of previous screening tests. The preclinical interval is the time required for a lesion to develop from first being potentially detectable by screening (for example, a 1-cm adenoma) to the appearance of signs and symptoms. The second probability is determined by the lesion's state of development when the screening test is applied (for example, its size), the random false-negative rate of the tests, the position of the lesion in the bowel, and the region of the bowel "reached" by the screening test. The third probability is determined by the lesion's rate of development, the history of previous screening tests, and the random false-negative rate of the tests. The fourth probability is determined by stage-specific relative survival rates, and the fifth probability is determined by age- and sex-specific rates of mortality from other causes. The model incorporates the following features:

Natural History

1. Colorectal cancers can develop from two sources: adenomatous polyps and de-novo mucosal lesions.
2. The pre-invasive stages of cancers from these two sources have different durations.
3. Not all adenomatous polyps develop into invasive cancers.
4. Both adenomatous polyps and de-novo cancers occur with different frequencies in different parts of the colon and rectum.

Screening Procedures

1. The three main types of screening tests are fecal occult blood tests, endoscopic procedures, and barium enemas.

2. The quality of a procedure can depend on the skill of the practitioner and the type of equipment available.
3. The procedures have two types of false-negative results, nonrandom and random. Nonrandom false-negative results are due to a lesion's biologic features, such as whether it has begun to bleed; immediate repetition of the examination will be negative. Random false-negative results are due to random or technical factors, such as bowel preparation, the examiner's technique, sampling, reporting, and intermittency of bleeding; immediate repetition of an examination could be positive, subject to the random false-negative rate.
4. Barium enemas and endoscopies might perforate the bowel; perforations might require surgery and might cause death.
5. The procedures can give false-positive test results, warranting follow-up diagnostic procedures (for example, colonoscopy).

Clinical History and Treatment

1. The effect of therapy for a colorectal cancer, as expressed by relative case-survival rates, depends on the stage of the cancer.
2. Signs or symptoms can cause patients to seek medical care in the interval between screening examinations.
3. Persons are subject to mortality from causes other than colorectal cancer.

The model also includes financial costs for the performance of screening tests, work-up of false-positive test results, initial and terminal care for patients with colorectal cancer, and terminal care for patients dying from other causes. The present value of a lifetime of expected costs can be calculated, taking into account the probabilities that each of these costs will occur at any time in the future. Any discount rate can be specified.

The model can calculate the outcomes of screening with any combination of tests in any order and frequency, starting and stopping at any age, in men or women, in any risk category. Outcomes include the probability that a person will develop an invasive colorectal cancer, the probability of dying from colorectal cancer, life expectancy, the chance of a false-positive test result, the chance of a specified risk (for example, a perforation), the chance of death associated with such a risk, the expected cost of screening, the expected cost of a false-positive test result, the expected savings in treatment costs, and the total costs.

Estimates of variables relating to the performance of screening tests (for example, reach, sensitivity) and the natural history of the disease (such as the proportion of invasive cancers arising from adenomas, the time for a 1-cm adenoma to become invasive) are based on questionnaires sent to 72 physicians, selected for their knowledge of colorectal cancer, and on the available literature, as interpreted by the Patient Care Subcommittee of the National Digestive Diseases Advisory Board in a process described elsewhere (9). The values assigned to the variables for the base case analysis are given in Appendix Table 1. The sources of the estimates are described elsewhere (9). The estimated false-negative, false-positive, and perforation rates of the screening procedures are based on the assumption that the procedures are being done by physicians with appropriate training and experience. Where the reported sources implied a range of values, where the external validity of reported data was in question, or where there were few empiric observations on which to base estimates, the subcommittee identified a parameter value as the most reasonable (the "base case") and defined a range of values to capture the range of uncertainty.

Because no clinical study using any of the strategies analyzed has been completed, comparing the mortality predictions of the model with the observed outcomes of randomized controlled trials is not possible. Comparing the predicted and observed proportions of lesions detected in various stages for one strategy, the annual fecal occult blood test, however, was possible. The predictions matched within 1% the observed proportion of adenomas and cancers found in various stages in an ongoing randomized controlled trial of the annual fecal occult blood test (Gilbertsen VA. Personal communication).

References

1. **Silverberg E, Boring CC, Squires TS.** Cancer statistics, 1990. *CA.* 1990;**40**:9-26.
2. **Seidman H, Mushinski MH, Gelb SK, Silverberg E.** Probabilities of eventually developing or dying of cancer—United States, 1985. *Ca-A Cancer J Clinic.* 1985;**35**:36-56.
3. **Winawer SJ, Fath RB Jr, Schottenfeld D, Herbert E.** Screening for cancer. In: Miller AB, ed. *Screening for Cancer.* New York: Academic Press; 1985.
4. **Devroede G.** Risk of cancer in inflammatory bowel disease. In: Winawer SJ, Schottenfeld D, Sherlock P, eds. *Progress in Cancer Research and Therapy.* v. 13. New York: Raven Press; 1980.
5. **Anderson DE, Strong LC.** Genetics of gastrointestinal tumors. In: *Cancer Epidemiology, Environmental Factors.* Excerpta Med Congr Ser No. 351. 1974;**3**:267-71.
6. **Lovett E.** Family studies in cancer of the colon and rectum. *Br J Surg.* 1976;**63**:13-8.
7. **Macklin MT.** Inheritance of cancer of the stomach and large intestine in man. *JNCI.* 1960;**24**:551-71.
8. **Woolf CM.** A genetic study of carcinoma of the large intestine. *Am J Hum Genet.* 1985;**10**:42-7.
9. **Eddy DM, Nugent FW, Eddy JF, et al.** Screening for colorectal cancer in a high-risk population. Results of a mathematical model. *Gastroenterology.* 1987;**92**:682-92.
10. **Winawer SJ, Cummins R, Baldwin MP, Ptak A.** A new flexible sigmoidoscope for the generalist. *Gastrointest Endosc.* 1982;**28**:233-6.
11. **Norfleet RG.** Effect of diet on fecal occult blood testing in patients with colorectal polyps. *Dig Dis Sci.* 1986;**31**:498-501.
12. **Kewenter J, Björk S, Haglind E, et al.** Screening and rescreening for colorectal cancer. A controlled trial of fecal occult blood testing in 27,700 subjects. *Cancer.* 1988;**62**:645-51.
13. **Songster CL, Barrows GH, Jarrett DP.** Immunochemical detection of fecal occult blood—the fecal smear punch-disc test: a noninvasive screening test for colorectal cancer. *Cancer.* 1980;**45**:1099-102.
14. **Bralow SP, Kopel J.** Hemoccult screening for colorectal cancer—impact study on Sarasota, Florida. *J Fla Med Assoc.* 1979;**66**:915-9.
15. **Frühmorgen P, Demling L.** Early detection of colorectal cancer—a modified guaiac test—a screening examination in 6,000 humans. In: Winawer SJ, Schottenfeld D, Sherlock P, eds. *Progress in Cancer Research and Therapy.* v. 13. New York: Raven Press; 1980.
16. **Glober GA, Peskoe SM.** Outpatient screening for gastrointestinal lesions using guaiac-impregnated slides. *Dig Dis.* 1974;**19**:399-403.
17. **Gnauck R.** Screening for colorectal cancer with the Hemoccult test. *Leber Magen Darm.* 1977;**7**:32-5.

18. **Hastings JB.** Mass screening for colorectal cancer. *Am J Surg.* 1974;**127:**228-33.
19. **Miller SF, Knight RA.** The early detection of colorectal cancer. *Cancer.* 1977;**40:**945-9.
20. **Schwartz FW, Holstein H, Brecht JG.** Preliminary report of fecal occult blood testing in Germany. In: Winawer SJ, Schottenfeld D, Sherlock P, eds. *Progress in Cancer Research and Therapy.* v. 13. New York: Raven Press, 1980.
21. **Gilbertsen VA, McHugh R, Schuman L, Williams SE.** The earlier detection of colorectal cancer. A preliminary report of the results of the occult blood study. *Cancer.* 1980;**45:**2899-901.
22. **Hardcastle JD, Thomas WM, Chamberlain J, et al.** Randomised, controlled trial of faecal occult blood screening for colorectal cancer. Results for first 107,349 subjects. *Lancet.* 1989;**1:**1160-4.
23. **Kronborg O, Fenger C, Sondergaard O, et al.** Initial mass screening for colorectal cancer with fecal occult blood test. A prospective randomized study at Funen in Denmark. *Scand J Gastroenterol.* 1987;**22:**677-86.
24. **Hertz RE, Deddish MR, Day E.** Value of periodic examinations in detecting cancer of the rectum and colon. *Postgrad Med.* 1960;**27:** 290-94.
25. **Gilbertsen VA.** Proctosigmoidoscopy and polypectomy in reducing the incidence of rectal cancer. *Cancer.* 1974;**34:**936-9.
26. **Selby JV, Friedman GD, Collen MF.** Sigmoidoscopy and mortality from colorectal cancer: the Kaiser Permanente Multiphasic Evaluation Study. *J Clin Epidemiol.* 1988;**41:**427-34.
27. **Friedman GD, Collen MF, Fireman BH.** Multiphasic health checkup evaluation: a 16-year follow-up. *J Chron Dis.* 1986;**39:**453-63.
28. **Keeler EB, Cretin S.** Discounting of life-saving and other nonmonetary effects. *Manage Sci.* 1983;**29:**300-6.
29. **U.S. Preventive Services Task Force.** Screening for colorectal cancer. *AFP.* 1989;**40:**119-26.
30. **Eddy DM.** Screening for breast cancer. *Ann Intern Med.* 1989;**111:** 389-99.
31. **Eddy DM.** Screening for cervical cancer. *Ann Intern Med.* 1990; **113:**214-26.
32. **Eddy DM.** *Screening for Cancer: Theory, Analysis and Design.* Englewood Cliffs, New Jersey: Prentice-Hall; 1980.
33. **Eddy DM.** A mathematical model for timing of repeated medical tests. *Med Decis Making.* 1983;**3:**45-62.
34. **Eddy DM.** Technology assessment: the role of mathematical modeling. In: *Assessing Medical Technologies.* Washington, DC: Institute of Medicine, National Academy Press; 1985.
35. **Eddy DM.** Estimating the effectiveness and risks of breast cancer screening: a mathematical model. In: Feig SA, McLelland R, eds. *Breast Carcinoma: Current Diagnostic Imaging and Therapeutic Update.* New York: Masson; 1983.
36. **Eddy DM.** The cost-effectiveness of colorectal cancer screening. In: Levin B, Riddell R, eds. *Gastrointestinal Cancer.* New York: Elsevier Science Publishing Co.; 1984.
37. **Sondik E, ed.** *Annual Cancer Statistics Review, 1988.* Washington, DC: Division of Cancer Prevention and Control, National Cancer Institute; 1989.
38. **Eddy DM.** Designing a practice policy-standards, guidelines, and options. *JAMA.* 1990;**263:**3077, 3081, 3084.
39. **Baker MS, Kessler LG, Smucker RC.** Analysis of the continuous medicare history sample file: the cost of treating cancer. *Proceedings of the Annual Meeting, Scientific Session. American Cancer Society, San Deigo California, May 1987.* New York: American Cancer Society; 1987.

Screening for Lung Cancer

DAVID M. EDDY, MD, PhD

There were approximately 152 000 new cases and about 139 000 deaths from lung cancer in 1988 (1). Most cases and deaths currently occur in men; however, incidence rates in women are increasing rapidly as more women begin to smoke. Lung cancer recently overtook breast cancer as the commonest cause of cancer death in women. Despite the lack of a satisfactory treatment, the very high incidence and poor prognosis of lung cancer prompt hopes that early detection will help to reduce mortality. This paper reviews the pertinent background for screening, the main screening tests available, and the evidence that screening reduces mortality.

Background

The probability that a person at average risk will develop lung cancer in a given year is shown for men and women of various ages in Table 1. In men the rate starts to rise at approximately age 40 and climbs rapidly until it peaks at a rate of about 470 per 100 000 at about age 75. In women, the incidence is lower but follows a similar pattern, starting to climb at age 40 and peaking at about 155 per 100 000 at approximately age 70 (2).

The most important risk factor for lung cancer by far is tobacco use. More than 80% of lung cancer cases occur in smokers (3), and incidence rates are approximately 10 times higher in smokers than non-smokers. When the proportion of smokers in the population is taken into account, smokers have a risk of developing lung cancer approximately 2.5 times the average rates listed in Table 1. The incidence of lung cancer in people who do not smoke is approximately 25% of the rates shown in the table.

Exposure to some industrial materials such as asbestos and hydrocarbons also increases the risk that a person will develop lung cancer, although these materials are responsible for only a small percentage of all cases of lung cancer (4).

▶ This chapter was originally published in *Annals of Internal Medicine*. 1989;111:232-7.

Table 1. *Annual Age-Specific Incidence Rates by Gender (per 100 000) for Cancers of the Lung and Bronchus**

Age	Males	Females
0 to 4	0.00	0.00
5 to 9	0.00	0.00
10 to 14	0.00	0.80
15 to 19	0.15	0.12
20 to 24	0.16	0.23
25 to 29	0.46	0.56
30 to 34	1.76	1.36
35 to 39	5.40	4.15
40 to 44	21.59	14.46
45 to 49	51.31	31.84
50 to 54	104.60	56.94
55 to 59	198.15	89.97
60 to 64	283.17	123.10
65 to 69	380.18	142.84
70 to 74	459.64	153.08
75 to 79	469.67	135.20
80 to 84	441.69	107.03
85 and over	314.12	75.17

* Data from reference 2.

Screening Tests

Two main screening tests have been proposed for lung cancer: chest roentgenograms and sputum cytology. Modern roentgenogram technology involves a 66 × 43-cm film taken at about 140 peak kV on medium-speed film and medium-speed screens. Two views are usually recommended: postero-anterior and lateral. The examination involves a small dose of radiation, takes only a few minutes, and costs approximately $50.

The modern technique of sputum cytology is based on a procedure developed by Saccomanno and colleagues (5). Sputum is collected in a special fixative, homogenized, and centrifuged. Slides are then prepared from the concentrated, resuspended sediment, and the material is stained with Papanicolaou stain. The current practice is to collect specimens (preferably morning sputum) on 3 days. These samples can be processed separately or "pooled" before processing.

Evidence of Effectiveness

Considerable research has been done to evaluate the effectiveness of various combinations of screening tests on lung cancer mortality. In the 1950s and 1960s, several uncontrolled and nonrandomized controlled studies (6-10) evaluated various combinations of roentgenograms and cytology given at various time intervals, ranging up to once every 6 months. These studies failed to show a benefit from lung cancer screening.

Since these studies were done, both the roentgenogram technique and cytology techniques have been improved, raising new questions about the potential effectiveness of lung cancer screening. Beginning in the early 1970s, three large randomized controlled trials were done in the United States to evaluate definitively the effectiveness of screening using modern techniques. In addition, a randomized controlled trial has been reported from Czechoslovakia and a case-control study reported from Germany.

Mayo Lung Project

Perhaps the most important of the new randomized controlled trials was done at the Mayo Clinic. Of the four, it compared the most intensive with the least intensive screening protocols. In this study, 10 933 men who smoked one pack or more of cigarettes a day were given initial examinations with chest roentgenograms and sputum cytology. The lung cancers that were found were analyzed as "prevalence cases." The 9211 men who tested negative for lung cancer on the initial screen and were otherwise acceptable were then randomized into two groups. One group of 4618 men was designated to receive chest roentgenograms and sputum cytology examinations every 4 months for 6 years (the "4-monthly group"). The other group of 4593 men (the "control group") did not receive any scheduled screening examinations but were given the "standard Mayo advice" to have an annual chest roentgenogram and annual sputum cytology. This advice was not repeated and no reminders were sent. All subjects and controls were contacted at least once a year to determine their status. When the trial was completed, it showed no effect of screening on the number of inoperable cases, the number of cases found in late stages, and–most importantly–the number of deaths from lung cancer.

At the time surveillance was ended in 1983, 206 cancers had been detected in the 4-monthly group and 160 in the control group. Forty-six percent of the cancers in the study group were resectable, compared with 32% in the control group. However, the death rate from lung cancer was slightly higher in the group offered roentgenograms and sputum cytology every 4

Table 2. *Effect of Screening on Percentage of Cancers Detected in Stages I and II**

Screening Results	Postsurgical Cancer Stage†		Total
	I and II	III and Nonresected	
	←——————— n (%) ———————→		
Cancers found			
4-Monthly group	71 (42)	96 (58)	167 (100)
Control group	32 (25)	99 (75)	131 (100)
5-Year survival			
4-Monthly group	47 (66)	4 (4)	53 (32)
Control group	13 (41)	4 (4)	17 (13)

* Data from reference 12.
† Cancer stage according to the guidelines of the American Joint Committee on Cancer.

months (3.2 per 1000 person-years) compared with the control group (3.0 per 1000 person-years) (11). The difference is not statistically significant.

An earlier report (12), based on 167 cancers in the study group and 131 in the control group, provided more detailed information on the proportion of lesions detected in various stages, 5-year survival rates by stage, number of late-stage cancers, number of nonresectable cancers, and number of deaths from lung cancer. This information highlights an apparent paradox that can confuse the interpretation of lung cancer screening studies if one focuses only on stage proportions and case-survival rates instead of the actual number of late-stage cancers or deaths from lung cancer.

Screening appeared to detect a higher proportion of cancers in early stages as classified by the American Joint Committee on Cancer postsurgical staging system (Table 2). It also appears that of the cancers diagnosed, patients classified as being in stages I and II of disease had a better 5-year survival than those classified as in stage III (Table 2). However, the ultimate indicators of the effectiveness of screening—deaths from lung cancer, the number of inoperable cases, and the number of late-stage cases—were unaffected by screening (Table 3).

Possible explanations for this apparent paradox are lead-time bias and "overdiagnosis" in the group offered screening compared with the control group. Lead-time bias occurs because screening allows earlier diagnosis, without necessarily delaying the time of death. Although moving forward the time of diagnosis

Table 3. *Results of Mayo Lung Project: Effect of Screening on Number of Late-Stage Cancers, Number of Nonresectable Cases, and Number of Deaths from Lung Cancer**

Result	Group	
	4-Monthly	Control
Late-stage lung cancers, *n*	123	119
Nonresectable lung cancers, *n*	112	109
Lung cancer deaths, *n*	122	115
Lung cancer death rate per 1000 person-years	3.2	3.0

* Data from reference 11.

increases 5-year survival rates calculated from that time, it does not necessarily change the actual mortality. Overdiagnosis occurs when a lesion is detected and labeled as a clinically important cancer, when in fact the lesion might not be a cancer at all, or might have an extremely long latent phase–so long that the study will be terminated or the patient will die from another cause before the cancer would ever become clinically evident.

Given the much greater number of lesions labeled as cancers in the 4-monthly group than in the control group, overdiagnosis in the 4-monthly group is a distinct possibility in the Mayo Lung Project. Insights into the potential effect of overdiagnosis can be gained by examining the results shown in Table 2 (12) and subtracting from the 4-monthly cases the "surplus" cases found in that group compared with the control group. In the screened group, 167 lesions were detected and labeled as lung cancer compared with 131 lesions in the control group, suggesting an excess of approximately 36 lesions in the screened group. If the data in the screened group are modified by subtracting 36 lesions from the 4-monthly group, assuming that each of these 36 lesions was staged a postsurgical stage I and assuming they would not have caused death even without surgery, then the data in Table 2 become as shown in Table 4. This revised table indicates that screening might have had no real effect on stage proportions of clinically relevant cancers or 5-year survival, which coincides precisely with the lack of an observed effect on mortality (Table 3). The data are thus consistent with the hypothesis that many of the lesions detected by screening and labeled as cancers were not clinically important in the sense that they would never have become clinically evident during the time of the trial and follow-up (approximately 12 years). If over-diagnosis is occurring as just speculated, its frequency over the 6 years of screening is about 0.8% (36 cases out of 4618 men offered screening), or about 0.1% per year of screening.

A factor to consider when evaluating the results of the Mayo Lung Project is that chest roentgenograms were widely available to patients in the control group. The investigators estimated that approximately 50% of the patients in the control group actually had roentgenograms (thus "contaminating" the control group), and approximately a third of the lung cancers in the control group were detected by nonstudy roentgenograms. The investigators believe, however, that most of these roentgenograms were not deliberate self-screening, but rather were received because of non-cancerous conditions, especially cardiovascular problems that are common in smokers. Thus, the detection of these cancers can be considered incidental findings on roentgenograms done for other reasons (11).

It is also worth noting that contamination of a control group, to the extent that it occurs, will only cause a proportional decrease in the observed effectiveness of screening, not eliminate it altogether. A rough way to adjust for the effect of contamination is to divide the effectiveness actually observed by a correction factor calculated as the reciprocal of the percentage of persons in the control group who did not receive any screening. In this case, the factor would be 2. The actual results of this trial indicate no effect at all (that

Table 4. *Effect of Screening on Proportion of Cancers Detected in Stages I and II, Adjusted for Potential Overdiagnosis*

Screening Results	Postsurgical Cancer Stage*		Total
	I and II	III and Nonresected	
	← *n (%)* →		
Cancers found†			
4-Monthly group	35 (27)	96 (73)	131 (100)
Control group	32 (25)	99 (75)	131 (100)
5-Year survival†			
4-Monthly group	11 (31)	4 (4)	15 (11)
Control group	13 (41)	4 (4)	17 (13)

* Cancer stage according to the guidelines of the American Joint Committee on Cancer.
† Data adjusted for potential overdiagnosis.

is, mortality rates of 3.2 per 1000 person-years in the 4-monthly group and 3.0 per 1000 person-years in the control group). Thus, even if the observed results were adjusted for possible contamination in the control group, the adjusted result is still zero effect.

Memorial Sloan-Kettering Project

This study was designed to determine the incremental effectiveness of sputum cytology when given in addition to annual chest roentgenograms. In this study, 10 040 men over age 45 who smoked were randomly assigned to one of two groups, a "dual-screened group" of 4985 men and a "roentgenogram-only group" of 5072 men. The dual-screened group received postero-anterior and lateral chest roentgenograms (140 peak kV) once a year and 3-day sputum cytology every 4 months. The roentgenogram-only group received annual postero-anterior and lateral chest roentgenograms. During the period of active screening, 288 lung cancers were diagnosed, split evenly between the two groups. Thus, if overdiagnosis occurred in this study, it was approximately equal in the two groups.

As with the Mayo Lung Project, data from this study published in 1984 (13) indicate that the screening tests can detect cancers in earlier stages and that cancers in earlier stages have better case-survival rates than cancers detected in later stages. However, there was virtually no difference between the dual-screened group and the roentgenogram-only group in the proportions of cancers found in various stages, "operable" cancers, 5-year case-survival rates, or actual mortality (13) (Table 5). Thus this trial indicates that adding sputum cytology, even as frequently as every 4 months, does not improve mortality rates compared with the use of annual chest roentgenograms alone.

Some of the investigators in the Sloan-Kettering study have argued (14) that, although there was no significant difference in lung cancer mortality in the two groups, the 5-year survival of nearly 35% in both groups was well above the national average (15). Furthermore, they believe that because approximately 40% of all lung cancers (in both groups) were found in American Joint Committee on Cancer postsurgical stage I and the case-survival rate for these patients who were treated by resection was 70% to 80%, screening may be beneficial:

> Either the screening is saving lives of some men who would otherwise have had disease undetected until it pro-

Table 5. *Results of the Memorial-Sloan Kettering Project: Effect of Screening on Number of Late-Stage Cancers, Number of Resectable Cancers, and Number of Deaths**

Result	Group	
	Dual Screen	Roentgenogram Only
	n	
Lung cancers		
Total	144	144
Late stage	78	75
Resectable	73	77
Deaths†	90	92

* Data from reference 13. The overall 5-year survival rate was 35%.
† Deaths from lung cancer, lung cancer-related diagnostic procedures, and other causes.

gressed to an advanced, symptomatic and incurable stage, or these men could have lived for many years unaware that they had lung cancer. To advise against efforts to detect lung cancer early, i.e. by screening asymptomatic high risk populations at least by annual chest X-ray films, is to assume the second explanation is true (14).

The principal investigator of the Mayo Lung Project has addressed this point:

[I] can appreciate the Memorial group's position. Today a decision not to test a high risk, asymptomatic patient does indeed seem tantamount to a decision not to treat for cure. Yet in the MLP screened group the 5-year survival and the proportion of stage I lung cancers were the same as at Memorial, while in the control group they were very much lower. Despite these striking differences in survival and staging, 4-monthly screening conferred no lung cancer mortality advantage. This observation, and the "missing" stage I lung cancers in the MLP control group, suggest that there may have been some control patients with asymptomatic, undetected lung cancers who "could have lived for many years unaware that they had lung cancer" (16).

Johns Hopkins Study

The design of the Johns Hopkins trial was virtually identical to that of the Memorial Sloan-Kettering Project. Lung cancers were detected in 396 men (dual-screen, 194; control, 202). Survival rates were similar in the two groups (approximately 20% at 8 years). Age-adjusted lung cancer mortality was not significantly lower in the dual-screen group (3.4 per 1000 person-years) than in the control group (3.8 per 1000 person-years). The investigators concluded:

This study showed no benefit (reduction in lung cancer mortality) from the addition of sputum cytology to an annual radiographic screening. Mass screening for lung cancer cannot be recommended based upon the findings of this study (17).

Czechoslovakian Study

A fourth randomized controlled trial was recently reported from Czechoslovakia. In this study, 6364 men who smoked, ages 40 to 64, were screened with postero-anterior chest photofluorograms and 1-day sputum cytology to identify prevalence cases. The remaining men were randomly assigned to either a screened group or control group. The screened group (3172 men) had a chest roentgenogram and sputum cytology every 6 months for 3 years; the control group (3174 men) had a single screen at the end of the 3-year study.

During the 3-year period, 39 "incidence" cancers were detected in the screened group and 27 were detected in the control group. The authors did not report overall mortality in the two groups over a fixed period, but did report the number of "5-year survivors"–nine and five in the screened and control groups, respectively. Given that 39 and 27 cancers were detected in the two groups, these data appear to imply 30 deaths in the screened group compared with 22 in the control group (18). However, this finding should be viewed with caution because of the unusual reporting method.

Case-Control Study from the German Democratic Republic

Ebeling and Nischan (19) took advantage of a tuberculosis control program involving screening with biennial chest roentgenograms to do a case-control study of the effect of screening roentgenograms on lung cancer mortality. One hundred and thirty men under 70 years of age who died from lung cancer during 1980 through 1985 in a district of Berlin were each matched by year of birth with four controls. Two controls were randomly selected from inhabitants of the same district and two were selected from the emergency surgical outpatient department of the general hospital. A screening history was obtained for all cases and controls. The relative risks of dying from lung cancer for screened participants compared with unscreened persons were 0.88 and 1.09 for the district group and the hospital group, respectively. Neither result was statistically significant nor was there a trend in relative risk with regard to the number of tests done or interval since the last test. Thus, this case-control study also failed to show any effect of screening roentgenograms on lung cancer mortality.

Risks

The main risk of lung cancer screening is a false-positive result. Chest roentgenograms and sputum cytology can both detect lesions that are not cancers, or that might grow so slowly that they would never surface clinically. Detection of such lesions can lead to work-ups with the concomitant inconvenience, discomfort, anxiety, and expenses, and possibly to unnecessary treatment. Definitive information on false-positive rates of either roentgenograms or sputum cytology in the three U.S. randomized controlled trials has not been published. An early report (20) of the initial (prevalence) screening at Sloan-Kettering indicated that about 10% of patients had abnormal chest roentgenograms leading to additional studies to rule out cancer. Approximately 5% of these patients had bronchoscopy, percutaneous needle aspiration, or thoracotomies, or all of these procedures. In all, 100 patients were evaluated for every cancer found. An evaluation of the "incidence" cases at the Hopkins Project revealed that approximately 18% of patients without cancer had "positive" or "suspicious" roentgenograms requiring close follow-up for 2 years, and approximately 3% of the patients without cancer had abnormal roentgenograms that led to further medical management.

Less information on false-positive results from sputum cytology screening is available. On the prevalence screen in the Memorial Project, sputum cytology showed marked atypia or cancer cells in seven patients who did not have cancer, indicating a false-positive rate of about 0.14%. The work-up for a positive sputum cytology test in a patient with a normal roentgenogram can be fairly extensive, because without an abnormal roentgenogram it is difficult to localize the lesion. The recommended evaluation at Memorial-Sloan Kettering is illustrative: If a comprehensive head and neck examination is normal, then a diagnostic bronchoscopic examination to segmental and subsegmental bronchi to sixth- and seventh-generation bronchi is done. If a lesion is located centrally in the main or lobar bronchus, it is readily visualized and doing a biopsy is easy. In many cases, the tracheo-bronchial tree appears normal. These cases require a meticulous sampling of each segmental bronchus by endobronchial brushing and cytologic analysis.

An additional risk of lung cancer screening is a false sense of security; smokers might believe that screening "protects" them from the consequences of lung cancer, and a negative examination might decrease their motivation to stop or reduce smoking. There have been no formal studies of this problem. Finally, chest roentgenograms involve delivering radiation to the chest. Because the amount of radiation is very small, however–approximately 20 millirems–the carcinogenic effect is negligible.

Costs

The costs of chest roentgenograms and sputum cytology vary widely. The average charge for a chest roentgenogram is approximately $50 and the charge for sputum cytology is approximately $60. If all smokers in the United States over the age of 40 were screened with annual chest roentgenograms, the annual cost for screening alone (not counting work-ups for false-positive examinations) would have been approximately $1.5 billion in 1988.

Discussion

The benefits, harms and costs of lung cancer screening are summarized in Table 6. The existing evidence does not indicate that sputum cytology every 4 months, when added to annual chest roentgenograms, or even that sputum cytology and roentgenograms every 4 months compared with "routine care" reduces the chance a smoker will die from lung cancer. On the other hand, screening can cause false-positive results, leading to needless work-ups and anxiety. If overdiagnosis does occur, it might affect approximately 1 of every 1000 smokers who receive intensive screening for a year.

Because of the available evidence, virtually all organizations concur that screening for lung cancer is not justified. For example, the American Cancer Society (21), the American College of Radiology (22), the National Cancer Institute (23), the U.S. Preventive Services Task Force (24), and the Canadian Task Force on the periodic health examination (25) all decline to recommend lung screening with any test at any frequency. Investigators of the Hopkins and Mayo and consider several problems the clinician may encounter when using them to formulate individualized plans for preventive care. In so doing, we hope to help individual physicians and other health care providers in deciding which preventive interventions to use for various patient subgroups; and to highlight not only areas of agreement and disagreement between organizations, but also recommendations that need to be clarified.

History of Practice Guidelines for Preventive Care

The characteristics of a beneficial screening program were elucidated as long ago as 1957, when a Federal Commission on Chronic Illness outlined a strategy for the control of chronic diseases (27). Salient considerations included the burden of suffering associated with the condition for which screening is being considered, the accuracy and acceptability of available screening tests, and the evidence that treatment of the disease at a preclinical stage is more effective than treatment after the disease manifests itself symptomatically. These criteria were intended to guide the development of mass screening programs.

In 1975, Frame and Carlson (2-5) suggested that the same criteria could be used to evaluate the usefulness of preventive services for individual patients. These investigators reviewed interventions to prevent 36 common diseases and suggested that physicians tailor their preventive practices to the age and gender of the individual patient (2-5). In 1986, Frame (9-12) wrote a series of articles updating the protocols he had proposed in 1975 and comparing his revised recommendations with the work of the CTF.

The CTF was established in 1976 with a mandate from the Canadian government to determine how the periodic health examination might enhance the health of the Canadian populace. A committee of experts from many health disciplines developed a highly organized process for evaluating the effectiveness of preventive services. This process included a review of the world's literature to identify important preventable conditions and to evaluate the strength of evidence supporting the use of various preventive interventions in physicians' offices. Evidence from randomized clinical trials was weighted heavily, whereas opinions or consensus statements from clinicians without accompanying objective evidence were considered to be less important. The first report of the CTF, in 1979, emphasized the distinctive needs and problems of high-risk groups (7). In 1982, the CTF established a working group that periodically reviewed existing CTF recommendations and appraised other interventions that had not been previously considered (14-16, 18-24, 142).

In the 1980s, two additional sets of preventive guidelines, one by the USPSTF and another by the ACP, were formulated. In 1984, the U.S. Department of Health and Human Services (DHHS) convened the USPSTF to develop recommendations about which preventive interventions should be used in asymptomatic persons who present in the clinical setting. The USPSTF included 20 health care professionals, was supported by a scientific staff from the DHHS' Office of Disease Prevention and Health Promotion, and was guided by more than 300 senior advisors. In formulating its recommendations, the USPSTF used the same methods as those developed by the CTF for rating the strength of its recommendations (Table 1). The resulting USPSTF report, *Guide to Clinical Preventive Services*, covered a wider range of preventive interventions than previous groups had considered (25). The *Guide* concluded that the greatest promise for preventing illness lay in changing patient behavior through effective counseling (28). The USPSTF also emphasized three considerations for the implementation of preventive health services: the need to use greater selectivity in ordering tests and providing services, the need to use the risk profile of each patient in determining which interventions are most important, and the need to use an illness visit as an opportunity for prevention. The cost of potential interventions was not explicitly considered in the formulation of USPSTF recommendations.

Through its Clinical Efficacy Assessment Project (CEAP), the ACP also has developed practice guidelines over the past decade (29). In formulating its recommendations, the CEAP has relied on detailed background papers prepared jointly by "content" and "methods" experts and reviewed thoroughly by clinical experts, including representatives of subspecialty societies and other interest groups (30, 31). The CEAP process has emphasized the use of quantitative methods (for example, decision analysis and cost-effectiveness analysis) to clarify the advantages and disadvantages of alternative practice strategies. From its background papers, the CEAP has developed position papers that have been reviewed and approved by the Health and Public Policy Committee and the Board of Regents of the ACP.

In 1986, National Blue Cross/Blue Shield (BC/BS)

Table 2. *(Continued)*

Area	USPSTF	Other
Height and Weight		
General	MF 18+ every 1-3 y†	Frame: MF 18+ every 4 y (12) 1989 Oboler and LaForce: MF 20+ every 4 y (43) 1989 IOM: MF 18+ every 5 y (84) 1978 AHA: MF 18+ every 5 y (85) 1987
Selective	No recommendation (25) p111 1989	
Blood Pressure Measurement		
General	MF 18+ every 2 y and at every visit for other reasons	Frame: MF 18+ every 2 y (9) 1986 IOM: MF 18+ every 5 y (84) 1978 JNC, AHA: MF 18+ every 2 y (85,86) 1988 Oboler and LaForce: MF 20+ every 2 y (43) 1989
Selective	MF 18+ every 1 y if diastolic BP is 85-89 mm Hg (25) p23 1989	JNC, AHA: MF 18+ every 1 y if diastolic BP is 80-89 mm Hg; measure BP more frequently if diastolic BP > 89 mm Hg (85,86) 1988
Assessment of Cognitive Impairment		
General	No recommendation§	NIH: MF clinical evaluation (87) 1987
Selective	No recommendation (25) p251 1989	

See end of table for footnotes.

Table 2. *History and Physical Examination (Continued)*

Area	ACP	CTF
Assessment of Depression and Suicidal Intent		
General	MF "elderly," functional assessment screening, including measures of emotional status	[D] Recommendation against
Selective	No recommendation (88) 1988	[C] MF 18+ for suicide risk if one or more: evidence of a psychiatric disorder, substance abuse, family history of suicide attempt (15) 1990
Assessment of Visual Impairment		
General	Not considered	[C] No recommendation
Selective	Not considered	No recommendation (7) 1979
Assessment of Hearing Impairment		
General	Not considered	[B] MF 18+ by history
Selective	Not considered	MF 18+ by history if one or more: exposure to jet engines or other noisy machinery, farm equipment, amplified music, gunfire, snowmobiles, or model airplanes for more than 2 hours several times per week (21) 1984

Table 2. *(Continued)*

Area	USPSTF	Other
Assessment of Depression and Suicidal Intent		
General	Recommendation against‖	Frame: recommendation against (12) 1986
Selective	MF 18+ for suicide risk if one or more: adolescent, young adult, personal or family history of depression, chronic illness, living alone, recent bereavement or separation or unemployment, sleep disturbance, multiple somatic complaints, drug or alcohol abuse (25,89) p261, 265 1989	
Assessment of Visual Impairment		
General	MF 18-39 recommendation against MF 40-64 no recommendation MF 65+ every 1 y	Oboler and LaForce: MF 60+ every 1 y by Snellen chart or similar test (43) 1989 AAO: MF 40-64 every 2-4 y, MF 65+ every 1-2 y
Selective	No recommendation (25) p181 1989	AAO: MF 20-39 every 3-5 y if black race (90) 1989
Assessment of Hearing Impairment		
General	MF 65+ by history	IOM: MF 40+ every 5 y (84) 1978 Oboler and LaForce: MF 60+ every 1 y by audioscope (43) 1989
Selective	MF 19-64 if regularly exposed to excessive noise (25) p193 1989	

See end of table for footnotes.

Table 2. *History and Physical Examination (Continued)*

Area	ACP	CTF
Examination of Oral Cavity to Detect Oral Cancer		
General	Not considered	[C] MF 65+ every 1 y
Selective	Not considered	[C] MF 18+ if tobacco use (7) 1979
Carotid Auscultation for Cervical Bruit		
General	Not considered	[C] No recommendation
Selective	Not considered	No recommendation (21) 1984
Thyroid Palpation		
General	Not considered	Not considered
Selective	Not considered	Not considered

Table 2. *(Continued)*

Area	USPSTF	Other
Examination of Oral Cavity to Detect Oral Cancer		
General	[C] Recommendation against	Frame: recommendation against (11) 1986¶ ACS, NCI: MF 20-39 every 3 y, MF 40+ every 1 y (13,91) 1988 Oboler and LaForce: recommendation against (43) 1989
Selective	MF 18+ if one or more: tobacco use, excessive alcohol exposure, suspicious lesions detected through self-examination (25,92) p91 1989	
Carotid Auscultation for Cervical Bruit		
General	No recommendation	Frame: recommendation against (9) 1986 Oboler and LaForce: recommendation against (43) 1989
Selective	MF 40+ if one or more: TIA symptoms, previous stroke, hypertension, smoking, CAD, atrial fibrillation, DM (25) p29 1989	
Thyroid Palpation		
General	No recommendation	ACS: M 20-39 every 3 y, M 40+ every 1 y (13) 1988 Oboler and LaForce: recommendation against (43) 1989
Selective	MF 18+ if personal history of upper body radiation (25) p108 1989	Oboler and LaForce: MF 18+ every 1 y if irradiation to the head, neck, or mediastinum during childhood (43) 1989

See end of table for footnotes.

Table 2. *History and Physical Examination (Continued)*

Area	ACP	CTF
Complete Skin Examination		
General	Not considered	[D] Recommendation against
Selective	Not considered	[B] MF 18+ if one or more: outdoor occupation, contact with polycyclic aromatic hydrocarbons [C] MF 18+ if personal or family history of dysplastic nevi (21) 1984
Breast Examination by Clinician		
General	F 40+ every 1 y	[C] F 40-49 every 1 y [A] F 50-59 every 1 y [B] F 60+ every 1 y
Selective	F 18+ every 1 y if personal history of breast cancer (38,49) 1989	F 35+ every 1 y if family history of premenopausal breast cancer in a first-degree relative or otherwise at "high risk" (20) 1986

Table 2. *(Continued)*

Area	USPSTF	Other
Pelvic Examination by Bimanual Palpation		
General	Recommendation against††	Frame: recommendation against (11) 1986 Oboler and LaForce: recommendation against (43) 1989 ACS, NCI: F 20-40 every 1 to 3 y, F 40+ every 1 y (13,91) 1988 ACOG: F 18+ every 1 y (93) 1989
Selective	No recommendation (25) p81 1989	
Testicular Examination		
General	No recommendation	Frame: recommendation against (11) 1986 ACS: M 20-39 every 3 y, M 40+ every 1 y (13) 1988 Oboler and LaForce: recommendation against (43) 1989
Selective	M 19-39 if one or more: cryptorchidism, orchiopexy, testicular atrophy (25) p77 1989	

See end of table for footnotes.

Table 2. *History and Physical Examination (Continued)*

Area	ACP	CTF
Digital Rectal Examination for Prostate Cancer		
General	Not considered	[C] No recommendation
Selective	Not considered	No recommendation (7) 1979‡‡

* "General" screening refers to routine testing of asymptomatic persons who have no risk factors, other than age or gender, associated with the target condition. "Selective" screening refers to testing of asymptomatic persons who are at increased risk for the target condition. Relevant risk factors are listed in columns for each authority. ACP = American College of Physicians; CTF = Canadian Task Force on the Periodic Health Examination; and USPSTF = U.S. Preventive Services Task Force. Other sources of preventive care guidelines are indicated by first author or a common abbreviation. BP = blood pressure; CAD = coronary artery disease; TIA = transient ischemic attacks; DM = diabetes mellitus; and first-degree relative = parent, sibling, or child. "Not considered" indicates that a health organization has not published a practice guideline about the preventive care intervention. "Recommendation against" means that the intervention should be excluded from routine preventive care for the age, sex, and risk status indicated. "No recommendation" indicates that an authority considered the intervention, but, for lack of convincing evidence, refrained from making a specific recommendation either for or against it. Square brackets enclose a one-letter "strength-of-recommendation" code, if available, as described in Table 1. Indicated next are gender (M, male; F, female; MF, both sexes), an age range to which the recommendation applies, and the frequency with which the test should be done (in years), if specified by the health organization. For selective screening strategies, risk factors are listed. Citations to original papers describing the practice guideline are given in parentheses. The year that the most recent practice guidelines were issued from the relevant authority appears last. In the case of the USPSTF *Guide to Clinical Preventive Services*, page numbers for relevant chapters are shown. For a preventive action to be recommended, the listed requirements for age, sex, and risk factors must be met. Recommendations are for nonpregnant adults 18 years of age or older. The relevant age range considered by the CTF is 16 to 44 years, whereas that considered by the USPSTF is 19 to 39 years. Other components of the clinical examination that were considered by fewer than two authorities include cardiac auscultation, abdominal palpation for aortic aneurysms, and examination for peripheral vascular disease.

Table 2. *(Continued)*

Area	USPSTF	Other
Digital Rectal Examination for Prostate Cancer		
General	No recommendation	Frame: recommendation against (11) 1986 ACS, NCI: M 40+ every 1 y (13,91) 1988 Oboler and LaForce: recommendation against (43) 1989 IOM: M 40+ every 2-5 y (84) 1978
Selective	No recommendation (25) p63 1989	

† The USPSTF recommends routine evaluation of height and weight using a table of desirable weights or a body mass index (body weight in kilograms divided by the square of height in meters) of more than 27.8 in men or 27.3 in women as a basis for further intervention.

‡ If diastolic blood pressure is < 90 mm Hg, blood pressure should be measured at least every 5 years and at every visit made for other reasons.

§ Clinicians should periodically inquire about the functional status of elderly patients at home and at work.

‖ Refers to use of formal instruments to screen for depression.

¶ All patients should be taught self-examination of the oral cavity for malignancy.

** Although routine screening for skin cancer by complete skin examination is not recommended, clinicians should be alert to skin lesions with malignant features when examining patients for other reasons.

†† Although the USPSTF states that screening of asymptomatic women for ovarian cancer is not recommended, they advise examination of the adnexa when doing gynecologic examinations for other reasons.

‡‡ The CTF is expected to issue new recommendations on screening for prostate cancer in 1991.

Table 3. *Laboratory Tests**

Test	ACP	CTF
Hemoglobin Measurement for Iron-Deficiency Anemia		
General	Recommendation against	[C] Recommendation against
Selective	F 18+ if one or more: recent immigrant from underdeveloped country, institutionalized elderly (95) 1987	[C] F 18-64 if of low socioeconomic status (7) 1979
Urine Analysis		
General	Recommendation against screening for bacteriuria	[D] Recommendation against screening for bacteriuria or for bladder cancer
Selective	Recommendation against (96) 1989	[B] MF 18+ urine cytology to screen for bladder cancer in smokers and persons occupationally exposed to bladder carcinogens (7) 1979
Fasting Plasma Glucose		
General	Recommendation against	[D] Recommendation against
Selective	F 18+ if intends to become pregnant and has risk factors for DM as listed below MF 18+ if one or more: DM in first-degree relative, age > 50 y, weight > 25% over ideal weight, personal history of gestational diabetes, membership in ethnic group with high prevalence of DM. MF 40+ once if obese and a diagnosis of DM would motivate weight loss (41,52) 1989	[B] MF 18+ if one or more: family history of DM, hyperglycemia associated with pregnancy, evidence of early occlusive vascular disease (7) 1979

Table 3. *(Continued)*

Test	USPSTF	Other
Hemoglobin Measurement for Iron-Deficiency Anemia		
General	Recommendation against	IOM: MF 40+ every 20 y (84) 1978
Selective	No recommendation (25) p163 1989	
Urine Analysis		
General	[C] MF 60+ screening for bacteriuria, hematuria, proteinuria	IOM: MF 40+ (84) 1978
Selective	[C] MF 18+ to screen for bacteriuria if diabetic (25,97,98) p95, 155 1989	
Fasting Plasma Glucose		
General	Recommendation against	Frame: recommendation against (12) 1986 IOM: MF 40+ every 5 y (84) 1978
Selective	MF 18+ if one or more: family history of DM, marked obesity, personal history of gestational DM (25,99) p95 1989	ADA: MF 18+ every 3 y if one or more: family history of DM in first-degree relative; > 20% over ideal body weight; American Indian, Hispanic, or black race; age ≥ 40; previously identified impaired glucose tolerance; hypertension, hypercholesterolemia or hyperlipidemia; personal history of gestational DM or birthweight of babies > 9 lb (100) 1989

See end of table for footnotes.

Table 3. *Laboratory Tests (Continued)*

Test	ACP	CTF
Nonfasting Cholesterol†		
General	MF 18-70 every 5 y	[C] M 30-59
Selective	MF 18+ more frequently if one or more: smoker, family history of hypercholesterolemia or premature cardiovascular disease in a parent or sibling, use of lipid-altering drugs, hypertension, CAD, or secondary cause of hyperlipidemia such as DM (34,45) 1989	No recommendation (24) 1991
Thyroid Function Testing§		
General	Recommendation against	[D] Recommendation against screening for hyperthyroidism [C] Recommendation against screening for hypothyroidism
Selective	F 50+ if one or more general symptoms that could be caused by thyroid disease (42,54) 1990	[C] F 40+ no recommendation if postmenopausal (14,101) 1990

Table 3. *(Continued)*

Test	USPSTF	Other
Nonfasting Cholesterol†		
General	[C] MF 18+ every 5 y‡	Frame: MF 18-70 every 4 y (9) 1986 AHA: MF 20-60 every 5 y (85) 1987 NCEP: MF 20+ every 5 y (55) 1987
Selective	MF 18+ more frequently if one or more: previous abnormal cholesterol, male, early CAD in a first-degree relative, smoker, hypertension, HDL < 35 mg/dL (0.91 mmol/L), DM, previous stroke or PVD, severe obesity (25) p11 1989	
Thyroid Function Testing§		
General	Recommendation against	Frame: recommendation against (12) 1986
Selective	F 65+ may be clinically prudent for populations at increased risk for hypothyroidism, such as older women (25) p105 1989	

See end of table for footnotes.

Table 3. *Laboratory Tests (Continued)*

Test	ACP	CTF
Human Immunodeficiency Virus (HIV) Serology‖		
General	Recommendation against	Not considered
Selective	MF 18+ if one or more: member of a high-risk population by virtue of sexual or drug-taking behavior, woman of childbearing age with any risks for HIV infection, received a blood transfusion between 1978 and 1985, person planning marriage who may be at increased risk (102) 1988	Not considered
Syphilis Serology		
General	Recommendation against	[D] Recommendation against
Selective	MF 18+ if one or more: sexual contact of known case; member of high-risk group, such as homosexuals; resident of area of high prevalence (105) 1987	[A] MF 18-64 if multiple sexual partners (7) 1979
Resting Electrocardiogram		
General	MF 18-65 recommendation against	[C] Recommendation against
Selective	MF 65+ no recommendation MF 18+ no recommendation if one or more cardiac risk factors are present (46) (risk factors include DM, hypertension, tobacco use, hypercholesterolemia) (32) 1990¶	No recommendation (21) 1984

Table 3. *(Continued)*

Test	USPSTF	Other
Human Immunodeficiency Virus (HIV) Serology‖		
General	[C] Recommendation against	CDC: recommendation against
Selective	[B] MF 18-64 if one or more: recently acquired STD, homosexual or bisexual man or partner of same, IV drug abuser or partner of same, prostitute, has multiple sexual contacts or partner of same, received blood transfusion between 1978 and 1985, long-term resident of high-prevalence area (25,103) p139 1989	CDC: MF 18+ if one or more: treated for STD, IV drug abuser or partner of same, prostitute, HIV-infected sexual partner, received blood transfusion between 1978 and 1985, resident of high-prevalence area, considers self at risk (104) 1987
Syphilis Serology		
General	Recommendation against	Frame: recommendation against (10) 1986
Selective	[B] MF 18-64 if one or more: sexual contact of proved case, prostitute, has multiple sexual partners, resident of area of high prevalence (25,103) p131 1989	Frame: MF 18+ if member of high-risk group, such as male homosexuals (10) 1986
Resting Electrocardiogram		
General	Recommendation against	Frame: recommendation against (9) 1986 IOM: MF 40-45 once (84) 1978 AHA: MF 20+ every 20 y (85) 1987
Selective	M 18+ if a cardiac event would endanger public safety M 40+ if sedentary and planning to begin vigorous exercise program M 40+ if two or more: hypercholesterolemia, smoker, DM, first-degree family history of early onset CAD (25) p3 1989**	

See end of table for footnotes.

Table 3. *Laboratory Tests (Continued)*

Test	ACP	CTF
Exercise Stress Test		
General	Recommendation against	[C] Recommendation against
Selective	No recommendation if one or more: occupation that puts others at risk, sedentary and about to begin a program of physical conditioning No recommendation if male, of "increased age," and one or more: family history of CAD, smoker, systolic BP > 140 mm Hg, DM, hypercholesterolemia, total:HDL cholesterol ratio > 6 (33,47) 1990	No recommendation (21) 1984
Assessment of Intraocular Pressure by Clinician††		
General	Not considered	[C] Recommendation against
Selective	Not considered	No recommendation (20) 1986

Table 3. *(Continued)*

Test	USPSTF	Other
Exercise Stress Test		
General	Recommendation against	Frame: recommendation against (9) 1986
Selective	M 18+ if a cardiac event would endanger public safety M 40+ if sedentary and planning to begin vigorous exercise program M 40+ if two or more: hypercholesterolemia, smoker, DM, first-degree family history of early-onset CAD (25) p3 1989**	Frame: MF once for high-risk groups, especially if planning exercise program (9) 1986 ACSM: MF 46+ once if planning exercise program (106) 1986 ACC, AHA: M 40+ once if occupation affecting public safety, sedentary and planning exercise, or two or more: hypercholesterolemia, hypertension, smoker, DM, family history of CAD before age 55 (107) 1986
Assessment of Intraocular Pressure by Clinician††		
General	MF 18-64 recommendation against MF 65+ by eye specialist	Frame: recommendation against (12) 1986 AAO: MF 20-39 every 2-4 y, MF 65+ every 1-2 y
Selective	No recommendation (25) p187 1989	AAO: MF 20-39 every 3-5 y if black race (90) 1989

See end of table for footnotes.

Table 3. *Laboratory Tests (Continued)*

Test	ACP	CTF
Tuberculin Skin Testing (PPD)		
General	Not considered	[E] Recommendation against
Selective	Not considered	[A] MF 18+ if exposed to TB at home or work or living in community with high infection rate (7) 1979
Chest Radiograph to Detect Lung Cancer		
General	Recommendation against	[D] Recommendation against
Selective	Recommendation against if smoker (37,50) 1989	[D] Recommendation against if smoker (22) 1990

Table 3. *(Continued)*

Test	USPSTF	Other
Tuberculin Skin Testing (PPD)		
General	Recommendation against	Frame: recommendation against (10) 1986
Selective	MF 18+ if one or more: exposed to TB case in the home, clinics or shelters for the homeless, nursing homes, substance abuse treatment centers, dialysis units, correctional institutions; recent immigrants or refugees from high-prevalence areas; migrant workers; HIV or renal failure, immunosuppressive drugs including steroids (25) p125 1989	Frame: MF 18+ for high-risk groups, including immigrants, alcoholics, contacts of TB cases, health care personnel, persons with a family history of TB, and persons living in institutions (10) 1986 CDC: MF 18+ if one or more: close contact with persons suspected to have TB; medical risks such as HIV infection, silicosis, previous gastrectomy, renal failure, DM, malignancy, prolonged corticosteroid use; foreign-born from area of high TB prevalence; member of high-risk racial, ethnic, or low income population; alcoholic or IV drug user; resident of long-term care facility (108) 1990
Chest Radiograph to Detect Lung Cancer		
General	Recommendation against	Frame: recommendation against (11) 1986 ACS: recommendation against (13) 1988 Oboler and LaForce: recommendation against (43) 1989
Selective	Recommendation against if smoker (25) p67 1989	

See end of table for footnotes.

Table 3. *Laboratory Tests (Continued)*

Test	ACP	CTF
Bone Mineral Content Testing‡‡		
General	F perimenopausal, recommendation against	[D] Recommendation against
Selective	MF 18+ no recommendation; risk factors: female, postmenopausal, white race, low body weight; roles of calcium intake and exercise in prevention are controversial; consider if decision to start long-term estrogen therapy will be based on knowledge of bone mass and related fracture risk (40,53) 1990	[C] F 40+ no recommendation if one or more: Caucasian, surgical menopause, early natural menopause, low body weight for height, immobile; uncertain roles for smoking, calcium intake, alcohol use, falls (19) 1988
Mammography		
General	F 50+ every 1 y	[A] F 50-59 every 1 y [B] F 60+ every 1 y
Selective	F 18+ every 1 y if personal history of breast cancer F 40+ every 1 y if family history of breast cancer or at increased risk after consideration of marital status, multiparity, late first pregnancy, early menarche, late menopause, history of benign breast conditions, high-fat diet (38,49) 1989	F 35+ every 1 y if "at high risk," especially if family history of premenopausal breast cancer in a first-degree relative (20) 1986

Table 3. *(Continued)*

Test	USPSTF	Other
Bone Mineral Content Testing‡‡		
General	Recommendation against	Frame: recommendation against (12) 1986
Selective	F 40-64 if one or more: perimenopausal, Caucasian, bilateral oophorectomy before menopause, slender build; and if estrogen therapy is being considered for prophylaxis against osteoporosis but would not otherwise be indicated (25,109) p239 1989	Frame: F 18+ no recommendation if one or more: Caucasian, early menopause, small body frame, family history of osteoporosis, sedentary lifestyle, low dietary calcium, steroid use (12) 1986
Mammography		
General	[A] F 50-59 every 1-2 y	Frame: F 50+ every 1 y (11) 1986
	[B] F 60-75 every 1-2 y	ACS, NCI, AMA, AAFP: F 40-50 every 1-2 y, F 50+ every 1 y (58,91,110-112) 1989
		ACOG: F 35-40 once, F 40-50 every 1-2 y, F 50+ every 1 y (93) 1989
		AGS: F 65-85 every 2-3 y (94) 1989
		Oboler and LaForce: F 40+ every 1 y (43) 1989
Selective	F 35+ every 1 y if family history of premenopausal breast cancer in a first-degree relative (25,67) p39 1989	

See end of table for footnotes.

Table 3. *Laboratory Tests (Continued)*

Test	ACP	CTF
Papanicolaou Smear (Cervical Cytology)§§		
General	F 20-65 every 3 y	[B] F 18-35 every 3 y
		[B] F 36-74 every 5 y
Selective	F 20-65 every 2 y if at increased risk after consideration of main risk factors (multiple sexual partners, early onset of sexual activity, smoking) and additional risk factors (black, Hispanic, Native American ethnic origins; certain partner characteristics, history of STD, oral contraceptive use) F 66-75 every 3 y if not screened in the 10 years before age 66 (39,48) 1989	[B] F 18-74 every 1 y if one or both: early onset of sexual activity, multiple sexual partners (7) 1979
Gonorrhea Culture¶¶		
General	Not considered	[D] Recommendation against
Selective	Not considered	[A] MF 18-64 if multiple sexual partners (7) 1979

Table 3. *(Continued)*

Test	USPSTF	Other
Papanicolaou Smear (Cervical Cytology)§§		
General	F 18-65 every 1-3 y	Frame: F 18-69 every 2 y (11) 1986 ACS, NCI, ACOG, AAFP: F 18+ every 1-3 y (13,58,93,113) 1989‖ ‖ Oboler and LaForce: F 20+ every 3 y (43) 1989 IOM: F 18+ every 5 y (84) 1978 AGS: F 60-70 every 3 y (57) 1989
Selective	F 18+ more frequently if one or more: early onset of sexual activity, multiple sexual partners, low socioeconomic status. F 65+ every 1-3 y if no documentation of consistently normal cervical cytology in the previous 10 years (25) p57 1989	ACS: F 18+ more frequently if one or more: early age at first intercourse, multiple sexual partners, other risk factors (8) 1980
Gonorrhea Culture¶¶		
General	Recommendation against	Frame: recommendation against (10) 1986 Oboler and LaForce: recommendation against (43) 1989 IOM: MF 18-24 once (84) 1978
Selective	[A] MF 18-64 if one or more: prostitute, multiple sexual partners, sexual contact with proved cases, history of repeated STDs (25,103) p135 1989	Oboler and LaForce: MF 18+ if one or more: prostitute, sexual contact with proved cases, history of repeated gonorrhea (43) 1989

See end of table for footnotes.

Table 3. *Laboratory Tests (Continued)*

Test	ACP	CTF
Chlamydia Testing***		
General	Not considered	[D] Recommendation against
Selective	Not considered	[C] MF 18+ if in high-risk group such as partners of persons with nongonococcal urethritis (21) 1984
Endometrial Aspirate or Biopsy		
General	Not considered	[D] Recommendation against
Selective	Not considered	No recommendation (19) 1988

Table 3. *(Continued)*

Test	USPSTF	Other
Chlamydia Testing*		
General	Recommendation against	Frame: recommendation against (10) 1986 Oboler and LaForce: recommendation against (43) 1989
Selective	MF 18-64 if one or more: attending STD clinic or other health care setting that sees high-risk patients, multiple sexual partners, partner with multiple sexual contacts, partner of persons with positive cultures (25, 103) p147 1989	CDC: MF 18+ if one or more: attending STD clinic or other health care setting that sees high-risk patients, low socioeconomic status, multiple sexual partners, partner with multiple sexual contacts, partner of persons with positive cultures (114) 1985
Endometrial Aspirate or Biopsy		
General	Not considered	Frame: recommendation against (11) 1986††††
Selective	Not considered	ACS: F at menopause, if one or more: history of infertility, obesity, anovulation, uterine bleeding, estrogen therapy (13) 1988 ACOG: F perimenopausal, if unexpected breakthrough bleeding during estrogen replacement therapy (93) 1989

See end of table for footnotes.

Table 3. *Laboratory Tests (Continued)*

Test	ACP	CTF
Stool Examination for Occult Blood		
General	MF 50+ every 1 y	MF 18-39 recommendation against [C] MF 40+ no recommendation
Selective	MF 40+ every 1 y if one or more: personal history of inflammatory bowel disease, familial polyposis coli, family history of colon cancer in first-degree relative (36,51) 1990	[C] MF 45+ every 1 y if family history of colorectal cancer detected after age 40 in a first-degree relative (16) 1989
Sigmoidoscopy		
General	MF 50+ every 3-5 y‡‡‡	[C] No recommendation
Selective	No recommendation (36,51) 1990	MF 18-29 if family history of familial polyposis [C] MF 40+ if family history of colorectal cancer detected after age 40 in one or more first-degree relatives [C] F 40+ if personal history of one or more: endometrial, ovarian, breast cancer (16) 1989

Table 3. *(Continued)*

Test	USPSTF	Other
Stool Examination for Occult Blood		
General	[C] No recommendation	Frame: MF 40-50 every 2 y, MF 50+ every 1 y (11) 1986 ACS, NCI, ACOG: MF 50+ every 1 y (13,91, 93) 1988 IOM: MF 40+ every 1 y (84) 1978
Selective	[C] MF 50+ every 1 y if one or more: personal history of adenomatous polyps or colorectal cancer or inflammatory bowel disease, first-degree relative with colorectal cancer [C] F 50+ every 1 y if personal history of one or more: endometrial, ovarian, breast cancer (25,115) p47 1989	
Sigmoidoscopy		
General	[C] MF 40+ no recommendation [D] MF 18-39 recommendation against	Frame: recommendation against (11) 1986 ACS, NCI, ACOG: MF 50+ every 3-5 y (93, 116) 1989
Selective	[C] MF 50+ every 3-5 y if one or more: personal history of adenomatous polyps or colorectal cancer or inflammatory bowel disease, first-degree relative with colorectal cancer after age 40. [C] F 50+ every 3-5 y if personal history of one or more: endometrial, ovarian, breast cancer (25,64) p47 1989	ACS: MF 18-49 more frequently if one or more: personal history of familial polyposis, the Gardner syndrome, ulcerative colitis, previous polyps or colon cancer; family history of colorectal cancer (8) 1980

See end of table for footnotes.

Table 3. *Laboratory Tests (Continued)*

Test	ACP	CTF
Colonoscopy		
General	Recommendation against	Recommendation against
Selective	MF 40+ every 3-5 y if one or more: personal history of inflammatory bowel disease, familial polyposis coli, family history of colon cancer in first-degree relative (36,51) 1990§§§	[C] MF 18+ if personal history of one or both: ulcerative colitis or adenomatous polyps of 10 years' duration, previous colorectal cancer [C] MF 30+ if family history of familial polyposis [C] MF 40+ if two or more first-degree relatives with colorectal cancer (16) 1989

* "General" screening refers to routine testing of asymptomatic persons who have no risk factors, other than age or gender, associated with the target condition. "Selective" screening refers to testing of asymptomatic persons who are at increased risk for the target condition. Relevant risk factors are listed in columns for each authority. ACP = American College of Physicians; CTF = Canadian Task Force on the Periodic Health Examination; and USPSTF = U.S. Preventive Services Task Force. Other sources of preventive care guidelines are indicated by first author or a common abbreviation. CAD = coronary artery disease; PVD = peripheral vascular disease; DM = diabetes mellitus; first-degree relative = parent, sibling, or child; HDL = high-density lipoprotein; and STD = sexually transmitted disease; IV = intravenous; BP = blood pressure; TB = tuberculosis; HIV = human immunodeficiency virus. "Not considered" indicates that a health organization has not published a practice guideline about the preventive care intervention. "Recommendation against" means that the intervention should be excluded from routine preventive care for the age, sex, and risk status indicated. "No recommendation" indicates that an authority considered the intervention, but, for lack of convincing evidence, refrained from making a specific recommendation either for or against it. Square brackets enclose a one-letter "strength-of-recommendation" code, if available, as described in Table 1. Indicated next are the gender (M, male; F, female; MF, both sexes) and the age range to which the test should be done (in years), if specified by the health organization. For selective screening strategies, risk factors are listed. Citations to original papers describing the practice guideline are given in parentheses. The year that the most recent practice guideline was issued from the relevant authority appears last. In the case of the USPSTF *Guide to Clinical Preventive Services*, page numbers for relevant chapters are shown. For a preventive action to be recommended, the listed requirements for age, sex, and risk factors must be met. Recommendations are for nonpregnant adults 18 years of age and older. The relevant age range considered by the CTF is 16 to 44 years, whereas that considered by the USPSTF is 19 to 39 years.

Table 3. *(Continued)*

Test	USPSTF	Other
Colonoscopy		
General	Recommendation against	
Selective	[A] MF 18+ if family history of hereditary polyposis syndromes [B] MF 18+ if personal history of 10 or more years of ulcerative colitis [B] MF 18+ if personal history of colorectal cancer or adenomatous polyps [B] MF 40+ if two or more first-degree relatives with colorectal cancer, particularly if age of onset is before 40 y (25,64) p47 1989	

† Measurement of nonfasting total serum cholesterol level by venipuncture. All authorities stress the importance of submitting samples to an accredited laboratory with good quality control. Abnormal results should be confirmed by a repeat test of nonfasting cholesterol level, and the mean of the two results should be used for decision making.

‡ Periodic total cholesterol screening is most important for middle-aged men and may be clinically prudent for others.

§ Sensitive thyrotropin (TSH) immunoradiometric assay or free thyroxin index.

‖ Most groups recommend testing with a Western blot test after repeatedly reactive results on enzyme immunoassay tests.

¶ Although no specific advice is given for the use of a resting electrocardiogram to screen for coronary artery disease in persons with risk factors for such disease, the ACP background paper states that general screening recommendations do not apply to persons with the characteristics listed.

** The USPSTF lists the same high-risk groups as possible candidates for exercise and resting electrocardiography, but observes that there is insufficient evidence to determine which is the better screening test for these persons.

†† Tonometry and ophthalmoscopy done by primary care provider.

‡‡ Methods for assessing the risk for osteoporosis-related fractures with bone mineral content testing include single-photon absorptiometry, dual-photon absorptiometry, dual energy x-ray absorptiometry, and quantitative computed tomography.

§§ The ACP, the ACS, the CTF, Frame, Oboler and LaForce, and the USPSTF suggest initiating screening with 2 to 3 annual smears at the onset of sexual activity. Recommendations pertain to women who are sexually active.

‖‖ After three normal annual examination results, the Papanicolaou test may be done less frequently at the discretion of the physician.

¶¶ Culture from urethral, rectal, throat, or endocervical swabs.

*** Culture or immunofluorescent assay of endocervical or urethral swabs.

††† All women should be taught to report postmenopausal bleeding.

‡‡‡ Air-contrast barium enema every 5 years may be substituted for sigmoidoscopy.

§§§ Air-contrast barium enema may be substituted for colonoscopy.

Table 4. *Adult Immunizations and Chemoprophylaxis**

Vaccine or Drug	ACP	CTF
Hepatitis B-Inactivated Virus Vaccine		
General	Recommendation against	Recommendation against
Selective	MF 18+ initial series if at increased risk for occupational, environmental, social, or family exposure; intimate family contact with infected persons, resident of institutions for the mentally retarded, prison inmate, homeless person, homosexual or bisexual man, person with multiple sexual partners, person with multiple sexually transmitted diseases or partner of same, intimate contact with persons from endemic areas, early renal disease or hemophilia, health care worker, IV drug abuser (117) 1990	[A] MF 18+ initial series if one or more: dialysis, blood product exposure, health care personnel, institutionalized mentally retarded person, IV drug abuser, homosexual, contact with patients with disease or carriers (21) 1984
Inactivated Influenza Vaccine		
General	MF 65+ every 1 y	[E] MF 18-64 recommendation against [A] MF 65+ every 1 y
Selective	MF 18-64 every 1 y if one or more: resident of nursing home or chronic care facility, health care occupation, chronic cardiopulmonary disorder or other chronic disease requiring regular medical care, HIV-infected patient, organ transplant recipient, alcoholic, cancer patient, person providing care to high-risk persons, or resident of area with increased risk for exposure (for example, dormitories, military barracks) (117) 1990	[A] MF 18+ every 1 y if chronic debilitating disease (7) 1979

Table 4. *(Continued)*

Vaccine or Drug	USPSTF	Others
Hepatitis B-Inactivated Virus Vaccine		
General	Recommendation against	
Selective	[A] MF 18+ initial series if one or more: homosexual man, IV drug user, blood product recipient, health care worker with blood product exposure (25,118) p363 1989	CDC: MF 18+ initial series if one or more: health care worker with blood product exposure, client or staff of institution for the developmentally disabled, staff of nonresidential day-care programs, hemodialysis patient, sexually active homosexual man, person with multiple sexual partners or recent STD, prostitute, user of illicit injectable drugs, household or sexual contact with HBV carriers, inmate of long-term correctional facilities, recipient of certain blood products (119) 1990
Inactivated Influenza Vaccine		
General	[A] MF 65+ every 1 y	Frame: recommendation against IOM: MF 60+ every 1 y (84) 1978 CDC: MF 65+ every 1 y
Selective	[A] MF 18+ every 1 y if one or more: resident of chronic care facility, chronic cardiopulmonary disease, hemoglobinopathy, diabetes, metabolic disease, renal dysfunction, immunosuppression; health care provider for high-risk patients (25,118) p363 1989	Frame: MF 18+ every 1 y if at high risk for lower respiratory tract infection (10) 1986 CDC: MF 18+ every 1 y if one or more: resident of nursing home or chronic care facility, chronic cardiovascular or pulmonary disease, person who has required regular medical care because of chronic metabolic or renal disease, person with hemoglobinopathy or immunosuppression; health care worker, home care provider, household member of high-risk persons (120) 1990

See end of table for footnotes.

Table 4. *Adult Immunizations and Chemoprophylaxis**

Vaccine or Drug	ACP	CTF
Measles Live Virus Vaccine†		
General	No recommendation	Not considered
Selective	MF 18+ two doses if born after 1956 and without documentation of receipt of live vaccine, physician-diagnosed measles, or laboratory evidence of immunity; revaccinate if college student or health care worker and previously given only one dose of vaccine or killed measles vaccine (117) 1990	Not considered
Pneumococcal Polysaccharide 23-Valent Vaccine		
General	MF 65+ once; consider revaccination after 6 years	[C] MF 55+ no recommendation
Selective	MF 18-64 once if one or more: chronic cardiac or pulmonary disease, asplenia, chronic liver disease, alcoholism, diabetes, chronic renal failure, hematologic malignancy, undergoing chemotherapy, organ transplant recipient, HIV infection, CSF leak, nursing home residence (117) 1990	[A] MF 18+ once if one or more: sickle cell anemia, asplenia [A] MF 55+ once if living in an institution [D] recommendation against if immunocompromised (142) 1991

Table 4. (*Continued*)

Vaccine or Drug	USPSTF	Others
Measles Live Virus Vaccine†		
General	No recommendation	
Selective	MF 18+ once if born after 1956 and no proof of immunity, documentation of receipt of live vaccine or physician-documented measles (25,121) p363 1989	CDC: MF 18+ if medical personnel or student born after 1956 and lacking evidence of two live measles vaccinations, physician-diagnosed measles disease, or laboratory evidence of measles immunity (122) 1989
Pneumococcal Polysaccharide 23-Valent Vaccine		
General	[B] MF 65+ once; consider revaccination after 6 years	Frame: recommendation against CDC: MF 65+ once
Selective	MF 18+ once if one or more: chronic cardiac or pulmonary disease, sickle cell disease, the nephrotic syndrome, Hodgkin disease, asplenia, diabetes, alcoholism, cirrhosis, multiple myeloma, renal disease, immunosuppression, HIV infection (25,118) p363 1989	Frame: MF 18+ once if sickle cell disease or asplenia (10) 1986 CDC: MF 18+ once; consider revaccination after 6 years if one or more: chronic illness such as cardiopulmonary disease, DM, alcoholism, cirrhosis, CSF leak; immunosuppression, such as splenic dysfunction, hematologic malignancy, renal failure, organ transplantation; HIV infection (123) 1989

See end of table for footnotes.

Table 4. *Adult Immunizations and Chemoprophylaxis**

Vaccine or Drug	ACP	CTF
Rubella Live Virus Vaccine		
General	Recommendation against	Recommendation against
Selective	MF 18+ once if lacking documentation of receipt of live vaccine on or after first birthday, particularly women of childbearing age and young adults studying or working in educational, health care, or military institutions (117) 1990	[A] F 18-44 once if lacking proof of immunity and agreeing not to become pregnant for 3 months (7) 1979
Tetanus-Diphtheria Toxoid		
General	MF 18+ every 10 y	[A] MF 18+ every 10 y
Selective	No recommendation (117) 1990	No recommendation (7) 1979
Chemoprophylaxis with Aspirin Therapy		
General	Not considered‡	Not considered§
Selective		

Table 4. *(Continued)*

Vaccine or Drug	USPSTF	Others
Rubella Live Virus Vaccine		
General	Recommendation against	
Selective	[A] F 18 to menopause once if lacking proof of vaccination or serologic evidence of immunity and agreeing not to become pregnant for 3 months (25) p215 1989	Frame: F 18+ once if non-pregnant and have had lack of immunity determined (10) 1986 CDC: MF 18+ once if nonpregnant and lacking adequate documentation of immunity, serologic laboratory evidence, or record of immunization on or after first birthday (124) 1990
Tetanus-Diphtheria Toxoid		
General	[A] MF 18+ every 10 y	Frame: MF 18+ every 10 y (10) 1986
Selective	No recommendation (25,118) p363 1989	
Chemoprophylaxis with Aspirin Therapy		
General	No recommendation	
Selective	M 40+ if risk factors for myocardial infarction such as high cholesterol, smoking, diabetes, family history of early onset of CAD, and no history of GI or other bleeding problems, other risks for bleeding, or cerebrovascular hemorrhage (25) p381 1989	

See end of table for footnotes.

Table 4. *Adult Immunizations and Chemoprophylaxis (Continued)*

Vaccine or Drug	ACP	CTF
Chemoprophylaxis with Estrogen Therapy		
General	Not considered‖	Recommendation against
Selective		[C] F 40+ consider if white race, perimenopausal, surgical or early menopause, low body weight for height, smoking, medication, alcohol use, inadequate dietary calcium (19) 1988

---

* "General" immunization or chemoprophylaxis refers to vaccination of asymptomatic persons who have no risk factors associated with the target condition. "Selective" immunization or chemoprophylaxis refers to vaccination of asymptomatic persons who are at increased risk for the target condition. Risk factors are listed in columns for each authority. ACP = American College of Physicians Task Force on Adult Immunization; CTF = Canadian Task Force on the Periodic Health Examination; and USPSTF = U.S. Preventive Services Task Force. Other sources of preventive care guidelines are indicated by first author or a common abbreviation. HIV = human immunodeficiency virus; HBV = hepatitis B virus; and CSF = cerebrospinal fluid; IV = intravenous; STD = sexually transmitted disease; DM = diabetes mellitus; CAD = coronary artery disease; GI = gastrointestinal. "Recommendation against" indicates that a recommendation was made to exclude the immunization from periodic preventive care for the age, sex, and risk status indicated. "No recommendation" indicates that an authority considered the intervention but refrained from making a specific recommendation either for or against it. "Not considered" indicates that a health organization has not published a practice guideline about the immunization. Square brackets enclose a one-letter "strength-of-recommendation" code, if available, as described in Table 1. Indicated next are the gender (M, male; F, female; MF, both sexes), the age range to which the recommendation applies, and the frequency with which immunization should be provided (in years), if specified by the health organization. For selective screening strategies, risk factors are listed. Citations to original papers describing the practice guideline are given in parentheses. The year that the most recent practice guideline was issued from the relevant authority is shown last together with a page number for the relevant manuscript chapter, if available. For a preventive action to be recommended, the listed requirements for age, sex, and risk factors must be met. Recommendations pertain to nonpregnant adults 18 years of age and older. Neither immunizations that may be appropriate for adults planning to travel nor postexposure prophylaxis are considered.

Table 4. *(Continued)*

Vaccine or Drug	USPSTF	Others
Chemoprophylaxis with Estrogen Therapy		
General	Recommendation against	
Selective	F 40+ at menopause; consider if perimenopausal and at risk because of white or Asian race, bilateral oophorectomy before menopause, early menopause, slender build and no abnormal vaginal bleeding, active liver disease, thromboembolic disorders, hormone-dependent cancer (25,109) p375 1989	Frame: F 40+ assess risk for osteoporosis at menopause and individualize therapy with estrogen and calcium (12) 1986

† Most authorities advise using a combined mumps, measles, and rubella vaccine.
‡ The ACP is expected to issue recommendations on aspirin therapy in 1991.
§ The CTF is expected to issue recommendations on aspirin therapy in 1991.
‖ The ACP is expected to issue recommendations on estrogen replacement therapy in perimenopausal women in 1991.

Table 5. *Healthy Lifestyles and Preventive Counseling**

Topic	CTF
Dietary Assessment and Nutritional Counseling	
Caloric balance	Not considered
Fat, cholesterol	Not considered
Fiber	Not considered
Sodium	Not considered
Calcium	[C] F 18+ maintain liberal intake of natural and supplemental calcium (19) 1987
Iron	[C] F 18-44 selective counseling for women of low socioeconomic status, food faddists (7) 1979

Table 5. *(Continued)*

USPSTF	ACP and Other
MF 18+ provide diet and exercise advice to all persons to achieve and maintain desirable weight by keeping caloric intake balanced with energy expenditures	ACP: MF 18+ provide guidelines for a healthful, well-balanced diet and encourage behavior modification to reduce and prevent obesity (125) 1985 NAS: MF 18+ advise to balance food intake and physical activity to maintain appropriate body weight (126) 1989
MF 18+ give dietary guidance on how to reduce total fat intake to less than 30% of total calories, saturated fat consumption to less than 10% of total calories, and dietary cholesterol to less than 300 mg/d [B] MF 18-59 advise to adopt low-fat diet for CAD prevention [C] MF 60+ advise to adopt low-fat diet for CAD prevention [A] MF 18+ repeated dietary change messages from multiple sources to effect decrease in fat content of diet	NAS: MF 18+ advise to reduce total fat intake to 30% or less of calories, saturated fatty acid intake to less than 10% of calories, and cholesterol intake to less than 300 mg/d (126) 1989 ACS: MF 18+ advise to reduce intake of calories from fat to 25% to 30% or less of total calorie intake (127) 1990
MF 18+ encourage patients to eat a variety of foods with emphasis on whole grain products, cereals, vegetables, and fruits	NAS: MF 18+ advise to eat five or more servings of vegetables and fruits daily and increase intake of complex carbohydrates (126) 1989 ACS: MF 18+ advise to eat more high-fiber foods such as whole grain cereals, legumes, vegetables, and fruits (127) 1990
MF 18+ advise patients to eat foods low in sodium and to limit salt added to food in preparation or consumption	NAS: MF 18+ advise to limit total intake of salt to 6 g/d or less by avoiding salty foods and limiting salt added to foods (126) 1989 ACS: MF 18+ advise to limit consumption of salt-cured, smoked, and nitrite-preserved foods (127) 1990
F 18+ counsel about methods to ensure adequate calcium intake	NAS: MF 18+ advise maintaining adequate calcium intake (126) 1989
F 18-64 all menstruating women, counsel about adequate iron intake (25,128) p305 1989	

See end of table for footnotes.

Table 5. *Healthy Lifestyles and Preventive Counseling (Continued)*

Topic	CTF
Physical Activity and Exercise	
Physical activity	[C] F 40+ teach effect of immobility on bone mass (19) 1987
Cancer Surveillance	
Skin self-examination	Not considered
Breast self-examination	[C] F 18-40 no recommendation (20) 1986
Testes self-examination	[C] No recommendation (7) 1979

Table 5. *(Continued)*

USPSTF	ACP and Other
[C] MF 18+ advise about seat belt use, alcohol- or drug-related risks with driving, general road safety, motorcycle helmet use (25) p318 1989	Frame: MF 18+ encourage use of seat belts (12) 1986 ACP: MF 18+ counsel patients to use seat belts (137) 1984
MF 18-64 teach injury prevention if one or more: previous back injury, high-risk body configuration, current or planned high-risk activities (25,138) p245 1989	Oboler and LaForce: MF 18+ if high-risk occupation: nursing, manual labor, driving (43) 1989
MF 18+ teach domestic safety to elderly adults and persons with elderly adults in the home (25) p326 1989	
MF 18+ encourage smoke detector installation and maintenance and discuss danger of smoking near bed or upholstery (25) p326 1989	
M 19-39 teach dangers of hand weapons, violent behavior; keep firearms in child-resistant containers (25,139) p321 1989	
[A] MF 18+ every 1 y (plaque) [C] MF 18+ every 1 y (caries), encourage regular tooth brushing, flossing, dental visits (25,92,140) p351 1989	Oboler and LaForce: MF 20+ every 1 y, teach about dental hygiene and importance of regular dental visits (43) 1989

See end of table for footnotes.

Table 5. *Healthy Lifestyles and Preventive Counseling (Continued)*

Topic	CTF
Stress and Bereavement	
Functional assessment	[C] MF 18-64 elicit history of marital and sexual problems
	[C] MF 46-64 preretirement counseling
	[B] MF 65+ every 1-2 y, assess physical, social, and psychologic function (7) 1979

* CTF = Canadian Task Force on the Periodic Health Examination; USPSTF = U.S. Preventive Services Task Force; ACP = American College of Physicians. Other sources of preventive care guidelines are indicated by first author or a common abbreviation. "Not considered" indicates that a health organization has not published a practice guideline about the particular form of counseling. "No recommendation" indicates that an authority considered the intervention but refrained from making a specific recommendation either for or against it. Square brackets enclose a one-letter "strength-of-recommendation" code, if available, as described in Table 1. Indicated next are the gender (M, male; F, female; MF, both sexes) and the age range to which the recommendation applies and the frequency with which the test should be done (in years), if specified by the health organization. The intervention is described, citations to original papers describing the practice guideline are given in parentheses, and the year that the most recent practice guideline was issued from the relevant authority is shown last.

† Although there is insufficient evidence to recommend for or against teaching testes self-examination, all young men should be advised to report testicular pain, swelling, or heaviness.

tables. Square brackets enclose a one-letter "strength-of-recommendation" code, as described in Table 1, if the strength was assessed by the issuer of the recommendation. Although ACP background papers describe the quality of the evidence supporting its recommendations, the ACP did not use any formal scheme for classifying the strength of its recommendations. Consequently, strength-of-recommendation codes are shown only for USPSTF and CTF guidelines.

The strength-of-recommendation code is followed by a letter indicating the gender (M = male; F = female; MF = both sexes) and the age range to which the recommendation applies and the frequency with which the intervention should be done, if specified by the issuer of the recommendation. Next, for selective preventive strategies, a series of risk factors that must be present for the intervention to be recommended are listed. Citations to original papers describing practice

Table 5. *(Continued)*

USPSTF	ACP and Other
MF 18+ remain alert for symptoms of abnormal bereavement, depression, physical abuse, and suicide risk in persons with recent bereavement, divorce, separation, unemployment, alcohol or other substance abuse, depression, living alone, serious medical illness (25,141) p257 1989	ACP: MF elderly, functional assessment screening including measures of emotional status and domestic adaptation (88) 1988

guidelines follow, and page numbers from the USPSTF report are provided (25, 26). The year that each practice guideline was most recently issued or updated by each authority appears last.

Several facts should be kept in mind when considering the recommendations we have summarized. First, only those interventions that were reviewed by one or more of the ACP, CTF, or USPSTF are included in the tables. Second, we have tried to present the exact wording with which each guideline was issued. Consequently, vague or incomplete entries in the tables likely reflect imprecision or incompleteness in the source documents themselves. Third, the ACP, CTF, and USPSTF anticipate further review and revision of their guidelines; these tables include the most recent updates, some of which currently are "in press." Fourth, we compare only guidelines applying to nonpregnant adults who are 18 years of age or older. The CTF advocates a lifelong prevention program based on age-specific health protection packages, four of which apply to adults (ages 16 to 44, 45 to 64, 65 to 74, and 75 years or older). The USPSTF also summarizes its recommendations in age-specific charts, three of which apply to adults (ages 19 to 39, 40 to 64, and 65 years or older). Finally, all preventive care recommendations listed in our tables pertain to "case finding" among all persons similar to North Americans who are not hospitalized or otherwise acutely ill and who present to a physician's office (62).

Interpreting Preventive Care Guidelines

The Institute of Medicine has identified eight attributes of good practice guidelines (63). These attributes include "clinical applicability"—guidelines should explicitly state the populations to which they apply; "clinical flexibility"—guidelines should identify the specifically known or generally expected exceptions to their recommendations; and "clarity"—guidelines should use unambiguous language, define terms precisely, and use logical, easy-to-follow modes of presentation. When we transformed the recommendations of various authorities into a table with specific entries for the age, sex, and health characteristics of the target population, the type of preventive intervention, and the frequency with which it should be applied, we were, in effect, testing for the presence of these three attributes of good guidelines.

For most preventive interventions listed in Tables 2 through 5, the age at which to begin and to stop providing the intervention and the frequency with which the intervention should be used for persons with different personal and family characteristics are clearly and specifically stated by the authorities recommending them. However, the strict demands of our tables expose deficiencies in some recommendations.

Descriptions of high-risk characteristics, for example, vary considerably. Some guidelines specify particular risks for preventable diseases, whereas others refer only to "high-risk patients." In other instances, risk factors are delineated clearly, but because of deficiencies in available empiric data, the practical implication of the presence of particular risk factors is unclear. For example, the USPSTF advises physicians to consider testing bone mineral content in women who are at increased risk for osteoporosis-related fractures and for whom long-term estrogen therapy is being considered (25). Risk factors for osteoporosis listed by the USPSTF include Caucasian race, bilateral oophorectomy before menopause, menopause, and slender build. The USPSTF guidelines, however, do not specify whether the presence of one of these conditions alone confers sufficient risk or whether some combination would be necessary to justify testing bone mineral content. For example, do all Caucasian women or all women at menopause merit a selective approach to bone mineral content testing? Similarly, the ACP advises against offering electrocardiograms to asymptomatic adults, but acknowledges that this advice may not be valid for smokers; men of "increased age"; persons with "a family history of coronary artery disease"; persons with hypertension, diabetes, or other cardiovascular risk factors; sedentary persons who plan to begin a vigorous exercise program; and persons whose occupation affects public safety (32, 33, 46, 47). Without evidence for guidance, the ACP has refrained from formulating a recommendation about these higher-risk persons, who, in total, likely account for a majority of internists' patients.

Overall, the guidelines issued by the ACP, CTF, and USPSTF are consistent with each other, and this consistency further strengthens them. This agreement is strongest for "general intervention" guidelines, in which inconsistencies are particularly infrequent and relate to the gender and age range for which an intervention is recommended (for example, cholesterol screening), the frequency with which tests should be done (for example, cervical cytology), and the grading of the recommendations' strength (for example, pneumococcal immunization) rather than to whether an intervention should ever be used as part of preventive care.

The various authorities more often differ in their specification of high-risk groups for selective interventions. For example, the ACP advises using colonoscopy or air-contrast barium enema instead of sigmoidoscopy for persons who are 40 years of age or older if a first-degree relative has had colon cancer (51). The CTF suggests colonoscopy for persons who are 40 years of age or older if two or more first-degree relatives have had colorectal cancer (16). The USPSTF recommends colonoscopic surveillance of persons who are 40 years of age or older if two or more first-degree relatives have developed colorectal cancer before 40 years of age (25, 64). Because considerably fewer persons have two or more first-degree relatives than have one first-degree relative with early colorectal cancer, the differences between these recommendations can substantially affect the number of colonoscopies proposed by primary care physicians.

Explaining Differences in Preventive Care Guidelines

How can differences among recommendations from different authorities be explained? Eddy (65) advises a search for three main sources of disagreement among practice policies: different targets, different objectives, and different rationales. Possible "targets" for preventive guidelines include particular health conditions, patient or provider populations, and specific preventive interventions. All of these factors are consistent for the major groups we have compared. Explanations for differences in the preventive practice guidelines that we have considered thus should be sought in differences among the authorities' objectives and the rationales they offer for endorsing an intervention or for recommending against the use of an intervention. Rationales are based on which evidence is considered, which methods are used to evaluate that evidence, and what values are assigned to the clinical outcomes associated with alternative practices.

In some instances, the authorities vary in their recommendations because they examined similar issues at different times and, thus, with different evidence available. In other cases, differences among sets of preventive practice recommendations derive from differences in the methods used to generate the recommendations. For example, various authorities have assigned differing levels of importance to the type and quality of reported studies and to the value of expert opinion. Subspecialty societies, for example, have tended to assign considerable importance to expert opinion, whereas the CTF has based its recommendations more strictly on the results of randomized controlled trials. When the results of randomized controlled trials are available, recommendations seldom differ. In many areas of inquiry, however, high-quality clinical trials have not been conducted, and committees must make recommendations with less than optimal data (66). A difference in willingness to rely on expert opinion in the face of such uncertainty may have led the ACS to recommend skin, testicular, ovarian, endometrial, and prostate cancer detection strategies that are more intensive than those advised by the CTF or USPSTF (13, 19, 25).

Another cause of variation in guidelines for preventive care derives from the differing value authorities place on potential outcomes, positive or negative, of preventive care interventions. For example, to maximize the detection of breast cancer at a stage when treatment is most effective, the ACS emphasizes the importance of teaching self-examination of the breasts. The CTF and USPSTF, in contrast, do not promote such programs because of a lack of rigorous evidence of effectiveness and because of concern about the high rate of false-positive results that may ensue among young women and the related anxiety and harm that could result from subsequent interventions done to evaluate lumps detected on self-examination (13, 20, 67).

Other differences in recommendations reflect differential consideration of the economic costs of different prevention strategies. Whereas the CTF and the USPSTF viewed these costs in general terms, the ACP used explicit cost-effectiveness models that considered the economic effect of different assumptions about the prevalence of target conditions, the cost of diagnosis and treatment, and the unintended costs associated with misdiagnosis and misadventure. Because they reflect an explicit consideration of costs, the ACP recommendations about Papanicolaou smears, mammography, and colonoscopy reflect value judgments about the trade-off between the increased number of cases of cancer that would be detected by more intensive surveillance and the increased economic cost that would be associated with such strategies. Although explicitly considering what levels of cost would be acceptable to achieve particular levels or types of clinical benefit is extremely difficult, doing so might increase consistency in how economic costs are considered across different sets of ACP recommendations as well as across recommendations made by other authorities.

Implementation of Selective Strategies for Preventive Care

Many physicians find implementing even the most rudimentary preventive services difficult. For example, ample data suggest that many physicians do not follow even relatively simple preventive guidelines based on consideration of patient age and sex (68-74), perhaps because the typical medical setting presents several barriers to the incorporation of activities that prevent disease and promote health: lack of reimbursement, time, and dedicated counselors; patient noncompliance; a lack of short-term benefit from preventive interventions; and a discordance between the anticipatory thinking required for effective preventive care and the more traditional focus on patients' immediate complaints. Moreover, preventive care is underemphasized in continuing medical education, and many physicians are skeptical of the quality of medical evidence underlying preventive care recommendations or frustrated by perceived inconsistency among recommendations from different professional groups (75, 76). Our analysis suggests that a high degree of consistency has been achieved in many preventive practice recommendations made by three independent authorities.

The time and effort required to incorporate into routine care the increased knowledge base and clinical data needed to individualize prevention are additional barriers to implementing selective preventive care. It is no small task to obtain and evaluate a medical history that is adequate for generating risk profiles and determining priorities for screening, counseling, and prophylaxis. Moreover, even when such clinical information is available, the clinician must synthesize it in light of contemporary preventive guidelines. Our tables are intended to make the latter task easier.

Despite these difficulties, opportunities to practice prevention in internal medicine have never been greater. Abundant evidence documents that the majority of deaths among North American adults younger than 65 years of age are preventable, many through interventions best offered in a clinician's office. Recent reductions in the incidence of cardiovascular disease suggest that prevention can be successful. The knowledge base and available recommendations for prevention have improved dramatically, the public's knowledge of and attitudes toward prevention have never been more favorable, and there is reason to believe that reasonable reimbursement for preventive services will be increasingly available.

We believe that physicians would be aided further by new tools to facilitate the assessment and documentation of health risks and the tailoring of preventive programs to individual patients. One approach for coping with the quantity and complexity of the information in contemporary guidelines is to use special flow sheets, automated systems, or dedicated personnel to remind physicians of when to use key preventive actions (77). To date, many such prompting systems have been studied and found useful. However, most of these systems have been restricted to general screening prompts because of a lack of convenient methods for recording and analyzing individual patients' health risks (78-81). Our tables are intended to facilitate the development of new computer software that can generate more selective reminders to physicians as well as to clarify areas of both agreement and disagreement in guidelines for selective screening. In some areas in which guidelines for selective screening are inconsistent, additional research on the effectiveness of selective preventive strategies is needed.

References

1. **American College of Physicians.** Periodic health examination: a guide for designing individualized preventive health care in the asymptomatic patients. Medical Practice Committee, American College of Physicians. Ann Intern Med. 1981;95:729-32.
2. **Frame PS, Carlson SJ.** A critical review of periodic health screening using specific screening criteria. Part 1: Selected diseases of respiratory, cardiovascular, and central nervous systems. J Fam Pract. 1975;2:29-36.
3. **Frame PS, Carlson SJ.** A critical review of periodic health screening using specific screening criteria. Part 2: Selected endocrine, metabolic, and gastrointestinal diseases. J Fam Pract. 1975;2:123-9.
4. **Frame PS, Carlson SJ.** A critical review of periodic health screening using specific screening criteria. Part 3: Selected diseases of the genitourinary system. J Fam Pract. 1975;2:189-94.
5. **Frame PS, Carlson SJ.** A critical review of periodic health screening using specific screening criteria. Part 4: Selected miscellaneous diseases. J Fam Pract. 1975;2:283-9.
6. **Breslow L, Somers AR.** The lifetime health-monitoring program. A practical approach to preventive medicine. N Engl J Med. 1977; 296:601-8.
7. **Canadian Task Force on the Periodic Health Examination.** The periodic health examination. Can Med Assoc J. 1979;121:1193-254.
8. **Eddy D.** ACS report on the cancer-related health checkup. CA. 1980;30:194-240.
9. **Frame PS.** A critical review of adult health maintenance. Part 1: Prevention of atherosclerotic diseases. J Fam Pract. 1986;22:341-6.
10. **Frame PS.** A critical review of adult health maintenance. Part 2: Prevention of infectious diseases. J Fam Pract. 1986;22:417-22.
11. **Frame PS.** A critical review of adult health maintenance. Part 3: Prevention of cancer. J Fam Pract. 1986;22:511-20.
12. **Frame PS.** A critical review of adult health maintenance: Part 4. Prevention of metabolic, behavioral, and miscellaneous conditions. J Fam Pract. 1986;23:29-39.
13. **American Cancer Society.** *Summary of Current Guidelines for the Cancer-Related Checkup: Recommendations.* Atlanta, Georgia: American Cancer Society; 1988.
14. **Canadian Task Force on the Periodic Health Examination.** Periodic health examination, 1990 update: 1. Early detection of hyperthyroidism and hypothyroidism in adults and screening of newborns for congenital hypothyroidism. Can Med Assoc J. 1990;142:955-61.
15. **Canadian Task Force on the Periodic Health Examination.** Periodic health examination, 1990 update: 2. Early detection of depression and prevention of suicide. Can Med Assoc J. 1990;142:1233-8.
16. **Canadian Task Force on the Periodic Health Examination.** The periodic health examination: 2. 1989 update. Can Med Assoc J. 1989;141:209-16.
17. **Canadian Task Force on the Periodic Health Examination.** Periodic health examination, 1989 update: 3. Preschool examination for developmental, visual and hearing problems. Can Med Assoc J. 1989;141:1136-40.
18. **Canadian Task Force on the Periodic Health Examination.** Periodic health examination, 1989 update: 4. Intrapartum electronic fetal monitoring and prevention of neonatal herpes simplex. Can Med Assoc J. 1989;141:1233-40.
19. **Canadian Task Force on the Periodic Health Examination.** The periodic health examination: 2. 1987 update. Can Med Assoc J. 1988;138:618-26.
20. **Canadian Task Force on the Periodic Health Examination.** The periodic health examination: 2. 1985 update. Can Med Assoc J. 1986;134:724-7.
21. **Canadian Task Force on the Periodic Health Examination.** The periodic health examination: 2. 1984 update. Can Med Assoc J. 1984;130:1278-85.

22. **Canadian Task Force on the Periodic Health Examination.** Periodic health examination, 1990 update: 3. Interventions to prevent lung cancer other than smoking cessation. Can Med Assoc J. 1990;143: 269-72.

23. **Canadian Task Force on the Periodic Health Examination.** Periodic health examination, 1991 update: 1. Screening for cognitive impairment in the elderly. Can Med Assoc J. 1991;144:425-31.

24. **Canadian Task Force on the Periodic Health Examination.** Periodic health examination. 1991 update. Lowering blood cholesterol to prevent coronary heart disease. Can Med Assoc J. 1991 [In press].

25. **U.S. Preventive Services Task Force.** Guide to Clinical Preventive Services: An Assessment of the Effectiveness of 169 Interventions. Baltimore: Williams and Wilkins; 1989.

26. **Eddy DM.** Common Screening Tests. Philadelphia: American College of Physicians; 1991.

27. **Commission on Chronic Illness.** Chronic Illness in the United States. Cambridge, Massachusetts: Harvard University Press; 1957.

28. **McGinnis JM, Woolf SH.** Background and objectives of the U.S. Preventive Services Task Force. J Gen Intern Med. 1990;5(Suppl): S11-3.

29. **Clinical Efficacy Project, American College of Physicians.** Clinical Efficacy Reports. Philadelphia: American College of Physicians; 1987.

30. **American College of Physicians.** Clinical Efficacy Assessment Project: Procedural Manual. Philadelphia: American College of Physicians; 1986.

31. **Steinberg EP.** Technology assessment—a physicians' perspective. In: Lohr KN, Rettig RA, eds. Quality of Care and Technology Assessment. Washington, DC: National Academy Press; 1988:79-88.

32. **Sox HC Jr, Garber AM, Littenberg B.** The resting electrocardiogram as a screening test. A clinical analysis. Ann Intern Med. 1989;111:489-502.

33. **Sox HC Jr, Littenberg B, Garber AM.** The role of exercise testing in screening for coronary artery disease. Ann Intern Med. 1989; 110:456-69.

34. **Garber AM, Sox HC Jr, Littenberg B.** Screening asymptomatic adults for cardiac risk factors: the serum cholesterol level. Ann Intern Med. 1989;110:622-39.

35. **Littenberg B, Garber AM, Sox HC Jr.** Screening for hypertension. Ann Intern Med. 1990;112:192-202.

36. **Eddy DM.** Screening for colorectal cancer. Ann Intern Med. 1990; 113:373-84.

37. **Eddy DM.** Screening for lung cancer. Ann Intern Med. 1989;111: 232-7.

38. **Eddy DM.** Screening for breast cancer. Ann Intern Med. 1989;111: 389-99.

39. **Eddy DM.** Screening for cervical cancer. Ann Intern Med. 1990; 113:214-26.

40. **Melton LJ III, Eddy DM, Johnston CC Jr.** Screening for osteoporosis. Ann Intern Med. 1990;112:516-28.

41. **Singer DE, Samet JH, Coley CM, Nathan DM.** Screening for diabetes mellitus. Ann Intern Med. 1988;109:639-49.

42. **Helfand M, Crapo LM.** Screening for thyroid disease. Ann Intern Med. 1990;112:840-9.

43. **Oboler SK, LaForce FM.** The periodic physical examination in asymptomatic adults. Ann Intern Med. 1989;110:214-26.

44. **American College of Physicians.** Screening for hypertension. In: Eddy DM, ed. Common Screening Tests. Philadelphia: American College of Physicians; 1991.

45. **American College of Physicians.** Screening low risk, asymptomatic adults for cardiac risk factors: serum cholesterol and triglycerides. In: Eddy DM, ed. Common Screening Tests. Philadelphia: American College of Physicians; 1991.

46. **American College of Physicians.** Screening for asymptomatic coronary artery disease: the resting electrocardiogram. In: Eddy DM, ed. Common Screening Tests. Philadelphia: American College of Physicians; 1991.
47. **American College of Physicians.** Screening for asymptomatic coronary artery disease: exercise stress testing. In: Eddy DM, ed. Common Screening Tests. Philadelphia: American College of Physicians; 1991.
48. **American College of Physicians.** Screening for cervical cancer. In: Eddy DM, ed. Common Screening Tests. Philadelphia: American College of Physicians; 1991.
49. **American College of Physicians.** Screening for breast cancer. In: Eddy DM, ed. Common Screening Tests. Philadelphia: American College of Physicians; 1991.
50. **American College of Physicians.** Screening for lung cancer. In: Eddy DM, ed. Common Screening Tests. Philadelphia: American College of Physicians; 1991.
51. **American College of Physicians.** Screening for colorectal cancer. In: Eddy DM, ed. Common Screening Tests. Philadelphia: American College of Physicians; 1991.
52. **American College of Physicians.** Screening for diabetes mellitus in apparently healthy, asymptomatic adults. In: Eddy DM, ed. Common Screening Tests. Philadelphia: American College of Physicians; 1991.
53. **American College of Physicians.** Screening for osteoporosis in perimenopausal women. In: Eddy DM, ed. Common Screening Tests. Philadelphia: American College of Physicians; 1991.
54. **American College of Physicians.** Screening for thyroid disease. In: Eddy DM, ed. Common Screening Tests. Philadelphia: American College of Physicians; 1991.
55. **National Cholesterol Education Program.** Report of the Expert Panel on Detection, Evaluation, and Treatment of High Blood Cholesterol in Adults. Washington, DC: U.S. Dept. of Health and Human Services; 1988.
56. **Woolf SH.** Practice guidelines: a new reality in medicine. I. Recent developments. Arch Intern Med. 1990;150:1811-8.
57. **American Geriatrics Society.** Screening for cervical carcinoma in elderly women. J Am Geriatr Soc. 1989;37:885-7.
58. **American Academy of Family Physicians.** Positions on the Clinical Aspects of Medical Practice. Kansas City, Missouri: American Academy of Family Physicians; 1991.
59. **Eddy DM.** How to think about screening. In: Eddy DM, ed. Common Screening Tests. Philadelphia: American College of Physicians; 1991.
60. **Feussner JR, Matchar DB.** When and how to study the carotid arteries. Ann Intern Med. 1988;109:805-18.
61. **Health and Public Policy Committee, American College of Physicians.** Diagnostic evaluation of the carotid arteries. Ann Intern Med. 1988;109:835-7.
62. **Sackett DL, Haynes RB, Tugwell P.** Clinical Epidemiology: a Basic Science for Clinical Medicine. Boston: Little, Brown and Co.; 1985.
63. **Field MJ, Lohr KN, eds.** Clinical Practice guidelines: Directions for a New Program. Washington, DC: National Academy Press; 1990.
64. **Selby JV, Friedman GD.** US Preventive Services Task Force. Sigmoidoscopy in the periodic health examination of asymptomatic adults. JAMA. 1989;261:594-601.
65. **Eddy DM.** Clinical decision making: from theory to practice. Resolving conflicts in practice policies. JAMA. 1990;264:389-91.
66. **Lederle FA.** Screening for snipers: the burden of proof. J Clin Epidemiol. 1990;43:101-4.
67. **O'Malley MS, Fletcher SW.** US Preventive Services Task Force. Screening for breast cancer with breast self-examination. A critical review. JAMA. 1987;257:2196-203.

68. **Lurie N, Manning WG, Peterson C, Goldberg GA, Phelps CA, Lillard L.** Preventive care: do we practice what we preach? Am J Public Health. 1987;77:801-4.

69. **Gemson DH, Elinson J.** Prevention in primary care: variability in physician practice patterns in New York City. Am J Prev Med. 1986;2:226-34.

70. **Romm FJ, Fletcher SW, Hulka BS.** The periodic health examination: comparison of recommendations and internists' performance. South Med J. 1981;74:265-71.

71. **Woo B, Woo B, Cook EF, Weisberg MC, Goldman L.** Screening procedures in the asymptomatic adult: comparison of physicians' recommendations, patients' desires, published guidelines, and actual practice. JAMA. 1985;254:1480-4.

72. **Schoenbaum SC.** Implementation of preventive services in an HMO practice. J Gen Intern Med. 1990;5(5 Suppl):S123-7.

73. **Lewis CE.** Disease prevention and health promotion practices of primary care physicians in the United States. Am J Prev Med. 1988;4(4 Suppl):S9-16.

74. **Fleming DM, Lawrence MS.** An evaluation of recorded information about preventive measures in 38 practices. J R Coll Gen Pract. 1981;31:615-20.

75. **Becker MH, Janz NK.** Practicing health promotion: the doctor's dilemma. Ann Intern Med. 1990;113:419-22.

76. **Schwartz JS, Lewis CE, Clancy C, Kinosian MS, Radany MH, Koplan JP.** Internists' practices in health promotion and disease prevention: a survey. Ann Intern Med. 1991;114:46-53.

77. **Davidson RA, Fletcher SW, Retchin S, Duh S.** A nurse-initiated reminder system for the periodic health examination: implementation and evaluation. Arch Intern Med. 1984;144:2167-70.

78. **Harris RP, O'Malley MS, Fletcher SW, Knight BP.** Prompting physicians for preventive procedures: a five-year study of manual and computer reminders. Am J Prev Med. 1990;6:145-52.

79. **Haynes RB, Walker CJ.** Computer-aided quality assurance. A critical appraisal. Arch Intern Med. 1987;147:1297-301.

80. **Frame PS.** Can computerized reminder systems have an impact on preventive services in practice? J Gen Intern Med. 1990;5(5 Suppl):S112-5.

81. **McPhee SJ, Bird JA.** Implementation of cancer prevention guidelines in clinical practice. J Gen Intern Med. 1990;5(5 Suppl):S116-22.

82. **Lawrence RS, Mickalide AD.** Preventive services in clinical practice: designing the periodic health examination. JAMA. 1987;257:2205-7.

83. **Goldbloom R, Battista RN.** The periodic health examination: 1. Introduction. Can Med Assoc J. 1986;134:721-3.

84. **National Academy of Sciences Institute of Medicine.** Preventive Services for the Well Population. Washington, DC: National Academy of Sciences; 1978.

85. **Grundy SM, Greenland P, Herd A, et al.** Cardiovascular and risk factor evaluation of healthy American adults. A statement for physicians by an ad hoc committee appointed by the Steering Committee, American Heart Association. Circulation. 1987;75:1340A-62A.

86. **1988 Joint National Committee.** The 1988 report of the Joint National Committee on detection, evaluation, and treatment of high blood pressure. Arch Intern Med. 1988;148:1023-38.

87. Consensus Conference. Differential diagnosis of dementing diseases. JAMA. 1987;258:3411-6.

88. **Health and Public Policy Committee, American College of Physicians.** Comprehensive functional assessment for elderly patients. Ann Intern Med. 1988;109:70-2.

89. **Haynes MA.** Preventing suicide: the physician's role. In: Goldbloom RB, Lawrence RS, eds. Preventing Disease: Beyond the Rhetoric. New York: Springer-Verlag; 1990.

90. **American Academy of Ophthalmology.** Preferred Practice Pattern: Comprehensive Adult Eye Examination. San Francisco, California: American Academy of Ophthalmology; 1989.

91. **National Cancer Institute.** Working Guidelines for Early Cancer Detection: Rationale and Supporting Evidence to Decrease Mortality. Bethesda, Maryland: National Cancer Institute; 1987.

92. **Greene JC, Louie R, Wycoff SJ.** Preventive dentistry. II. Periodontal diseases, malocclusion, trauma, and oral cancer. JAMA. 1990;263:421-5.

93. **American College of Obstetricians and Gynecologists. Committee on Professional Standards.** Report of Task Force on Routine Cancer Screening. In: Standards for Obstetric-Gynecologic Services. 7th ed. Washington, DC: American College of Obstetricians and Gynecologists; 1989:97-104.

94. **American Geriatrics Society.** Screening for breast cancer in elderly women. J Am Geriatr Soc. 1989;37:883-4.

95. **Shapiro MF, Greenfield S.** The complete blood count and leukocyte differential count. An approach to their rational application. In: Sox HC Jr, ed. Common Diagnostic Tests: Use and Interpretation. 2d ed. Philadelphia: American College of Physicians; 1990: 183-203.

96. **Komaroff AL.** Urinalysis and urine culture in women with dysuria. In: Sox HC Jr, ed. Common Diagnostic Tests: Use and Interpretation. 2d ed. Philadelphia: American College of Physicians; 1990: 286-301.

97. **Woolhandler S, Pels RJ, Bor DH.** Screening asymptomatic adults for hematuria and proteinuria: dipstick urinalysis. In: Goldbloom RB, Lawrence RS, eds. Preventing Disease: Beyond the Rhetoric. New York: Springer-Verlag; 1990.

98. **Pels RJ, Bor DH, Woolhandler S.** Screening asymptomatic adults for bacteriuria. In: Goldbloom RB, Lawrence RS, eds. Preventing Disease: Beyond the Rhetoric. New York: Springer-Verlag; 1990.

99. **Singer DE, Samet JH, Coley CM.** Screening for diabetes mellitus. In: Goldbloom RB, Lawrence RS, eds. Preventing Disease: Beyond the Rhetoric. New York: Springer-Verlag; 1990.

100. **American Diabetes Association.** Screening for diabetes. Diabetes Care. 1989;12:588-90.

101. **Goldbloom R.** Periodic health examination, 1990 update: 1. Early detection of hyperthyroidism and hypothyroidism in adults and screening of newborns for congenital hypothyroidism [Letter]. Can Med Assoc J. 1990;143:259-60.

102. **Health and Public Policy Committee, American College of Physicians; and the Infectious Diseases Society of America.** The acquired immunodeficiency syndrome (AIDS) and infection with the human immunodeficiency virus (HIV). Ann Intern Med. 1988;108:460-9.

103. **Horsburgh CR Jr, Douglas JM, LaForce FM.** Preventive strategies in sexually transmitted diseases for the primary care physician. JAMA. 1987;258:814-21.

104. **Centers for Disease Control.** Public Health Service guidelines for counseling and antibody testing to prevent HIV infection and AIDS. MMWR. 1987;36:509-15.

105. **Hart G.** Syphilis tests in diagnostic and therapeutic decision making. In: Sox HC Jr, ed. Common Diagnostic Tests: Use and Interpretation. 2d ed. Philadelphia: American College of Physicians; 1990:302-26.

106. **American College of Sports Medicine.** Guidelines for Exercise Testing and Prescription. 3d ed. Philadelphia: Lea & Febiger; 1986.

107. **American College of Cardiology/American Heart Association Task Force on Assessment of Cardiovascular Procedures.** Guidelines for exercise testing. J Am Coll Cardiol. 1986;8:725-38.

108. **Advisory Committee for Elimination of Tuberculosis.** Screening for tuberculosis and tuberculous infection in high-risk populations. MMWR. 1990;39 RR 8:1-7.

109. **Mann K, Wiese WH, Stachenchko S.** Preventing postmenopausal osteoporosis and related fractures. In: Goldbloom RB, Lawrence RS, eds. Preventing Disease: Beyond the Rhetoric. New York: Springer-Verlag; 1990.

110. **Gordillo C.** Breast cancer screening guidelines agreed on by AMA, other medically related organizations. JAMA. 1989;262:1155.

111. **American Medical Association Council on Scientific Affairs.** Mammographic screening in asymptomatic women aged 40 years and older. JAMA. 1989;261:2535-42.

112. **American Medical Association.** Mammography Screening in Asymptomatic Women 40 Years and Older (Resolution 93 I-87). Report of the Council on Scientific Affairs, Report F (A-88). Chicago: American Medical Association; 1988.

113. **Fink DJ.** Change in American Cancer Society Checkup Guidelines for detection of cervical cancer. CA. 1988;38:127-8.

114. **Centers for Disease Control.** Chlamydia trachomatis infections: policy guidelines for prevention and control. MMWR. 1985;34(Suppl): 53S-74S.

115. **Knight KK, Fielding JE, Battista RN.** US Preventive Services Task Force. Occult blood screening for colorectal cancer. JAMA. 1989; 261:586-93.

116. **American Cancer Society.** Update of American Cancer Society guidelines for detection of colorectal cancer: sigmoidoscopy. CA. 1989;39:317.

117. **American College of Physicians Task Force on Adult Immunization.** Guide for Adult Immunization. 2d ed. Philadelphia: American College of Physicians; 1990.

118. **LaForce FM.** Immunizations, immunoprophylaxis, and chemoprophylaxis to prevent selected infections. JAMA. 1987;257:2464-70.

119. **Immunization Practices Advisory Committee.** Protection against viral hepatitis. MMWR. 1990;39 RR 2:1-26.

120. **Immunization Practices Advisory Committee.** Prevention and control of influenza. Recommendations of the Immunization Practices Advisory Committee (ACIP). MMWR. 1990;39 RR 7:1-15.

121. **Skinner HA, Allen BA, McIntosh MC, Palmer WH.** Lifestyle assessment: applying microcomputers in family practice. Br Med J [Clin Res]. 1985;290:212-4.

122. **Immunization Practices Advisory Committee.** Measles prevention. MMWR. 1989;38(Suppl 9):1-18.

123. **Immunization Practices Advisory Committee.** Pneumococcal polysaccharide vaccine. MMWR. 1989;38:64-8, 73-6.

124. **Immunization Practices Advisory Committee.** Rubella prevention. MMWR. 1990;39 RR 15:1-18.

125. **American College of Physicians.** Nutrition. Philadelphia: American College of Physicians; 1985.

126. **National Academy of Sciences.** National Academy of Sciences report on diet and health. Nutr Rev. 1989;47:142-9.

127. **American Cancer Society.** The American Cancer Society Guidelines on Nutrition and Cancer. Atlanta: American Cancer Society; 1990.

128. **Goldbloom RB, Lawrence RS, eds.** Preventing Disease: Beyond the Rhetoric. New York: Springer-Verlag; 1990:407.

129. **Harris SS, Caspersen CJ, DeFriese GH, Estes EH Jr.** Physical activity counseling for healthy adults as a primary preventive intervention in the clinical setting. Report for the US Preventive Services Task Force. JAMA. 1989;261:3588-98.

130. **World Health Organization.** Self-examination in the early detection of breast cancer: memorandum from a WHO meeting. Bull World Health Organ. 1984;62:861-9.

131. **American Cancer Society.** For Men Only—Testicular Cancer and How To Do Testicular Self-Examination. New York: American Cancer Society; 1984.

132. **National Cancer Institute.** Testicular Self-Examination. Washington, DC: Government Printing Office; 1986.

133. **Fielding JE, Williams CA.** Preventing unwanted teenage pregnancy in the United States. In: Goldbloom RB, Lawrence RS, eds. Preventing Disease: Beyond the Rhetoric. New York: Springer-Verlag; 1990.

134. **Health and Public Policy Committee, American College of Physicians.** Methods for stopping cigarette smoking. Ann Intern Med. 1986;105:281-91.

135. **American College of Physicians.** Chemical Dependence. Philadelphia: American College of Physicians; 1984.

136. **Kottke TE, Battista RN, DeFriese GH, Brekke ML.** Attributes of successful smoking cessation interventions in medical practice. A meta-analysis of 39 controlled trials. JAMA. 1988;259:2882-9.

137. **American College of Physicians.** Health Promotion/Disease Prevention: Seat Belt Use. Philadelphia: American College of Physicians; 1984.

138. **Gross G.** Preventing low back pain. In: Goldbloom RB, Lawrence RS, eds. Preventing Disease: Beyond the Rhetoric. New York: Springer-Verlag; 1990.

139. **Polen MR, Friedman GD.** Automobile injury—Selected risk factors and prevention in the health care setting. JAMA. 1988;259:76-80.

140. **Greene JC, Louie R, Wycoff SJ.** Preventive dentistry. I. Dental caries. JAMA. 1989;262:3459-63.

141. **Medalie JH.** Bereavement: health consequences and preventive strategies. In: Goldbloom RB, Lawrence RS, eds. Preventing Disease: Beyond the Rhetoric. New York: Springer-Verlag; 1990.

142. **Canadian Task Force on the Periodic Health Examination.** Periodic health examination, 1991 update: 2. Administration of pneumococcal vaccine. Can Med Assoc J. 1991;144:665-71.

APPENDIXES

Introduction to the Guidelines

DOUGLAS S. PETERS, SENIOR VICE PRESIDENT
BLUE CROSS AND BLUE SHIELD ASSOCIATION

This book is the latest product of a long-standing, successful collaboration between the American College of Physicians and the Blue Cross and Blue Shield Association's Medical Necessity Program. In 1987, the Blue Cross and Blue Shield Association (BCBSA) commissioned leading clinical researchers to analyze clinical evidence on the effectiveness of common screening tests in detecting disease in asymptomatic adults. The researchers were asked to consider the efficient use of health care resources in developing their recommendations on screening tests for subsets of the general population at clinically indicated frequencies. The recommendations are designed to maximize the cost-effectiveness of screening.

The American College of Physicians, through its Clinical Efficacy Assessment Project (CEAP) Subcommittee and through *Annals of Internal Medicine*, rigorously reviewed the commissioned papers as did the BCBSA Medical Advisory Panel. The revised papers were published in *Annals of Internal Medicine*. The summary recommendations at the end of this book were rigorously reviewed by the CEAP Subcommittee and ultimately approved by the College's Board of Regents.

The papers were commissioned by BCBSA to determine which common adult screening tests should be included in a model screening benefit. This represented a significant departure from traditional insurance practices, which had their origins in covering the unpredictable and potentially catastrophic costs of acute inpatient care. Historically, private insurers have not viewed routine, low-cost screening and preventive services as insurable risks. Moreover, group and individual purchasers of health insurance, until recently, expressed little demand for screening and preventive benefits.

This situation is changing, however. Efforts of the federal government and voluntary and professional societies to promote screening and preventive care are succeeding. Health-conscious employers and individuals are increasingly seeking benefits that cover wellness care as well as illness care. The role of screening in early disease detection, and in reducing mortality, morbidity, and health care costs associated with these diseases, is becoming more widely understood among purchasers of insurance.

Managed care plans such as health maintenance organizations (HMOs) and preferred provider organizations (PPOs) have been at the forefront in providing coverage for screening and preventive services. Offerings of traditional fee-for-service insurance coverage are now incorporating benefits for screening and prevention to meet account and subscriber demand. Broad coverage for screening and preventive services is now offered by many Blue Cross and Blue Shield HMOs and PPOs. Over half of the Blue Cross and Blue Shield Plans are also marketing benefits for periodic physical examinations, and 40% are offering benefits for disease-specific screening through traditional insurance products.

The guidelines in this book, and the BCBSA coverage recommendations based on the guidelines, will aid these plans and managed-care programs in determining which screening tests to cover, for which populations, and at what frequencies. Because the guidelines attest to the clinical efficacy and cost-effectiveness of the recommended screening tests, they may encourage all health insurers to offer wider coverage for screening. The recommendations will also be used by BCBSA plans in provider education.

We at the Association owe a large debt to David Eddy, MD, PhD, for his critical role in the evolution of this publication. His innovative methods for evaluating clinical evidence and comparing the benefits and harms of medical interventions have shaped the direction of the entire guideline development process. He has ably served as advisor to the BCBSA and editor of this book in addition to writing many of the papers. We also thank all the authors of the papers and the staff of the American College of Physicians.

Common Screening Tests is an important contribution to the evaluation and use of screening tests. We hope the guidelines and coverage recommendations will foster and support the trend of increasing third party coverage for efficacious screening tests. Working together, the medical community, insurers, and the federal government can make early disease detection a reality for the American people. The Blue Cross and Blue Shield Association is proud to be a part of this effort.

Screening for Hypertension

Disease

Classifications of primary hypertension, based on severity of disease, include: malignant and accelerated hypertension; and mild, moderate, and severe hypertension. Hypertension is common among Americans, and is among the most important causes of disease and disability in the population. A significant proportion of the hypertensive population are not under adequate treatment.

Risk factors for primary hypertension include race, family history, age and body weight.

Screening Test

Sphygmomanometry is the only screening test for hypertension.

Recommendations

1. Screening for hypertension is recommended. Normotensive persons should be screened for hypertension every 1 to 2 years if their blood pressure is below 140/85 mm Hg, or yearly if their diastolic pressure is between 85 and 89 mg Hg.
2. Patients with risk factors for hypertension should be tested at least annually. These risk factors include black race, history of hypertension in parents or siblings, previous hypertension, and moderate and extreme obesity.

Rationale

There is considerable evidence that the detection and treatment of hypertension before it becomes symptomatic reduces the risks of stroke, and renal and heart disease.

There currently are insufficient data to be certain of the most efficacious screening interval. The average adult visits a physician about five times per year. The inclusion of blood pressure recording within a visit for other purposes is a reasonable screening approach. Younger adults do not visit physicians at this average frequency. Therefore, clinicians should make particular efforts to take blood pressure recordings in young adults. Education programs should be aimed at these groups. The availability of community facilities for blood pressure assessment should be emphasized within educational programs.

Individuals at high risk for hypertension, including those with a family history of hypertension, diabetes, previous hypertension, known coronary artery disease or risk factors for cardiovascular disease, should be tested more frequently than those without risk factors.

Patients with diastolic blood pressure between 90 and 104 mm Hg should be checked with repeat measurements over the course of several weeks before a diagnosis of mild hypertension is made.

There are no risks directly associated with sphygmomanometry.

Screening for Asymptomatic Coronary Artery Disease: The Resting Electrocardiogram

Disease

The test most commonly used to screen for coronary artery disease is the resting electrocardiogram. Many physicians obtain a resting electrocardiogram when they do a complete health appraisal. The definition and frequency of occurrence of asymptomatic coronary artery disease has been introduced in the guideline on exercise stress testing.

The effect of early detection on the outcome of coronary artery disease is unknown. Also unknown is the prognosis of disease in asymptomatic persons. Although there is an epidemic of coronary artery disease, its annual incidence in men with no or average risk factors is low. For example, 996 of 1000 40-year-old men, and 982 of 1000 60-year-old men will not show clinical signs of disease.

Screening Tests

A test commonly used in persons suspected of having coronary artery disease is the resting electrocardiogram (ECG). An electrocardiogram is a recording of emitted cardiac electrical activity from the vantages of standardized limb and chest locations, corresponding to lead placements.

Recommendation

The resting ECG is not recommended as a routine practice in people who are under age 65 and do not have evidence for cardiovascular disease or its risk factors. However, it may be appropriate in selected patients, especially in situations where the published evidence is not decisive.

The rationale for using an ECG to screen for the presence of coronary artery disease is weak, especially if the person has already had a normal resting ECG. The evidence about the value of a baseline ECG in deciding about admission of a patient with chest pain is inconclusive. A baseline ECG may have value in a small proportion of patients and may be worthwhile in patients who because of advancing age may be especially likely to visit an emergency room because of chest pain.

There is too little information on the prognostic value of ECG findings in men over age 65 to know if this recommendation should apply to them. This recommendation probably applies to women. Although there is comparatively little information on the prognostic value of resting ECG findings in women, the prevalence of coronary artery disease is lower in women, and its overall prognosis is better than in men.

Rationale

Some ECG findings increase the probability that an apparently healthy person will die from coronary artery disease. However, these findings are uncommon, and the risk for death attributable to them is small. There is no evidence that early detection of such findings leads to a clinical intervention that improves health outcome.

Frequent ventricular premature beats appear to be a risk factor for death from coronary artery disease. However, there are no studies on the effect of anti-arrhythmic therapy on survival in people without clinical evidence of coronary heart disease. Effective anti-arrhythmic drugs have significant potential side effects, including death. Treatment of ventricular premature beats is not generally recommended in people without evidence of heart disease.

Bifascicular block (including left bundle branch block) occurs in apparently healthy persons but progresses to complete heart block relatively infrequently and almost always after warning symptoms (usually syncope). Preventive treatment of bifascicular block in healthy persons is not indicated.

Q-waves, T-wave inversion, and ST segment abnormalities are associated with increased mortality from coronary artery disease. The effect of bypass surgery on mortality from asymptomatic coronary artery disease is unknown. However, there is no good evidence that pharmacologic or surgical treatment of coronary artery disease prolongs life in asymptomatic persons.

Left axis deviation is a marker for coronary artery disease, but has no management implications in itself. First degree atrioventricular block is not associated with increased risk for coronary artery disease or for complete heart block. There is no evidence that early detection of left ventricular hypertrophy shown by ECG in a normotensive person would prolong life.

Screening for Asymptomatic Coronary Artery Disease: Exercise Stress Testing

Disease

Asymptomatic coronary disease is atherosclerosis in the coronary arteries without clinical manifestations. Based on autopsy findings after accidental deaths, 4% of men under age 50 had asymptomatic coronary artery disease and 11% of men over age 50 had disease. For women, 0.7% of those under 50 years and 5% over 50 had disease. The prevalence of disease in asymptomatic persons without risk factors is unknown, but has been estimated to be 5%. Risk factors have been shown to be associated with nearly a threefold increase in disease prevalence.

Asymptomatic coronary artery disease is an important cause of premature death in the United States. Sudden death was reported in 1971 to be the first and only manifestation of disease in about 18% of persons with coronary artery disease in the Framingham study.

Screening Tests

Exercise stress testing usually entails use of graded exercise on a treadmill or bicycle ergometer, with a gradual increase in workload. Patients exercise until they are exhausted or develop angina or other abnormalities, including ST-segment deviation, a fall in blood pressure, or a failure to raise the heart rate.

A normal result occurs when the patient attains the target heart rate without having any of the events that define an abnormal test. An indeterminate result is one in which the patient fails to attain the target heart rate and does not have any of the events that define an abnormal result.

Myocardial scintigraphy with thallium-201 imaging measures myocardial perfusion. In most protocols for myocardial scintigraphy, thallium-201 is injected at the time of maximal stress during a multistage protocol for exercise testing. The patient's heart is scanned immediately and several hours later. An ischemic region is defined as a defect that appears on the first scan but not on the second.

Recommendation

Exercise testing is not recommended as a routine procedure in screening for coronary artery disease in asymptomatic adults.

Rationale

Screening for coronary artery disease is not a good application of exercise testing for several reasons. First, most asymptomatic people do not have the disease. Second, most patients with a positive test would have false-positive results. When arteriography is done in asymptomatic people with a positive result on their exercise electrocardiogram, only about 20% have the disease. Third, the types of coronary artery disease that might be treated by bypass surgery occur infrequently in asymptomatic persons. The most frequent type of coronary artery disease in such persons is single-vessel or double-vessel disease.

Some asymptomatic persons may have particular reasons to consider exercise stress testing for coronary artery disease. Some persons are especially likely to have the disease because of increased age, male gender, and at least one other risk factor (for example, family history of coronary artery disease, cigarette smoking, diabetes mellitus, systolic blood pressure greater than 140 mm Hg, hypercholesterolemia, or a cholesterol:high-density lipoprotein ratio of more than 6.0). Other persons have an occupation that puts others at risk (for example, bus drivers or airline pilots) or are sedentary and about to begin a program of physical conditioning. There is insufficient evidence to make a strong recommendation for or against use of routine stress testing in these groups.

Screening Low Risk, Asymptomatic Adults for Cardiac Risk Factors: Serum Cholesterol and Triglycerides

Disease

Coronary artery disease is associated with atherosclerotic plaques which, by decreasing the lumen of the coronary arteries, significantly reduce the oxygen supply to the myocardium. This reduction may result in angina pectoris, ischemia-induced arrhythmias, or myocardial infarction.

Undisputed risk factors for coronary artery disease include age, male gender, smoking, hypercholesterolemia, low levels of high-density lipoprotein (HDL) cholesterol, diabetes, menopause, hypertension, and family history; questionable risk factors include obesity, personality type, hypertriglyceridemia, oral contraceptives, and physical activity.

Although several studies have suggested that hypertriglyceridemia is associated with increased risk of coronary artery disease, others have provided evidence to the contrary. The balance of the evidence indicates that hypertriglyceridemia in asymptomatic individuals may not be a risk factor.

Screening Tests

Cholesterol and triglyceride measurements are obtained by submitting a blood sample for analysis.

Epidemiologic studies show that HDL and low-density lipoprotein (LDL) cholesterol levels are better predictors of cardiac risk than total cholesterol. However, HDL and LDL levels are less reliably measured in day-to-day laboratory practice than total cholesterol.

Measurement of total cholesterol may be inaccurate. One study of total cholesterol levels reported by the College of American Pathologists found levels reported in the range of 197 to 379 mg/dL among 5000 laboratories when the actual value was 262.6 mg/dL.

The following screening recommendations apply only to asymptomatic, non-smoking persons without a family history of hypercholesterolemia or premature cardiovascular disease in a parent or sibling, who are not undergoing treatment with lipid-altering medications, and are not known to have hypertension, coronary heart disease, or a cause of secondary hyperlipidemia such as diabetes. The recommendations should be considered a minimum for persons at risk of coronary artery disease.

Recommendations

1. Screening for cardiac risk factors with a total serum cholesterol measurement is recommended at least once in early adulthood and at intervals of 5 or more years up to age 70.
   1.1 The LDL and HDL cholesterol and serum triglyceride levels should be measured in persons with an elevated total serum cholesterol level. The decision to perform these additional tests should be individualized. Factors to be taken into account include: age, gender, number of other cardiovascular risks factors, and the patient's willingness to comply with drug and dietary treatment of hypercholesterolemia.
2. Screening for cardiac risk factors with a serum triglyceride measurement is not recommended.

Rationale

Because hypercholesterolemia usually does not cause symptoms until blood vessels have become damaged, early detection of the condition is best accomplished by screening asymptomatic persons before age 70.

Although direct evidence is limited, indirect evidence supports the benefit of treating individuals with hypercholesterolemia. Many studies have confirmed the association between extreme elevations of cholesterol and increased prevalence of ischemic heart disease and overall mortality rates; markedly elevated serum cholesterol levels can be reduced with treatment, leading to decreased morbidity and mortality from coronary artery disease.

Risks and discomfort associated with these tests are limited to those of venipuncture. Occasional patients are treated with medications unnecessarily due to false-positive test results and some are made needlessly anxious.

Screening for Diabetes Mellitus in Apparently Healthy, Asymptomatic Adults

Disease

Diabetes mellitus is a heterogeneous disorder characterized by hyperglycemia and abnormalities in fat and protein metabolism that are due to impaired insulin secretion or insulin resistance. The two major types are insulin dependent (type I), and non-insulin dependent (type II). Other categories are gestational diabetes, which occurs with pregnancy and usually remits after delivery, and secondary diabetes, associated with other illnesses, such as acromegaly, hemochromatosis, and chronic pancreatitis. The National Diabetes Data Group criteria for diabetes mellitus include repeated casual plasma glucose values equal to or greater than 200 mg/dL, or fasting plasma glucose level equal to or greater than 140 mg/dL, or oral glucose tolerance test results meeting the criteria.

Type II diabetes is estimated to occur at the rate of 1.6 per 1000 school-age children. Type I diabetes is rarer. Gestational diabetes occurs in 3% of pregnancies.

Risk factors have been established for Type II diabetes. These include age over 50 years, diabetes in a first degree relative, personal history of gestational diabetes, body weight that exceeds generally accepted standards of ideal weight by at least 25%, or belonging to an ethnic group that has a high prevalence of diabetes.

Screening Tests

The principal test used to screen for gestational diabetes mellitus is the plasma glucose level obtained 1 hour after a 50-g glucose load. For other types of diabetes, screening may be done via fasting or casual plasma glucose, glycated hemoglobin, or oral glucose tolerance testing after a 75-g glucose load.

Recommendations

1. Screening for diabetes in healthy, asymptomatic persons is not recommended. Screening is reasonable in obese adults over age 40 if knowl-

edge of the diagnosis would motivate weight loss.

2. Screening for gestational diabetes is recommended for all pregnant women.

3. Screening for diabetes mellitus may be indicated in women planning to become pregnant who are at increased risk of diabetes mellitus and in other persons with risk factors as listed above.

Rationale

The prevalence of asymptomatic, Type I diabetes detected by screening is small, and the benefits of early hypoglycemic therapy have not been shown.

Although the prevalence of undiagnosed Type II diabetes mellitus is substantial, the benefits of early diagnosis and therapy in preventing disease progression or complications have not been shown. Although treatment is available for diabetic retinopathy, retinopathy threatening to vision rarely precedes the diagnosis of Type II diabetes mellitus. The detection of Type II diabetes in an obese person may strengthen efforts to lose weight.

Gestational diabetes mellitus, which may be "silent," occurs in approximately 3% of pregnancies. Studies have confirmed an association between gestational diabetes and large birth weight (macrosomia), which is associated with neonatal morbidity; glycemic control appears to reduce these neonatal complications. Some studies have also reported an association between gestational diabetes and neonatal mortality.

Risks and discomfort associated with glucose screening tests are limited to venipuncture and to ingestion of a potentially distasteful liquid.

Screening for Thyroid Disease

Disease

Thyroid dysfunction includes hypothyroidism and thyrotoxicosis. The signs and symptoms of hypothyroidism and thyrotoxicosis can be subtle and easily mistaken by patient or physician for evidence of other illnesses, or simply for "old age" in elderly patients. New overt hypothyroidism or hyperthyroidism occurs in approximately 25 of 1000 members of unselected general populations. From 2% to 5% of elderly patients admitted to specialized geriatric units for general disability, failure to thrive, and other admission diagnoses have treatable thyroid disease. The incidence of thyroid dysfunction is higher for women than for men, and increases with age, particularly in women age 50 and above.

The following guidelines do not address the screening of infants, nor do they apply to the surveillance of patients known to be at increased risk of thyroid disease due to previous illnesses or procedures.

Potential Screening Tests

Thyroid function tests include the total thyroxine (TT4), T3 resin uptake (T3 uptake), free thyroxine (FT4), triiodothyronine (TT3), free triiodothyronine (FT3), and thyrotropin (TSH). Newer, sensitive thyrotropin assays (sTSH) are distinguished from older TSH assays by their ability to detect low concentrations of TSH and by their usefulness in diagnosing thyrotoxicosis. An FT4 is most commonly estimated as a free thyroxine index (FT4I), which is calculated as the product of the TT4 and the thyroid hormone binding ratio (THBR). (The ratio is the T3 uptake of the patient divided by the mean T3 uptake of a group of normal patients). The FT3I is the product of the TT3 and the THBR.

Recommendations

1. Routine screening for thyroid disease is not indicated in asymptomatic persons.
2. Routine testing for thyroid disease is not indicated in patients admitted to the hospital for acute medical or psychiatric illnesses.

3. Testing may be indicated to identify unsuspected disease in women over 50 years who have general symptoms that could be caused by thyroid disease.

   3.1 The TT4, FT4I, or sTSH can be used as the initial test. The TT4 or FT4I are preferred because there is better evidence available regarding their use, and because the sTSH is far more costly even if it were equally effective.

   3.2 The sTSH is indicated as the initial test in populations of patients with conditions (for example, pregnant women or certain patients with renal disease) that affect the accuracy of the TT4 or FT4I.

Rationale

Thyroid function tests are reliable when used to confirm clinically suspected thyroid disease. However, routine testing in patients with little clinical evidence of thyroid disease or in patients with systemic illnesses can lead to misleading test results, inappropriate consultation, and even unnecessary treatment.

To avoid these problems, the physician should use the principle that the meaning of an abnormal test result depends on the reason for testing, the strength of the clinical picture, and the presence of factors that affect the accuracy of thyroid function tests.

A structured approach in interpretation of tests, including clinical examinations, can minimize the risks of false-positive and false-negative tests. If test findings are unexpected with regard to the initial clinical findings, reevaluation of the patient may be indicated.

Discriminating and efficient use of these tests also can be assured by explicit arrangements between the ordering physician and the laboratory. Testing sequences can be done according to the results of the initial test. In this way, costs are minimized and the frequency of false-positive results is reduced.

Risks and discomforts associated with these tests are limited to those of venipuncture, and the extensive diagnostic tests associated with false-positive results.

(For detailed discussion of appropriate follow-up testing sequences and supporting documentation for this guideline, *see* Helfand M, Crapo L. Testing for suspected thyroid disease. In: Sox HC Jr, ed. *Com-*

mon Diagnostic Tests: Use and Interpretation. 2nd ed. Philadelphia: American College of Physicians; 1990:148-82; and, Medical necessity guidelines: thyroid function tests. In: Sox HC Jr, ed. *Common Diagnostic Tests: Use and Interpretation.* 2nd ed. Philadelphia: American College of Physicians; 1990: 407-10.)

Screening for Osteoporosis in Perimenopausal Women

Disease

Osteoporosis is metabolic bone disease, characterized by a decrease in the amount of bone, which leads to an increase in the risk of fractures, especially of the hip, distal radius, or vertebral body. An estimated 1.3 million fractures occur annually due to osteoporosis—250 000 of the hip, 250 000 of the wrist, and 500 000 vertebral. Because the fracture rate increases with age, these numbers are expected to increase over the next 20 to 30 years.

Osteoporosis is associated with low peak bone mass, accelerated postmenopausal bone loss, age-related bone loss in both sexes, and various conditions causing secondary osteoporosis. Specific risk factors include female sex, white race, and low body weight; the roles of calcium intake and exercise remain controversial.

Screening Tests

The main techniques to screen for osteoporosis include single-photon absorptiometry, dual-photon absorptiometry, dual energy x-ray absorptiometry, and quantitative computed tomography. Neutron activation is considered the "gold standard" for measuring total body calcium but is not in widespread use for detecting osteoporosis.

Single-photon absorptiometry entails calculation of bone mineral content (g/cm) at sites in the appendicular skeleton. Single-photon absorptiometry cannot measure bone density in the hip or spine, nor can it distinguish between cortical and trabecular bone.

Dual-photon absorptiometry entails the direct measurement of bone mineral content (g/cm) or area density (g/cm^2) in the total body or specific regions, including the hip and spine. Dual-photon absorptiometry cannot discriminate between cortical and trabecular bone.

Dual-energy x-ray absorptiometry entails the direct measurement of bone mineral content (g/cm) or area density (g/cm^2) in the total body or specific regions, including the hip, spine, and others. Dual-energy x-ray absorptiometry cannot discriminate between cortical and trabecular bone.

Quantitative computed tomography entails the calculation of bone mineral equivalents to estimate bone mineral density (g/cm³). Quantitative computed tomography can discriminate between cortical and trabecular bone in the axial or appendicular skeleton.

Recommendation

Routine screening of all perimenopausal women for osteoporosis is not recommended.

Rationale

Preliminary evidence suggests that screening for osteoporosis has the potential to reduce the probability of fractures in postmenopausal women: The tests can safely measure bone mass, one of the main factors in pathogenesis, and there is a treatment (estrogen) that can reduce bone loss and prevent fractures. Although measurement of bone density might affect the choice of treatment, additional evidence is necessary before widespread screening for osteoporosis in all perimenopausal women can be recommended: Specific screening protocols must be defined and various risk groups classified on the basis of bone mass measured through screening; treatment protocols based on these risk categories must be formulated; and there should be evidence that treatment decisions will be based on the results of screening.

Because there is no alternative to direct assessment, however, bone mass measurements may be indicated in specific clinical situations where the decision to treat must be based on knowledge of bone mass and related fracture risk.

Screening for Breast Cancer

Disease

Most breast cancers are infiltrating ductal carcinomas; the remainder are of various pathologic types. Although prognosis varies slightly with pathologic type, the principles of screening and management do not differ.

In 1989 approximately 114 000 women were diagnosed with new primary breast cancer in the United States, and nearly half are likely to die of the disease.

Risk factors for breast cancer include personal or family history, marital status, multiparity, age at first pregnancy, age at menarche and menopause, history of benign breast conditions, and diet.

Screening Tests

Two main tests are used for breast cancer screening: breast physical examination and mammography.

A breast physical examination done by a trained practitioner entails visual inspection and manual palpation of the breast.

Two types of mammography are used for breast cancer screening: plain-film and xeromammography. Xeromammography is effective in identifying microcalcifications associated with early breast cancers; plain-film mammography is more effective at detecting poorly defined lesions.

Recommendations

1. Screening with breast physical examination is recommended annually for asymptomatic women 40 years and older.
2. Screening with breast physical examination and mammography is recommended annually for asymptomatic women 50 years and older.
3. Screening with breast physical examination and mammography is recommended annually for women at any age who have a personal history of breast cancer.
4. Screening with breast physical examination and mammography is recommended annually for women 40 years and older who have a family

history of breast cancer or who are otherwise at increased risk.

Rationale

There is substantial direct evidence that breast cancer screening with breast physical examination and mammography reduces mortality from breast cancer in women over 50 years. The evidence of effectiveness of mammography for women under 50 years is conflicting; however, the natural history of breast cancer in women under 50 years is such that annual screening with mammography in women who are at increased risk is strongly recommended. All women should be counselled regarding the benefits, risks, and costs so they might choose the screening strategy that suits their personal history and preferences.

The risks associated with breast cancer screening are primarily due to false-positive results which can lead to further diagnostic tests, including breast biopsy. Although radiation might increase the risk of a new cancer, the carcinogenic effect of the radiation from mammography is extremely small.

Screening for Cervical Cancer

Disease

Most cervical cancers are of the squamous cell type, arising in the transition zone of squamocolumnar cells, near the junction of the cervical canal and ectocervix. The development of cervical cancer is associated with a long latency period, ranging up to 30 years.

Screening for cervical cancer increases the average life expectancy of women nearly 100 days. The 13 000 cases expected in 1988 and 7000 deaths may have been more directly affected by more extended and effective screening programs.

The main risk factors for cervical cancer are multiple sexual partners, early age at first intercourse, and smoking; additional risk factors include black, Hispanic, and native American ethnic origins; characteristics of partner; a history of sexually transmitted diseases; and use of oral contraceptives.

Screening Tests

The main screening test is the Papanicolaou smear. The cytologic specimen is obtained by gently scraping the os and transitional zone of the cervix with a spatula and spreading and fixing the material on a glass slide. The slide is stained with Papanicolaou stain and examined under a microscope for cell morphology. Recommended practice is to take two smears per examination.

Recommendations

1. Screening with a Papanicolaou smear is recommended every 3 years in sexually active women 20 to 65 years.
2. Screening with a Papanicolaou smear is recommended every 3 years for women 66 to 75 years who have not been screened within the 10 years before age 66.
3. Screening with a Papanicolaou smear is recommended every 2 years for women at increased risk of cervical cancer.
4. Initial screening tests may be done as frequently as annually for two or three examinations to ensure diagnostic accuracy.

Rationale

There is overwhelming indirect evidence, including numerous epidemiologic studies, the natural history of the disease, mathematical models, and data from large screening programs, that indicate the effectiveness of cervical cancer screening.

Precursor lesions, including dysplasia and carcinoma in situ (or cervical intraepithelial neoplasia), are potentially detectable an average of 10 years before the development of invasive cancers. These precursor lesions are detectable with a Papanicolaou smear and are treatable, resulting in significant reduction in mortality.

For most women, a 3-year screening frequency will be appropriate. However, some women may prefer more intensive screening (every 2 years, or annually), and longer intervals between screening may be appropriate for women who are not sexually active. All women should be given information on the expected benefits, risks, and costs, and allowed to choose the screening strategy that reflects their preferences.

There are virtually no risks associated with a Papanicolaou smear. False-negative and false-positive results can be reduced with appropriate sampling, slide preparation, and quality control of laboratory methods and reporting.

Screening for Colorectal Cancer

Disease

Invasive colorectal cancers arise from adenomas or originate (de novo) from the mucosa of the colon. Progression from adenoma to invasive cancer takes about 5 years.

Colorectal cancer accounts for 150 000 new cases each year and 61 000 deaths. It is the second most common form of cancer in the United States. On the average, it deprives patients of nearly 10% of their expected life span.

Risk factors for colorectal cancer include inflammatory bowel disease, familial polyposis syndromes, family history, and a previous history of neoplasms. A diagnosis of familial polyposis syndrome or inflammatory bowel disease requires monitoring.

Screening Tests

Several tests and procedures have been proposed for colorectal cancer screening; the most common are digital examination, fecal occult blood tests, and sigmoidoscopy. Air-contrast barium enemas and colonoscopy have been proposed for screening persons at high risk of developing colorectal cancer.

The digital rectal examination entails a manual exploration of the rectum.

Fecal occult blood tests entail smearing a stool specimen on a slide and submitting the specimen for analysis. Recommended practice is to take two samples on each of 3 consecutive days, while on a diet designed to reduce the frequency of false-positive results.

Sigmoidoscopy is the inspection of the interior of the colon through an endoscope inserted via the rectum. Sigmoidoscopes vary in length and may be rigid or flexible. When available, use of a flexible scope is preferred; otherwise, a rigid scope is acceptable.

Air-contrast barium enema and colonoscopy allow the inspection of the entire colon. The first method involves the administration of barium into the rectum, followed by roentgenographic study of the entire intestine; the second, introduction of a fiberoptic instrument.

Recommendations

1. Screening with fecal occult blood tests is recommended annually for persons 50 years and older.
2. Screening with sigmoidoscopy is recommended every 3 to 5 years or with air-contrast barium enema every 5 years for persons 50 years and older.
3. For persons 40 years and older who have familial polyposis coli, inflammatory bowel disease, or a history of colon cancer in a first degree relative (parent or sibling), screening with air-contrast barium enema or colonoscopy in addition to annual fecal occult blood tests, is recommended every 3 to 5 years.

Rationale

Although there is little direct evidence of the effectiveness of colorectal cancer screening, there is indirect evidence, based on the natural history of the disease and the effectiveness of screening tests, that screening should reduce colorectal cancer incidence and mortality.

Risks associated with colorectal cancer screening include perforations from sigmoidoscopy, colonoscopy, and barium enema, and the extensive diagnostic tests associated with false-positive results of fecal occult blood testing.

Persons at high risk for colorectal cancer due to familial polyposis coli or inflammatory bowel disease, or a history of colorectal cancer in a first degree relative should be encouraged to have a complete examination of the colon. Factors influencing the choice between air-contrast barium enema and colonoscopy include cost and access to qualified physicians able to perform safe and accurate studies.

Screening for Lung Cancer

Disease

The four main pathologic types of lung cancer are squamous (epidermoid) carcinoma, adenocarcinoma, large-cell undifferentiated carcinoma, and small-cell undifferentiated carcinoma. Prognosis and response to treatment differ with pathologic type.

The most important risk factor for lung cancer is a history of smoking.

Screening Tests

Two tests have been used to screen for lung cancer: chest roentgenogram and sputum cytologic examination. Chest roentgenograms usually entail two views taken on full-size film; sputum cytologic examination entails the collection and processing of sputum specimens.

Recommendation

Screening for lung cancer is not recommended in the asymptomatic adult.

Rationale

Several randomized clinical trials have shown that screening for lung cancer with chest roentgenogram and sputum cytologic examination does not decrease mortality from this disease. Although screening can detect cancers in earlier stages and appears to increase 5-year survival rates, these rates are apparently due to the detection of lesions that would never surface clinically.

There are no risks directly associated with chest roentgenograms or sputum cytologic examinations. False-positive results of screening tests, however, may lead to performance of additional tests.

0116364

Common Screening Tests

P172
2270
HNH T (Edd)

SEVEN DAY LOAN

This book is due for return on or before the last date shown below.

.td., London, N.21   Cat. No. 1208   DG 02242/71

0943126197

Also Available from the American College of Physicians

Clinical Efficacy Reports
    (evaluations of medical tests and procedures; in looseleaf form)
Common Diagnostic Tests: Use and Interpretation—Second Edition
Diagnostic Strategies for Common Medical Problems
Guide for Adult Immunization—Second Edition
Providing Quality Care: The Challenge to Clinicians

Publications from the *British Medical Journal* are now distributed in North America by the American College of Physicians.

Publications catalogue and ordering information for American College of Physicians and *British Medical Journal* publications are available from:

Subscriber Services
American College of Physicians
Independence Mall West
Sixth Street at Race
Philadelphia, PA 19106-1572
(215) 351-2600
(800) 523-1546